Heart Transplantation

Hashim Talib Hashim · Naseer Ahmed ·
Giuseppe Faggian · Martí Manyalich ·
Francesco Onorati
Editors

Heart Transplantation

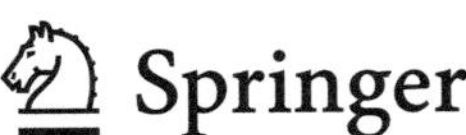 Springer

Editors
Hashim Talib Hashim
College of Medicine
University of Baghdad
Baghdad, Iraq

Giuseppe Faggian
Department of Cardiac Surgery
Azienda Ospedaliera Universitaria Integrata
Verona
Verona, Italy

Francesco Onorati
Division of Cardiac Surgery
University of Verona
Verona, Italy

Naseer Ahmed
Rehman Medical Institute
Hayatabad, Peshawar, Pakistan

Martí Manyalich
Parc Científic de Barcelona
President of Donation and Transplantation
Barcelona, Spain

ISBN 978-3-031-17313-4   ISBN 978-3-031-17311-0   (eBook)
https://doi.org/10.1007/978-3-031-17311-0

This Springer imprint is published by the registered company Springer Nature Switzerland AG
The registered company address is: Gewerbestrasse 11, 6330 Cham, Switzerland

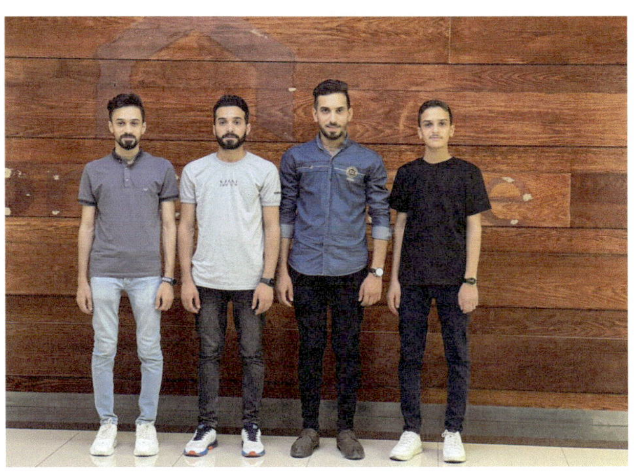

To my family: my father (Talib), my mother (Jawaher), and my grandmothers (Hamdia and Alya).
To my grandfathers (Hashim and Mutar), hoping they are resting in peace.
To my uncle (Abbas) and aunts (Shafaa and Rasha).

To all my friends and especially Mustafa, Mohammed, Ahmed, Zanyar, Mahdi, and Abdalla.
Finally, to those who supported me and be with me all the times passed and still being my support, my brothers (Ali, Mustafa, Mujtaba, Hussein, and Mortada), my sister (Noor Alhuda), my nephew (Razan), and my brother's wife (Zainab).

Preface

Heart Transplantation: Theory and Practice is a translational and comprehensive reference which broadly covers a range of topics within Heart Transplantation including surgical procedure, requirements, potential complications, and follows up with the most up-to-date research and literature review. The book first lay out the anatomy, physiology, embryology, and pathology of the heart as an introduction, then goes into the details of cardiac transplantation including the surgical procedure, the potential complications, and cardio-immunology. It also delves into other aspects of heart transplantation including organ procurement, religious aspects, the ethical issues that can emerge prior or during the surgery, and artificial heart. Then it explores multi-organ transplantations including transplants that have been done in the specialized centers and their outcomes and complications. All these topics are discussed in a scientific medical language with illustrations and charts to aid understanding, allowing readers to gain a full understanding of the whole procedure easily.

This book is—to our knowledge—the first book that vastly focuses on cardiosurgical and medical aspects of heart transplantation, emerging from the significant need to fill a defect in the related cardiology and surgical resource map and incorporate meaningful updates regarding all aspects of the procedures. Many books were dedicated to the subject over the years, but those were rather superficial, immunological, or pathological.

"Heart Transplantation Surgery: Theory and Practice" is composed of 12 chapters, containing concise and up-to-date information within about 200 pages.

The book contains around 100 diagrams, tables, illustrations, and figures attempting to make it more interesting and easier to memorize by readers.

More than 70 single-best-answer multiple choice questions (MCQs), distributed along the chapters, cover important aspects of heart transplantation surgery, from the basic sciences to ultimately surgery.

Authors believe that heart transplantation has many aspects that should be more widely discussed, and through this proposed book the authors hope to stimulate further research and clinical trials for heart transplantation, as well as more discussion in the field especially related to the ethical and religious aspects. The book also focuses on multi-organ transplantations including heart and artificial heart, and how this could be developed to solve the problem of lack of donors. At the end of each chapter, a list of MCQs related to the topics of that chapter and a list of references that readers can look up for additional information are provided. What makes our book novel is that the book looks at heart transplantation from all the aspects of medicine and surgery in addition to the ethical issues. It is written in simple medical language that makes it possible for various medical healthcare workers and students to build their knowledge base about the topic.

It talks about these topics from the surgical perspective and covers the details of heart transplantation surgery in a step-by-step fashion. In this book, we are presenting new, unique, and sequenced surgical guidelines in heart transplantation surgery either in childhood or adulthood with pros and cons. Detailed ways with highly organized, attractive graphs and photos will make this book easily understandable for medical students, surgical residents, and surgeons alike. Finally, we have put more than 30 multiple-choice questions at the end of each chapter that cover all the topics and subjects discussed within that chapter. These could serve to boost the question banks for medical schools and residency programs.

Baghdad, Iraq   Hashim Talib Hashim
Peshawar, Pakistan   Naseer Ahmed
Verona, Italy   Giuseppe Faggian
Barcelona, Spain   Martí Manyalich
Verona, Italy   Francesco Onorati
25 October 2022

Contents

Anatomy of the Heart

Rema Yousif Bakose, Ahmed Dheyaa Al-Obaidi, Mustafa Najah Al-Obaidi,
Hasan Al-Abbasi, Mohammed Omer AL-Bayati, Ali Talib Hashim,
Abdullah Muhanned, Adil Alhaideri, and Jaafar Dhiaa Al-Dabagh

Abstract The heart is a unique organ in the human body; it is a muscular pump with
independent electrical activity that is governed by central innervation; also, unlike
other organs such as the gut, its cells are not amenable to repair or division. The heart
is around the size of a human fist, weighing around 310 g for males and 225 g for
females on average. The heart is situated in the midline of the mediastinal cavity,
somewhat to the left turned posteriorly, with the right ventricle occupying the majority
of the anterior surface. It is surrounded by the lungs laterally and the diaphragm inferiorly and is encased by a bony structure; the ribs and sternum, extending along the
left second to fifth intercostal spaces, at which the most inferio-lateral part of the
heart is roughly localized; the apex; at the fifth intercostal space mid-clavicular line
as the point of maximal impulse. It is made up of three layers: Endocardium: lining
the cardiac chambers, myocardium: a thick striated muscle layer that pumps blood,
and pericardium: two-layer sac with roughly 10–20 cc of pericardial fluid in between;
acts as a shock absorber. Upper chambers: right and left atria separated by interatrial septum; lower chambers: right and left ventricles separated by interventricular
septum; upper and lower chambers separated by atrioventricular septum; atrioventricular valves: mitral and tricuspid valve; semilunar valves: aortic and pulmonary
valves connect the heart to systemic and pulmonary circulation. The cardiac cycle
is governed by a network that runs from the sino-atrial node (SA node) down to the
purkinje fibers and is influenced by hormones, sympathetic, and parasympathetic
innervation. The hearts measure 12 cm (434 inches) in length, 9 cm (312 inches) in
breadth, and 6 cm (212 inches) in depth. A complex network of arteries, arterioles,
and capillaries pumps around 4–6 L of blood every minute, which is returned to the

R. Y. Bakose · A. D. Al-Obaidi · M. N. Al-Obaidi · H. Al-Abbasi · A. Muhanned · A. Alhaideri ·
J. D. Al-Dabagh
College of Medicine, University of Baghdad, Baghdad, Iraq
e-mail: adel.ferras1700b@comed.uobaghdad.edu.iq

M. O. AL-Bayati
College of Veterinary Medicine, University of Diyala, Diyala, Iraq

A. T. Hashim (✉)
Golestan University for Medical Sciences, Gorgan, Iran
e-mail: talibhashim42@gmail.com

H. T. Hashim et al. (eds.), *Heart Transplantation*,
https://doi.org/10.1007/978-3-031-17311-0_1

heart via venules and veins. Blood transports oxygen and nutrition to all of the body's major organs, as well as carbon dioxide and metabolic waste products.

Keywords Heart · Valves · Champers · Atrium · Ventricles · Myocardium · Pericardium · Endocardium veins · Arteries · Coronary · Conduction system · Bundle of His · Aorta · Pulmonary circuit · Systemic circuit

1 Introduction

The exact anatomy of the heart is best determined intraoperatively via a midline sternotomy that shows the surgical anatomy that the surgeon is concerned about while doing any cardiac intervention or after the human being has deceased in what is known as an autopsy that shows the basic anatomy. The superior vena cava, inferior vena cava, aorta and the pulmonary artery and veins connect the heart to the systemic circuit and the pulmonary circuit, respectively. The heart contracts around 2.5 billion times in a person's lifetime, or nearly 100,000 times per day. The heart is placed in the mediastinum, between the lungs, and is encased by the pericardial sac, which has a posterior border near the spinal column and an anterior border near the sternum, with the diaphragmatic crurae on the inferior surface [1].

2 Structure of the Heart

The heart is made up of contiguous layers that are closely adherent to one other, as seen in a cross-section:

1. *Pericardium*: This is the layer that surrounds the heart and is made up of two layers: parietal pericardium (a serous and fibrous layer that provide strength and elasticity) and visceral pericardium, also known as epicardium (fibroelastic layer and a broad layer of adipose tissue that connects it to the underlying myocardium) [2].
2. *Myocardium*: the spiral-shaped cardiac muscle which contracts and makes the heartbeat.
3. *Endocardium*: the cardiac chambers and valves are lined with a thin layer of endothelial cells sitting on the connective tissue basement membrane.

3   Cardiac Chambers

The heart has four champers divided by two on each side [3].

A. *Right Atrium*

The right atrium takes deoxygenated blood from the superior and inferior vena cava, as well as the coronary sinus, and sends it through the tricuspid valve to the right ventricle. Both the inferior vena cava and coronary sinus have valves to prevent blood backflow: the eustachian valve of the inferior vena cava and the besian valve of the coronary sinus are positioned within the inferior surface of the right atrium, the latter being anterior and inferior to the former [3].

B. *Left Atrium*

The left atrium lies superior to the left ventricles and posterior to the right atrium [4]. The foramen ovalis flap is seen on the septal surface, whereas the left atrial appendage covers the coronary sinus on the anterior surface and is utilized as a landmark to distinguish the left from the right atrium, which is typically narrow and extended [4, 5] (Fig. 1).

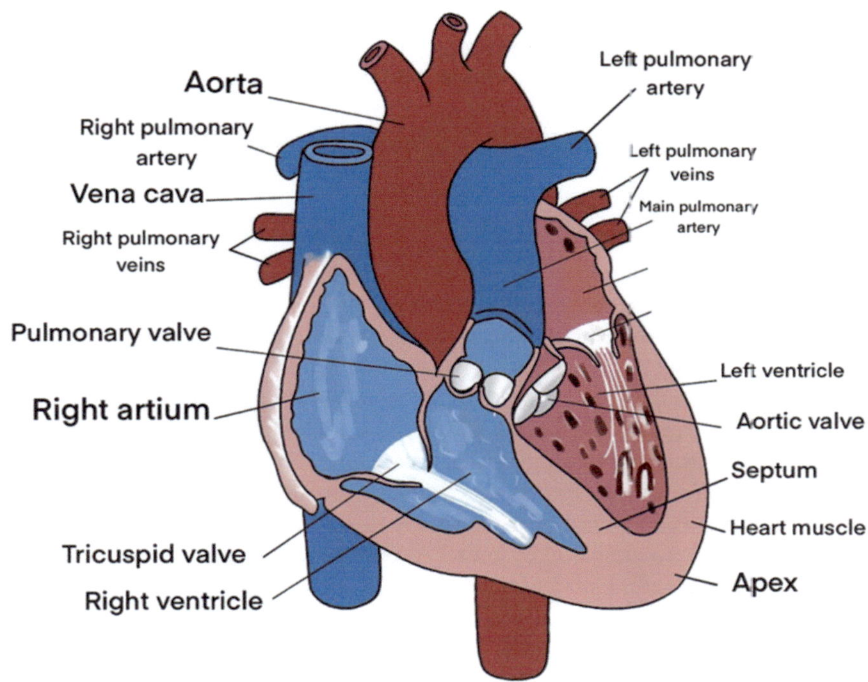

Fig. 1 Structure of the heart including the cardiac chambers

C. *Right Ventricle*

The right ventricle receives deoxygenated blood throughout the tricuspid valve and then the conus arteriosus, also known as the infundibulum which represents the outflow tract, delivers the blood to the pulmonary circulation throughout the pulmonary valve.

The papillary muscles keep the tricuspid valve leaflets from relapsing back into the atrium when the ventricles contract and they are connected to the leaflets by a tendinous band called chordee tendinae.

D. *Left Ventricle*

The left ventricle's free wall possesses fine internal trabeculations, and the septal surface is divided into a trabecular septum and a smooth part right beneath the mitral valve [6].

4 Cardiac Valves

Blood flow between the pulmonary and systemic circulations must be coordinated during each cardiac cycle. The heart valves are responsible for synchronizing the systolic and diastolic phases of the cardiac cycle. Two semilunar valves, the aortic and pulmonary valves, and two atrioventricular valves, the mitral and tricuspid valves, make up the heart's four valves. The semilunar valves separate the ventricles from the major arteries, while the atrioventricular valves separate the atria from the ventricles (Fig. 2).

A. *Tricuspid Valve*

The tricuspid valve apparatus is a complex dynamic system made up of several unique and closely linked components: the fibrous ring (annulus) and the three leaflets (anterior, septal, and posterior). It has a triangle aperture that is broader than the mitral orifice [4]. The leaflet bases are held together by a fibrous ring. "The largest anterior leaflet extends from the medial border of the ventricular septum to the anterior free wall, partially separating the inflow and outflow tracts of the right ventricle; the posterior leaflet extends from the lateral free wall to the posterior portion of the ventricular septum, and the septal leaflet extends from the annulus to the medial side of the interventricular septum". The chordae tendineae's fibrous strands connect the leaflets' free edges to the papillary muscles, preventing the cusps from separating during ventricular contraction and maintaining the valve closed [6].

B. *Mitral Valve*

The mitral valve is also known as the bicuspid valve because it has two cusps, one anterior and one posterior. The front cusp, also known as the aortic or septal cusp, is nearly triangular, whereas the posterior cusp, also known as the ventricular or mural

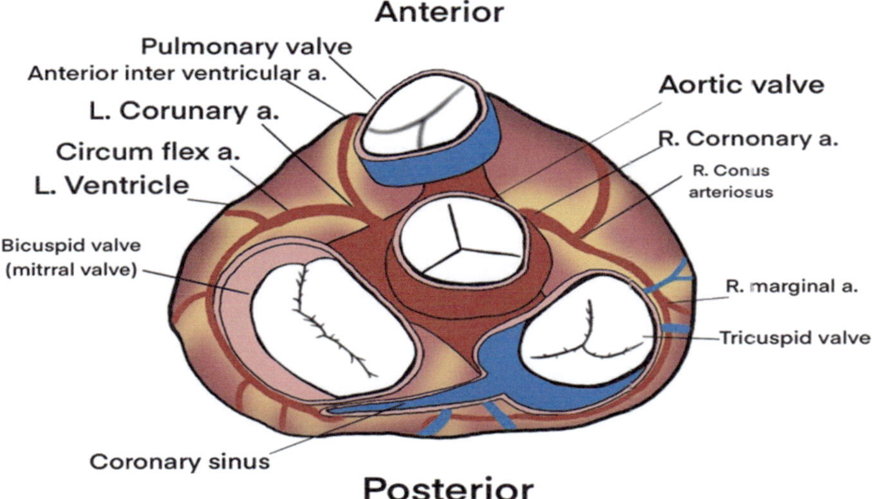

Fig. 2 The cardiac valves

cusp, is scalloped. The annulus, two cusps, papillary muscles, and chordae tendinae make up the mitral valve apparatus, which work together to maintain the valve's integrity during systole, preventing backflow of blood while permitting blood flow during diastole.

C. *Pulmonary Valve*

The pulmonary valve is made up of three cusps: anterior (nonseptal), left, and right, each having a midline nodule at the free end and lunulas that extend upward into the lumen of the pulmonary trunk through their free edges. The pulmonary valve has thinner cusps than the aortic valve, not connected to the ccronary arteries and not continuous with the corresponding (anterior) leaflet of the tricuspid valve [7].

D. *Aortic Valve*

This valve has a structure that is comparable to that of the pulmonary valve. It consists of three semilunar cusps, each with a midway nodule and lunulus at the free end. They arise from the aortic root, with each cusp's free edge projecting upward into the ascending aorta lumen, and they are connected to the membranous septum and anterior mitral leaflet. There are three anatomical dilations between the semilunar cusps and aortic wall known as the right, left, and posterior aortic sinuses, named for their relative placements (Fig. 3). [7].

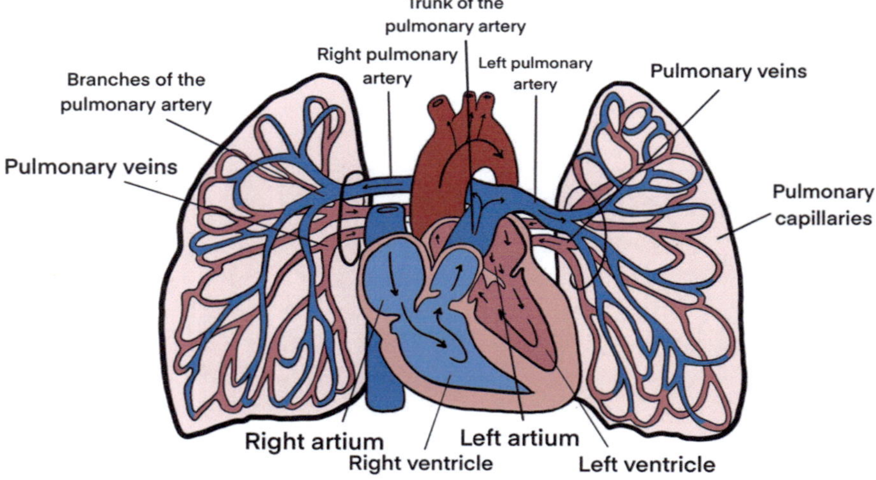

Fig. 3 The great vessels

5   The Great Vessels

A. *Aorta*

The aorta, which is the largest artery in the cardiovascular system, originates from the left ventricle of the heart carrying oxygen rich blood to the systemic circulation to ensure oxygen supply for all body tissues. "This great vessel can be divided into the ascending part, which gives coronary arteries that supply the cardiac muscle just above the aortic valve near its origin, the aortic arch, which gives rise to the right brachiocephalic trunk, left common carotid, left subclavian arteries, and the descending part which continues as the thoracic aorta in the thoracic cavity and as the abdominal aorta in the abdominal cavity" [8].

B. *Pulmonary Artery*

This is the only artery in the cardiovascular system that transports deoxygenated blood from the heart to the lungs, where it undergoes gas exchange and becomes oxygenated. The primary pulmonary trunk emerges from the right ventricle before branching into two major blood vessels, the right and left pulmonary arteries. This branching occurs below the aortic arch in typical human anatomy. The "Ductus Arteriosus," a short connecting blood vessel that connects the proximal descending aorta and pulmonary trunk, is advantageous to the fetus because it directs blood away from the immature fetal lung. Because it is no longer needed, the ductus arteriosus generally closes within a few days of birth. The ductus arteriosus's patency can have major consequences for the infant, and it needs to be closed either medically or surgically if it is not closed spontaneously [9].

C. *Pulmonary Veins*

These veins are the superior and inferior veins on each side. Superior pulmonary veins travel in an oblique direction, while inferior pulmonary veins travel horizontally.

D. *The Superior Vena Cava (SVC)*

SVC is "the largest vein in the body, and it collects deoxygenated blood from the upper body. It begins with the union of the right and left brachiocephalic trunks beyond the lower border of the first right costal cartilage and terminates in the upper and posterior section of the sinus venarum as it enters the right atrium". This large vessel is important in clinical practice since it is the location of central venous access, either through a central venous catheter or peripheral venous catheter [10].

E. *The Inferior Vena Cava (IVC)*

IVC is the main vein that drains blood from the organs below the diaphragm. "At the level of the fourth lumbar vertebrae, it is formed by the union of the left and right common iliac veins", and it continues its path toward the diaphragm, passing anterolateral to the vertebral column until it pierces the diaphragm's central tendon at the level of the eighth thoracic vertebra. At its infero-posterior boundary, the IVC enters the right atrium. The inferior vena cava, unlike many other veins in the human venous system, is devoid of valves. The inferior vena cava possesses a "Eustachian valve" that functions throughout embryonic life, which is one of the many variations of fetal body structure. This valve, which diverts oxygenated blood from the inferior vena cava to the right atrium through the foramen ovale to avoid pulmonary circulation of the fetus, normally regresses in the first few years after birth since it is no longer needed. The presence of the Eustachian remnant, if not linked with the patent foramen ovale, does not always necessitate surgical excision. It can, however, increase the chances of thrombus development, paradoxical embolism with foramen ovale patency, and endocarditis of the Eustachian valve remnant [10].

6 The Conduction System of the Heart

The hear is electrically controlled by special types of cells and electricity. This coordination is what causes both atria to contract at the same time and before the ventricles (Fig. 4).

A. *Sinoatrial Node (SA)*

The sinoatrial node is a "cigar-shaped structure located at the junction between the superior vena cava and right atrium". The SA node can occasionally extend across the atrial appendage and into the interatrial groove. The sinoatrial node (the heart's pacemaker) is the major impulse generating center in the heart (the heart's pacemaker). The cardiac impulses that flow from the sinoatrial node are discharged at

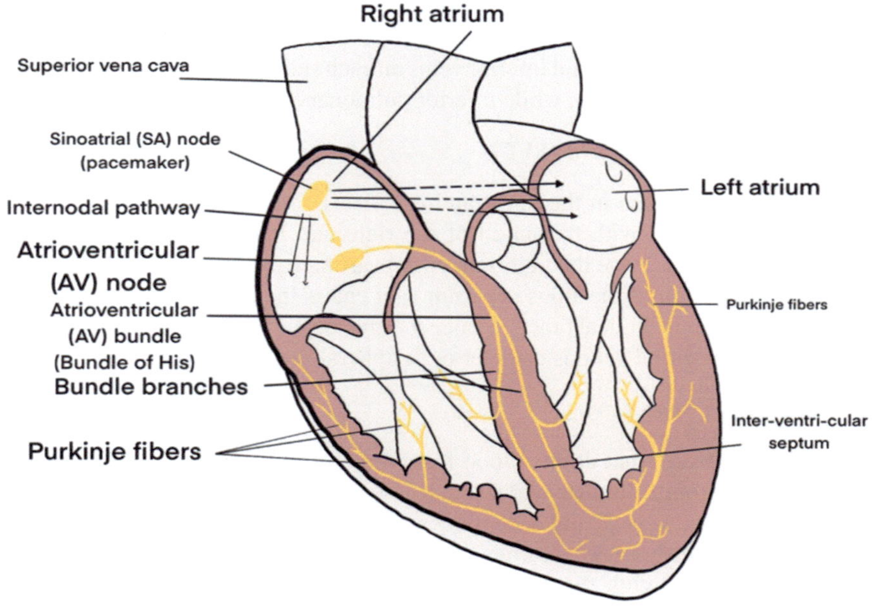

Fig. 4 Conduction system of the heart

a regular rate and rhythm in the normal cardiac conduction system due to continuous action potential [11].

B. *Internodal Conduction*

The intermodal conduction of the electrical impulses is carried out by plain myocardial cells and not by specialized cells. Although there is no evidence that specific cardiac conducting tracts transmit impulses between the SA node and AV node, tests imply that there exist "routes," which are pathways where the majority of impulses are considered to be conveyed. "The terminal crest, front lip of the oval fossa, and sinus septum are among the conspicuous muscle bundles along which these channels run". To avoid postoperative atrial conduction problems, at least one of these pathways should be preserved after atrial surgery [12].

C. *Atrioventricular Node*

The Koch triangle completely encloses the atrioventricular node. The right coronary artery supplies blood to the atrioventricular node in 80–90% of cases, and the left circumflex artery in the remaining cases. The atrioventricular node is in charge of the conduction and coordination of excitation waves from the sinoatrial node, which travels through the atria via specific conduction tracts until they reach the atrioventricular node, where they are delayed. This 0.09 second delay in the transmission of impulses is required to ensure that the atria have expelled all of the blood to the ventricles before ventricular contraction [12].

D. *His Bundle*

The His Bundle is a complicated architecture of cells grouped into "an elongated segment that connects the AV node to the left and right bundle branches". In an adult's heart, this segment is around 1.8 cm long and deeply entrenched in connective tissue. In contrast to the previously stated conduction pathways in the atria, there is a specific insulated conduction system that transmits impulses through the ventricles [13].

E. *Bundle Branches*

At the junction between the membranous and muscular parts of the ventricular septum or in the left ventricular aspect of the ventricular septum, the bundle of His branches into the right and left bundle branches. The right bundle branch descends intramyocardially as a cord structure to reach the right side of the septum and then continues beneath the medial papillary muscle complex, extending until it ramifies at the right ventricular apex [14].

F. *Terminal Purkinje Fibers*

Purkinje fibers are unique end-organ made up of specialized excitable tissue that are located just beneath the endocardium and are referred to as "subendocardial branches." These fibers are responsible for carrying electrical impulses from both the right and left bundle branches to the ventricular myocytes. Another function of the purkinje fibers is that they can act as a pacemaker, but this occurs only when the upstream conduction system is disrupted. 1.5. AV node, bundle of His, and ventricular myocardium innervation: A complex branching system of cholinergic and adrenergic fibers innervates the heart's conduction system and ventricular myocardium. The variation in heart rate as a result of the body's response to varied stimuli is caused by this distribution of neuronal input to the cardiac conduction system [14].

7 Coronary Circulation

Despite the fact that the left and right cardiac chambers contain blood with differing levels of oxygen saturation, heart muscles cannot rely solely on diffusion. Instead, the coronary circulation, which emerges from the aortic root, supplies the heart with blood. The right and left coronary arteries branch from the ostia of the aortic semilunar valves' sinuses (right and left) and run through the epicardium, supplying the entire heart through a complicated network formed by the right coronary artery and left coronary artery along with its branches (left anterior descending artery and left circumflex coronary artery). Deoxygenated blood is returned to the right atrium via the cardiac veins (Fig. 5).

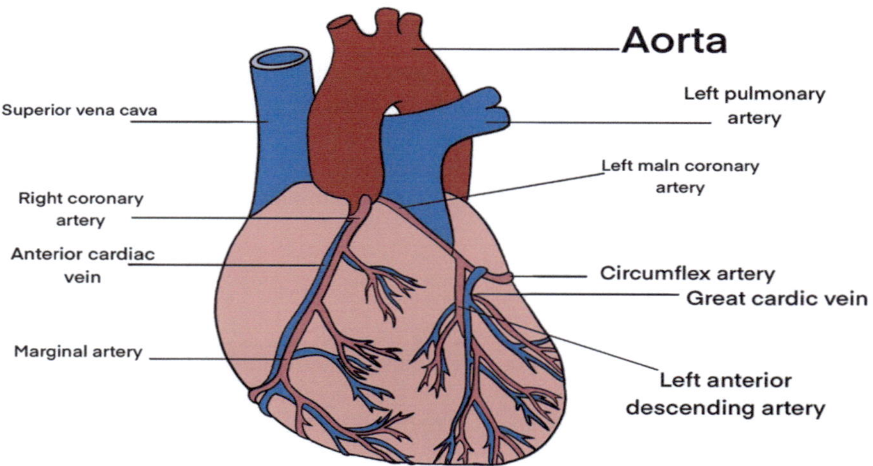

Fig. 5 Cardiac vasculature (arteries and veins)

8   Coronary Arteries

A. *Left Main Coronary Artery*

"The left main coronary artery (LCA) emerges from the aorta through the ostia of the left aortic sinus and runs for about $1-2$ cm between the left atrial appendage and pulmonary artery until it splits into two branches in the left atrioventicular groove: 1-left anterior descending artery (LAD) and 2-left circumflex coronary artery (LCX)". The LCA is sometimes not present; instead, its branches emerge straight from the aorta, frequently from separate ostia [15].

1. *Anterior Descending Artery (LAD)*

As a continuation of the left main artery (LCA), the left anterior descending artery (LAD) runs along the anterior interventricular groove and supplies both ventricles. The LAD gives branches to the anterior papillary muscle of tricuspid and bicuspid valves and the free wall of the left ventricle via diagonal arteries. It also forms a collateral supply known as the circle of Vieussens by anastomosing with another RCA branch, the conus artery [4, 15].

2. *Left Circumflex Artery*

The left atrium is supplied by the atrial circumflex artery, which is a branch of the LCX artery. The LCX artery gives another branch, the obtuse marginal (OM) artery, that supplies the left ventricle's postero-lateral surface and another branch to supply bicuspid valves posterior papillary muscle. In less than 40% of people, The LCX artery provides blood to the sinoatrial node [4].

B. *Right Coronary Artery*

It is a large artery that originates from the aorta and runs along the atrioventricular groove between the right auricle and right ventricle before it bends posteriorly at the crux to enter the posterior interventricular groove [1, 3]. At the heart's crux, the RCA provides the atrioventricular nodal artery, which supplies the atrioventricular node in 50–60% of people and sections of the proximal bundle of His [16–18].

The RCA provides an important collateral supply to the anterior surface of the heart, the left ventricle, and the anterior 2\3 of the interventricular septum via the conus artery and communicating arteries [2, 19].

9 Coronary Veins

"The great, middle, and small cardiac veins that merge to form the coronary sinus and anterior cardiac veins. The great cardiac vein is the principal tributary of the coronary sinus that drains the heart areas supplied by the LCA" [19]. The majority of the RCA that supplies the heart is drained by the middle and small cardiac veins. Starting at the apex, the middle cardiac vein ascends in the posterior interventricular groove parallel to the posterior interventricular artery before emptying into the right side of the sinus. Except for that carried by the anterior cardiac veins, all venous blood from the heart is drained by the coronary sinus. Two to four anterior cardiac veins drain the anterior right ventricular wall, pass through the right atrioventricular sulcus, and empty straight into the right atrium without passing via the coronary sinus [20]. The anterior cardiac veins and right coronary artery (RCA) lie perpendicular to each other at a right angle as the veins cross the RCA artery in this sulcus, which is filled with adipose tissue. The besian veins are small intramural veins that drain the myocardium into the cardiac channels, primarily the right atrium [2, 4, 21].

Multiple Choice Questions

1. **Intra-operatively, by medial rotation, you can reveal the following:**

    A. Left ventricle apex.
    B. Left atrium.
    C. Left pulmonary veins.
    D. All of the above.

2. **You can differentiate between the right atrium and right auricle through:**

    A. Fossa ovalis septum primum.
    B. Sulcus terminalis.
    C. Crista terminalis.
    D. Both B & C.

3. **The most accurate way to distinguish left atrium from right atrium is the existence of:**

A. Mitral valve.
B. Tricuspid valve.
C. Wall thickness.
D. Left atrial appendage.

4. **The right ventricular inner surface is characterized by:**

A. Increased in the thickness compared to the left ventricle.
B. Presence of fewer papillary muscles compared to the left ventricle.
C. Absence of chorda tendane.
D. Coarse trabeculation of the apical part.

5. **Which one of the following subdivisions is clinically important?**

A. Conal septum.
B. Interventricular septum.
C. Septal band.
D. Trabecular septum.

6. **The following can be used to differentiate between the right ventricle and left ventricle:**

A. The vascular resistance is tenfold different between these two.
B. Interventricular septum.
C. Shape of the ventricle.
D. Both A & C.

7. **Unlike tricuspid and pulmonary valves, the inflow and outflow sections in the left ventricle are:**

A. Absent.
B. Fused.
C. Widely separated.
D. Closely juxtaposed.

8. **The cardiac conducting system is made of:**

A. Nerve tissue.
B. Cardiac muscle cells.
C. Conducting fibers.
D. Both B and C.

9. **The main pacemaker of the heart is:**

A. Cardiac muscle tissue.
B. Fibrous skeleton.
C. Purkinji fibers.
D. Sinoatrial node.

10. **In most people, the blood supply to the Sinoatrial node comes from:**

A. Left coronary artery.

   B. Right coronary artery.

   C. Left anterior descending artery.

   D. Circumflex artery.

11. The Bachmann bundle is:

   A. A branch from the fibrous skeleton that is responsible for cutting off electrical conductance.

   B. A pathway that conducts electricity from the sinoatrial node to the ventricle.

   C. A large muscle bundle that conducts electricity from the right atrium to the left atrium.

   D. A branch of vagus nerve to supply the heart.

12. The number of pathways that conduct electricity from the Sinoatrial node to the atria is:

   A. One.

   B. Ten.

   C. Three.

   D. Seven.

13. The atrioventricular node tends to get blood supply from:

   A. Left anterior descending.

   B. Circumflex artery.

   C. Right coronary artery.

   D. Posterior descending artery.

14. What makes the atrioventricular node special is:

   A. It's location.

   B. Presence of more than one node.

   C. Delay in the conduction of the impulse.

   D. It's ability to proliferate.

15. One of the things that makes the atrioventricular node delay the conductance of electricity:

   A. Getting depolarized by Calcium.

   B. Containing too many cells.

   C. Arrangement of the cells.

   D. All of the above.

16. The reason why bundle of his is impervious to ischemic injury at the upper interventricular septum is:

   A. Absence of any blood supply.

   B. The difficulty of forming atherosclerosis.

   C. The presence of more than one artery.

   D. Surrounded by a thick layer protecting it.

17. **Bundle of his arise from:**

    A. Right atrium.
    B. Directly below the membranous part of the interventricular septum.
    C. Fibrous skeleton.
    D. Sinoatrial node.

18. **Valves that conduct blood to the ventricles are:**

    A. Tricuspid and pulmonary valves.
    B. Aortic and pulmonary valves.
    C. Pulmonary and mitral valves.
    D. Mitral and tricuspid valves.

19. **Of the following, which one is responsible for maintaining closure of mitral valve during systole:**

    A. Sinoatrial node.
    B. Coronary artery.
    C. Endocardium.
    D. Papillary muscles.

20. **Left Ventricle thickness is:**

    A. 2 cm.
    B. 5 cm.
    C. 1.3–1.5 cm.
    D. 10 mm.

21. **The heart of any person can be considered right dominant in the case of:**

    A. Left anterior descending is 1 cm in diameter.
    B. Left circumflex artery is 5 mm in diameter.
    C. Presence of a third coronary artery.
    D. The posterior descending artery comes from the right coronary artery.

22. **Main supply of left ventricle is:**

    A. Right coronary artery.
    B. Left anterior descending.
    C. Left coronary artery.
    D. Left Circumflex artery.

23. **In the atrioventricular groove, which one of the following runs:**

    A. Left circumflex artery.
    B. Right coronary artery.
    C. Posterior descending artery.
    D. Left anterior descending artery.

24. **The first branch that arises from right coronary artery is:**

    A. Septal branches.
    B. Branch to the heart's apex.
    C. Posterior descending artery.
    D. Branch to sinus node.

25. **Which one of the following is responsible for the drainage of the blood from the heart?**

    A. Right coronary artery.
    B. Left coronary artery.
    C. Left anterior descending.
    D. Coronary sinus.

Answers

1. D. "The medial rotation from the left reveals the apex of the left ventricle, the left pulmonary veins, and the left atrium".
2. D. A slight posterior vertical indentation (the sulcus terminalis) on the right atrium and an inner vertical crest separate the right auricle from the right atrium (the crista terminalis).
3. D. The most accurate approach to distinguish the left and right atriums is to identify this appendage. "The left atrial appendage is the only trabecular structure in the left atrium since it lacks the crista terminalis, unlike the right atrium".
4. D.
5. A. The conal septum, septal band division, and trabecular septum are the three sections of the outflow tract. The conal septum is the most clinically relevant of these three sections because it can be misplaced in people with congenital defects.
6. D.
7. D. Unlike the right ventricle, where the tricuspid and pulmonary valves are far apart, the input and outflow sections of the left ventricle are close together.
8. D.
9. D. The sinoatrial node, atrioventricular node, and purkinji cells are the three pacemakers for the conductive system of the heart, from above to below. When one stops working, the other begins to work.
10. B. "In 55–60% of hearts, the artery that supplies the sinus node branches from the right coronary artery, while in 40–45% of hearts, it branches from the left circumflex artery".
11. C.
12. C. "The Anatomical evidence suggests the existence of three intra-atrial pathways: the anterior internodal direction, middle internodal tract, and posterior internodal tract".
13. C. "The AV node is fed by a branch of the right coronary artery that originates near the posterior intersection of the AV and interventricular grooves in 85–90% of human hearts (crux)".
14. C. "The main function of the AV node is to control atrial impulse transmission to the ventricles in order to coordinate atrial and ventricular contractions".

15. D. The atrioventricular node's delay in impulse conduction is due to the fact that it is depolarized by calcium, and calcium channels are slower than sodium channels, in addition to the presence of too many cells arranged in an unorganized manner with too many gab junctions, unlike the sinoatrial node.
16. C.
17. B.
18. D. "Cardiac valves are classified into two groups based on their function and anatomy. The mitral and tricuspid valves, which conduct blood to the ventricles, are part of the AV group; the aortic and pulmonary valves, which conduct blood out of the ventricles, are part of the semilunar group".
19. D. A structure made up of papillary muscles, chorda tendon, leaflets, and annuls is responsible for the valve's stability.
20. C. The left ventricle is 1.3–1.5 cm thick, whereas the right ventricle is 0.3–0.5 cm thick.
21. D. The root of the posterior descending artery is referred to as supremacy (PDA). "The heart is said to be right-dominant when the PDA is formed from the terminal branch of the RCA (>85% of cases)".
22. B.
23. B. "The right coronary artery (RCA) is a single large artery that runs along the right AV groove. The right atrium, right ventricle, interventricular septum, and SA and AV nodes all receive blood from the RCA".
24. B.
25. D.

References

1. Kenny, T. The nuts and bolts of implantable device therapy pacemakers, 1st ed. Wiley; 2015.
2. Weinhaus AJ, Roberts KP. Anatomy of the human heart. In: Iaizzo, P. editor. Handbook of cardiac anatomy, physiology, and devices. Humana Press; 2009. https://doi.org/10.1007/978-1-60327-372-5_5.
3. Hinton RB, Yutzey KE. Heart valve structure and function in development and disease. Annu Rev Physiol. 2011;73:29–46. https://doi.org/10.1146/annurev-physiol-012110-142145.
4. Iaizzo, PA, editor. Handbook of cardiac anatomy, physiology, and devices. Springer Science and Business Media; 2010.
5. Sundjaja JH, Bordoni B. Anatomy, thorax, heart pulmonic valve. In: StatPearls. Treasure Island (FL): StatPearls Publishing; 2021.
6. Lama P, Tamang BK, Kulkarni J. Morphometry and aberrant morphology of the adult human tricuspid valve leaflets. Anat Sci Int. 2016;91(2):143–50. https://doi.org/10.1007/s12565-015-0275-0.
7. Bauer M. Cardiovascular anatomy and pharmacology. Basic Sci Anesth. 2017;3:195–228. https://doi.org/10.1007/978-3-319-62067-1_11.PMCID:PMC7121118.
8. Drake R, Vogl W, Mitchell A, Drake R. Gray's atlas of anatomy. 3rd ed. London: Churchill Livingstone Elsevier; 2014.
9. Lee CH, Laurence DW, Ross CJ, et al. Mechanics of the Tricuspid Valve-From Clinical Diagnosis/Treatment, In-Vivo and In-Vitro Investigations, to Patient-Specific Biomechanical

Modeling. Bioengineering (Basel). 2019;6(2):47. Published 2019 May 22. https://doi.org/10.3390/bioengineering6020047.

10. Sanchez Vaca F, Bordoni B. Anatomy, thorax, mitral valve. In: StatPearls. Treasure Island (FL): StatPearls Publishing; 2021.

11. Thorp J, Rogers D. Thorp and Covich's Freshwater invertebrates. 4th ed. London: Academic Press; 2015.

12. Rich NL, Khan YS. Anatomy, thorax, heart papillary muscles. In: StatPearls. Treasure Island (FL): StatPearls Publishing; 2021.

13. Tucker WD, Shrestha R, Burns B. Anatomy, abdomen and pelvis, inferior vena cava. In: StatPearls. Treasure Island (FL): StatPearls Publishing; 2021.

14. Padala SK, Cabrera JA, Ellenbogen KA. Anatomy of the cardiac conduction system. Pacing Clin Electrophysiol. 2021;44(1):15–25. https://doi.org/10.1111/pace.14107.

15. Hazekamp M. Coronary anatomy in congenital heart disease: the important contributions of Professor Dr. Adriana Gittenberger-de Groot. J Cardiovasc Dev Dis. 2021;8(3). https://doi.org/10.3390/jcdd8030027. PMID: 33803117; PMCID: PMC8000438.

16. Whiteman S, Alimi Y, Carrasco M, Gielecki J, Zurada A, Loukas M. Anatomy of the cardiac chambers: a review of the left ventricle, Translational Research in Anatomy. ScienceDirect; 2021.

17. Bravo-Valenzuela NJ, Peixoto AB, Araujo JE. Prenatal diagnosis of congenital heart disease: a review of current knowledge. Indian Heart J. 2018;70(1):150–64. https://doi.org/10.1016/j.ihj.2017.12.005.

18. Parkhomenko RA, et al. SIOP ABSTRACTS. Pediatr Blood Cancer. 2020;67(S4):1294–1294.

19. Anderson RH, Franklin RCG, Spicer DE. Anatomy of the functionally univentricular heart. World J Pediatr Congenit Heart Surg. 2018;9(6):677–84. https://doi.org/10.1177/2150135118800694.

20. Gaasedelen E, Deakyne A, Iles T, Iaizzo P. Using Smartphone-Based Virtual Reality to Explore Internal Anatomy of 3D Heart Models. In: Proceedings of the 2017 design of medical devices conference. Minneapolis, Minnesota, USA; 2017. 10–13 April 2017. V001T09A009. ASME. https://doi.org/10.1115/DMD2017-3472.

21. Jarvis S, Saman S. Cardiac system 1: anatomy and physiology. Nursing Times [online]. 2018;114:2, 34–37.

Physiology of the Heart

Mustafa Raad Kamil

Abstract It is essential for the maintenance of hemostasis that fundamental materials, such as oxygen and nutrients, are continuously picked up from the external environment and delivered to cells, while waste is eliminated. Hemostasis requires the regulation of body temperature, which is accomplished by transporting generated heat to the skin and releasing it at the body's surface, so that muscle heat activity is maintained. The blood also carries hormones, the chemical messengers of the body. The bloodstream transports it from the site of production to tissues or organs, and it is essential for regulating physiology and behavior. The cardiovascular system includes the heart, blood vessels, and blood.

Keywords Stroke volume · Cardiac output · Peripheral resistance · Blood pressure · Heart rate · Pulse rate · Apex beat · Bruit · Carotid · Pacemaker · Excitation fibers · Cardiac cycle

1 Introduction

The heart is the primary component of this system. The blood contains oxygen and other nutrients that our bodies need to survive. The body takes nutrients and oxygen from the blood and gives to the blood waste products for it to get rid of (Fig. 1).

2 Relationships of the CVS to Homeostasis

Humans have trillions of cells that need oxygen and nutrients to continue working, so the body requires a more sophisticated system to help maintain homeostasis [1, 2].

By transporting nutrients and waste products, preventing blood loss, distributing heat, and containing white blood cells that protect the body as part of the immune

M. R. Kamil (✉)
College of Medicine, Thi Qar University, Nassiryah, Iraq
e-mail: musta-faraad70@gmail.com

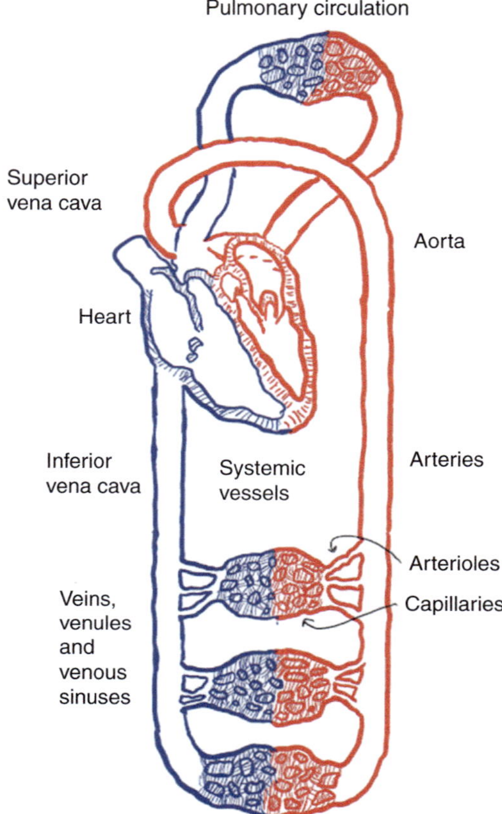

Fig. 1 The circulatory system

system, the blood maintains hemostasis. Without these safeguards, death or infection will occur, which could be fatal [3].

3 The Cardiac Muscles

The heart is located in the front and center of the chest cavity, slightly behind and to the left of the breastbone, and directly above the diaphragm [4]. The endocardium is a thin membrane that lines the inside of the heart and separates the myocardium from the blood flow through the heart [5]. The endocardium also lines the blood-flow-regulating valves and, as a service to the conduction system, regulates the heart's activity and rhythm via nerves embedded within it.

The heart's pumping action is caused by the rhythmic contraction and relaxation of the myocardium. The contraction pumps the blood, which raises the blood's pressure

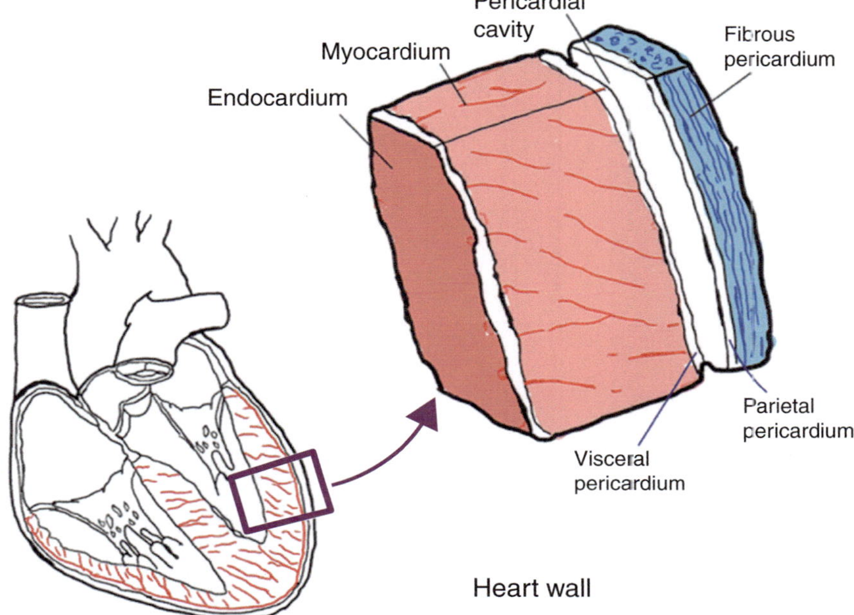

Fig. 2 The heart muscles

and forces it out. When the muscle relaxes, the chamber enlarges and blood fills it (Fig. 2).

4   Coronary Circulation

See Fig. 3.

Functions of the Atria

The atria serve the following functions. (1) They receive and store the venous return during ventricular systole before delivering it to the ventricles during ventricular diastole. (2) The atrial walls contain stretch receptors that monitor changes in intra-atrial pressure and initiate several cardiovascular regulatory reflexes. (3) Certain atrial cells secrete the atrial natriuretic peptide, which promotes the kidney's excretion of sodium and water.

Fig. 3 Heart valves

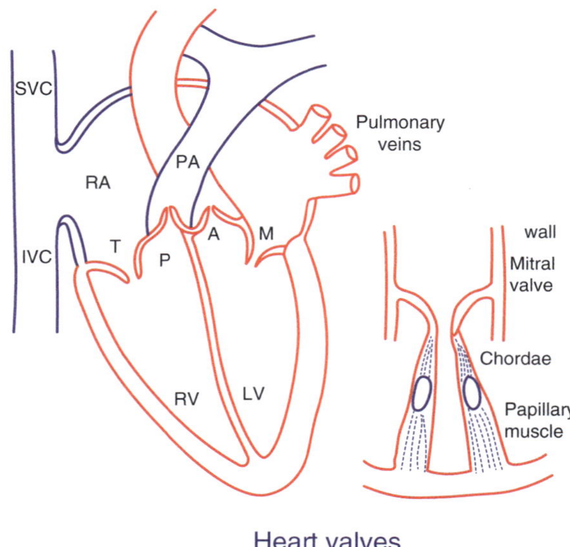

Types of Cardiac Muscle Fibers

(A) Contractile Fiber (99%)

Atrial and ventricular walls are composed of these fibers.
  They are characterized by the following:

(1) Similar to skeletal muscles, they are striated and contract via a similar mech-
     anism. The T-system is located at the Z lines. Additionally, they contain the
     protein dystrophin, a deficiency of which causes cardiomyopathy, a serious
     form of heart disease.
(2) Along the muscle fibers, there are intercalated disks (Fig. 4), which are always
     present at the Z lines. These disks are cell membranes that separate individual
     fibers [1, 6].

  Accordingly, from a functional point of view, the cardiac muscle is a syncytium
that follows the all-or-nothing rule and causes its contraction as a single unit resulting
in an efficient pumping force. The heart contains two functional syncytia, one formed
by the walls of the two atriums and the other by the walls of the two ventricles. The
fibrous A-V ring fully separates these syncytia.

(B) Autorhythmic Fibers (1%)

These are converted into nearly non-contractile cardiac muscle fibers that are unique
for the production, conduction, and distribution of cardiac action potentials that
stimulate contractile muscle fibers. They form a network of wires known as the heart's
conducting system and connect contractile muscle fibers through gap junctions.

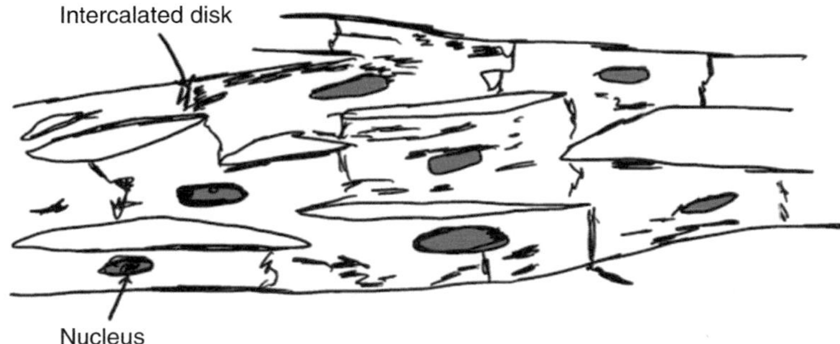

Fig. 4 Cardiac muscles fibers

5 Mechanism of the Beating of the Heart

A specialized muscular conducting system in the heart is responsible for initiating and propagating action potentials to the ventricles, which then induce ventricular contraction.

6 Heart Conduction System

See Fig. 5.

7 Electrical Activity of the Heart

Cardiac action potential

See Figs. 6, 7 and 8.

Phases of cardiac muscle action potential [6]
See Figs. 9 and 10.

Frank-Starling's Law of the Heart
See Figs. 11 and 12.

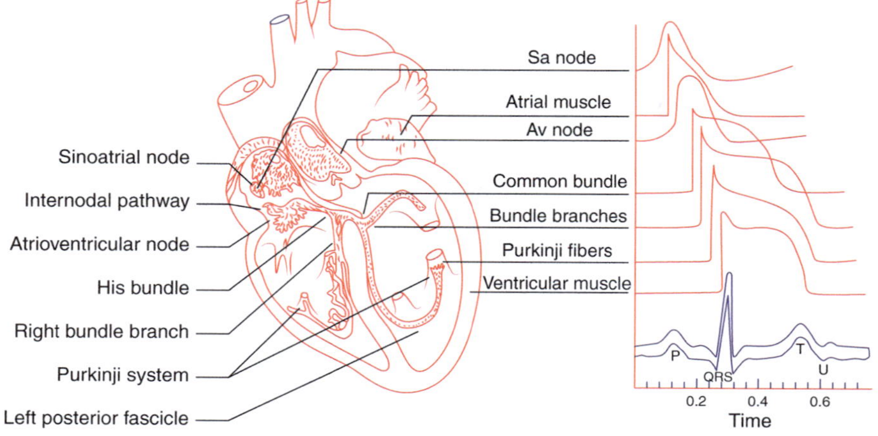

The conducting system of the heart
and their actions potentials

Fig. 5 The conduction system of the heart and its action potentials

Fig. 6 Action potential of
the heart

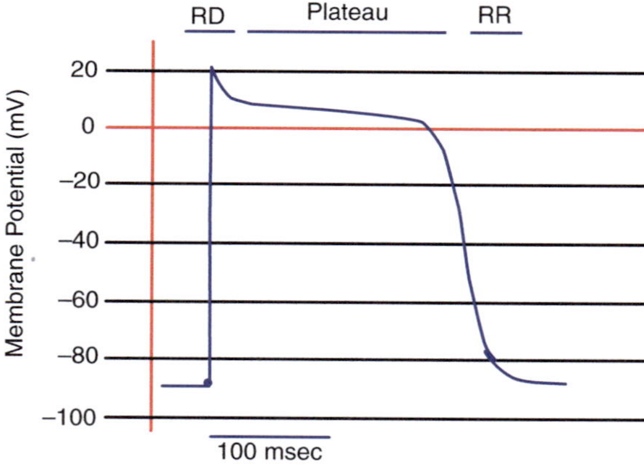

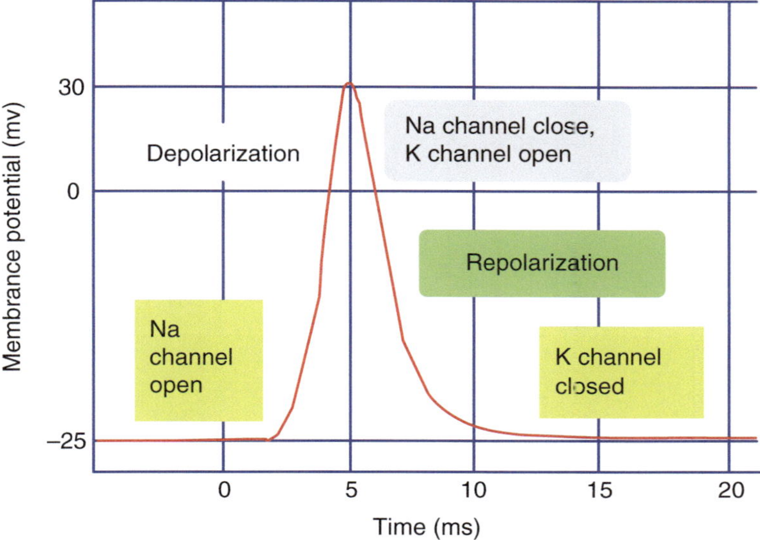

Fig. 7 Depolarization and repolarization of the heart

Fig. 8 Comparison between
the action potential of the
cardiac and skeletal muscles

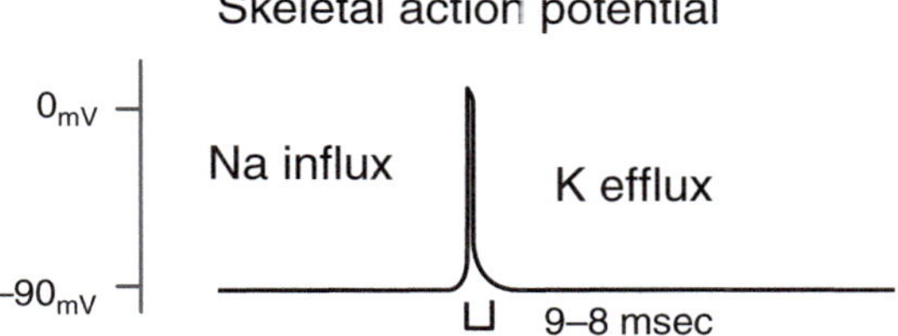

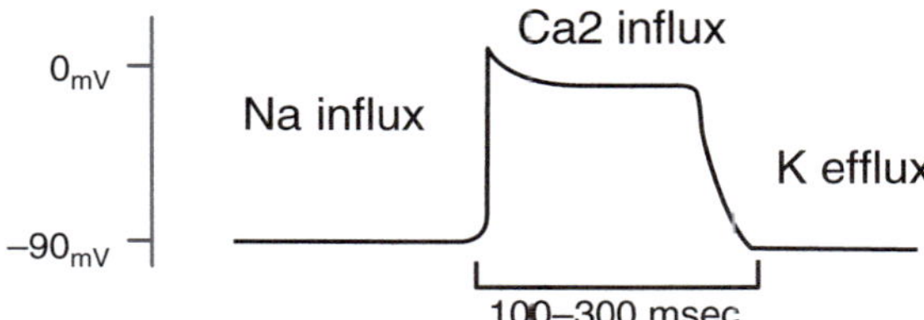

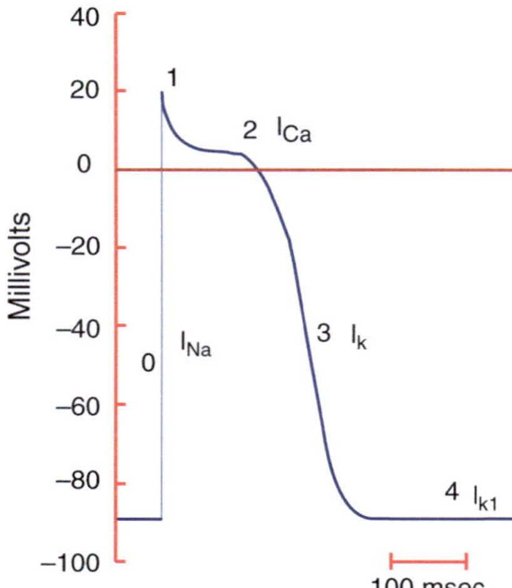

Fig. 9 The phases of the cardiac muscle action potential

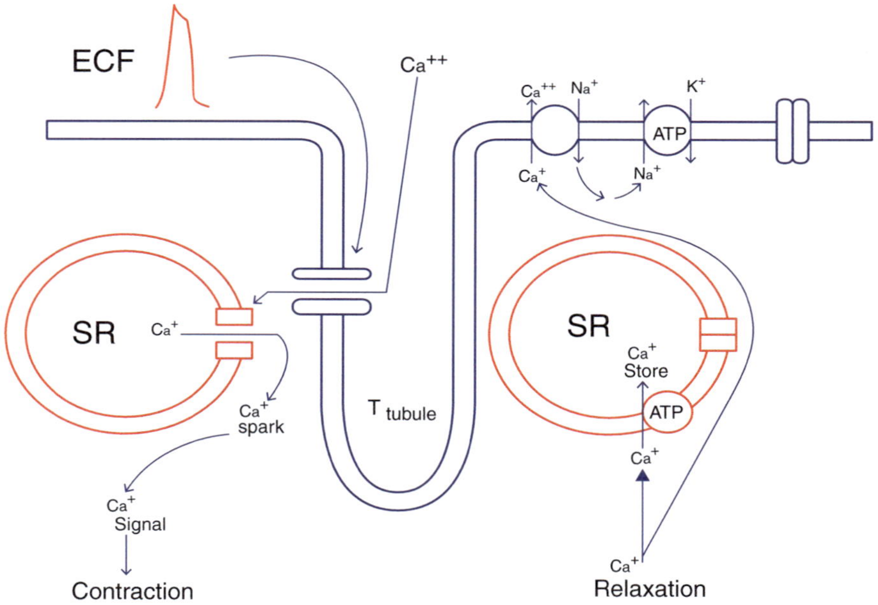

Fig. 10 Action potential stimulation

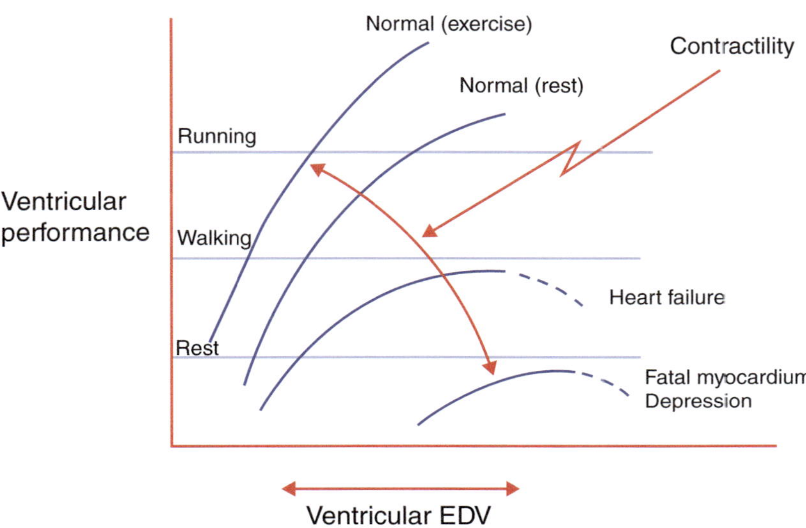

Fig. 11 Frank-Starling law

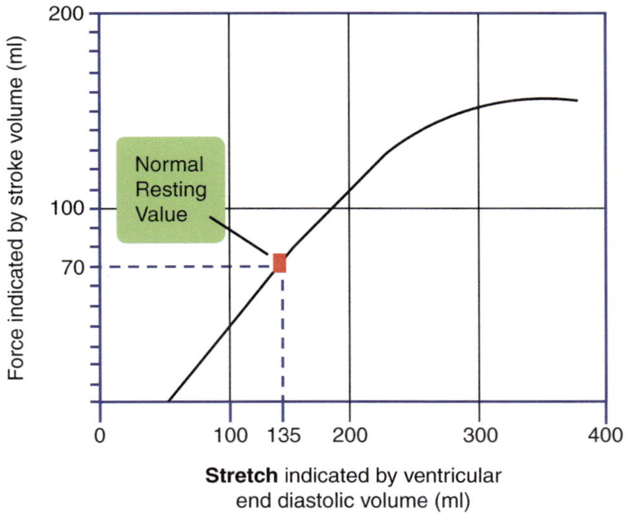

Fig. 12 Frank-Starling relationship

8   Control of the Heart by Sympathetic and Parasympathetic Nerves

Extrasystoles (Premature Beats)

These are abnormal contractions caused by the discharge of impulses from an ectopic focus that is hyperexcitable. These foci may originate in the ventricle, causing ventricular extrasystoles, or the atria or atrioventricular node, causing supraventricular extrasystoles. They may arise physiologically, as in the case of smoking, or pathologically, as in myocardial ischemia. Extrasystoles occur only when an ectopic focus discharges during diastole, as impulses discharged during systole fall within the absolute refractory period and are therefore ineffective. They are called premature beats because they do not increase the heart rate, cause irregular heart rate, and are frequently associated with pulse deficit.

9   ECG: Recording the Heart's Electrical Activity

See Fig. 13.

"A standard ECG is obtained by setting an electrode on each limb and at six specific locations on the anterior chest wall. In a lead, one electrode is regarded as the positive side of a voltmeter and another is the negative side" [7].

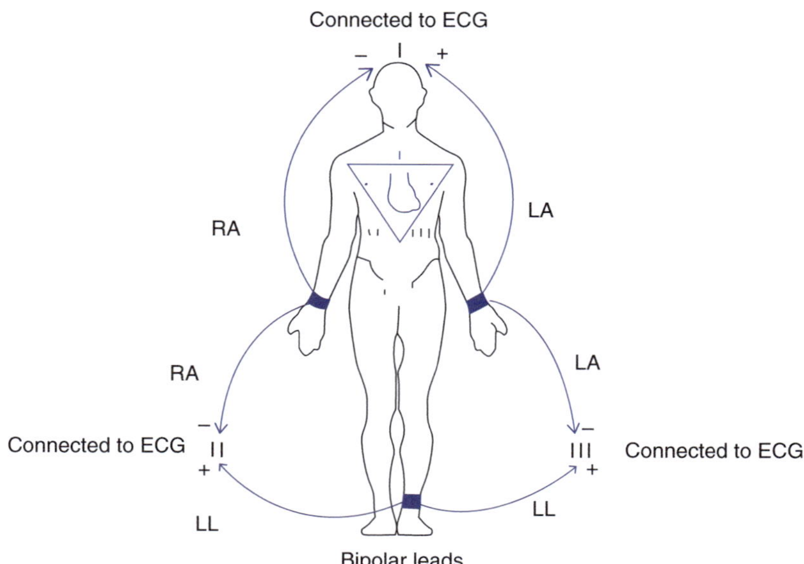

Fig. 13 ECG leads distribution

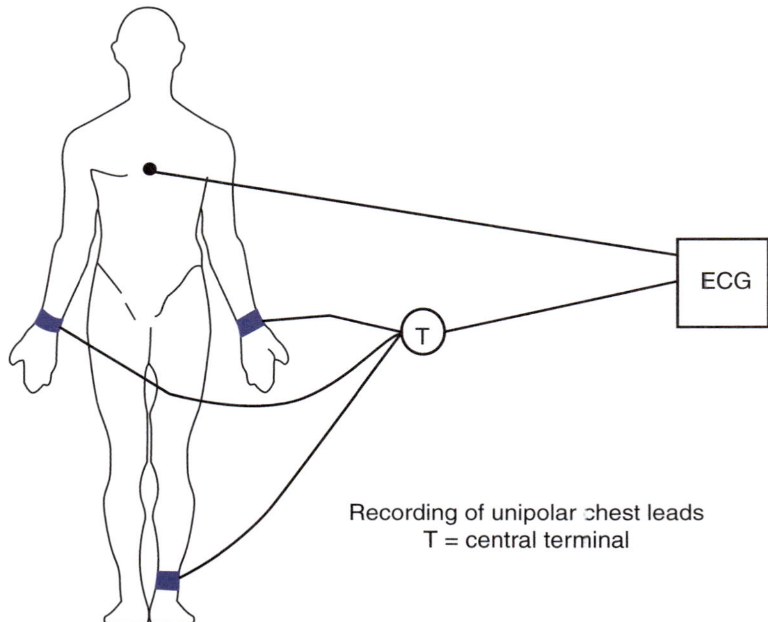

Fig. 14 ECG upper and lower limbs lead

The ECG Lead

The 12 electrodes that record the ECG can be applied at many areas of the skin, and any particular positioning of these electrodes is called a lead. Typically, 12 leads are used to record electric cardiac events from various situations.

(B) *Unipolar Leads*

See Fig. 14.

How can an ECG electrode be made indifferent (at 0 potential)?

In a locked circuit, the potentials cancel each other out, so their algebraic sum is zero. Electrodes from three limbs connected to a central terminal form a closed circuit, so the terminal's potential will be zero. Consequently, when the central terminal is connected to the negative pole of the electrocardiograph, it will constitute an indifferent electrode with zero potential, known as Wilson's electrode, and applying the exploring electrode, which is the electrode that is connected to the positive pole of the electrocardiograph, at a certain point will record the absolute potential at that point (Fig. 15).

The Augmented Unipolar Limb Leads (Goldberger's Leads)

By separating the electrode from the central terminal, a unipolar limb lead can be augmented. The augmented lead then measures the difference between the potential

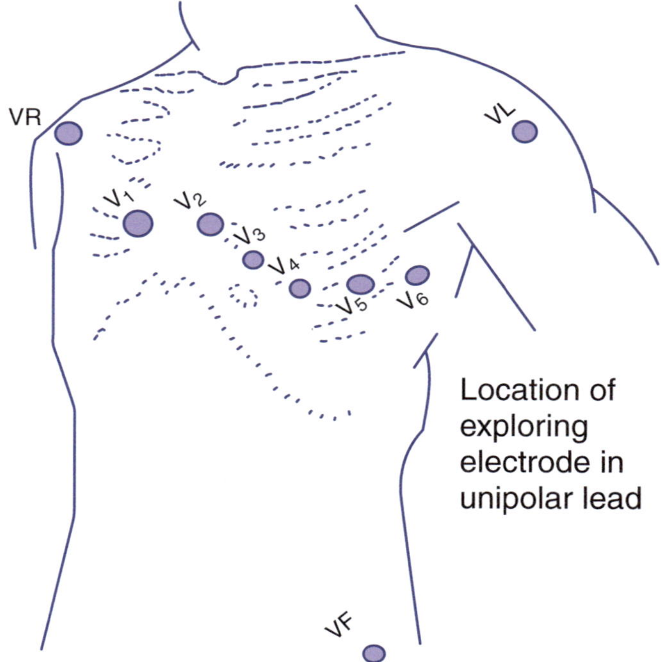

Fig. 15 ECG chest leads

of one limb and the sum of the potentials of the other two limbs; for example, to record a VR, the electrode of the central terminal in the right arm is detached (Fig. 16).

Calibration of the Electrocardiograph

This is arranged such that a charge of 1 mV results in a deflection of 10 mm amplitude, so each millimeter in the vertical lines of the tracing paper (a side of a small square) corresponds to 0.1 mV. In contrast, the typical recording speed is 25 mm per second, so the duration of each millimeter in the horizontal lines of the tracing paper (side of a small square) is 0.04 s and the duration of each 5 mm (side of a large square) is 0.20 s.

The heart rate is then determined by the number of cardiac cycles per minute. For example, if the measured distance was 15 mm, the duration of a single cardiac cycle would be $15 \times 0.04 = 0.6$ s, and the heart rate would be $60/0.6 = 100$ beats per minute [8].

Additionally, the heart rate can be determined by counting the number of smaller, larger squares on the ECG paper. When the recording speed is 25 mm per second, one minute will be represented by $25 \times 60 = 1500$ mm on the ECG paper (i.e. 1500 small squares or 300 big squares). In this example, if the duration of one cardiac cycle was 15 mm (i.e. 15 small squares or 3 large squares), the heart rate would be $= 1500/15$ or $300/3 = 100$ beats per minute (Fig. 17).

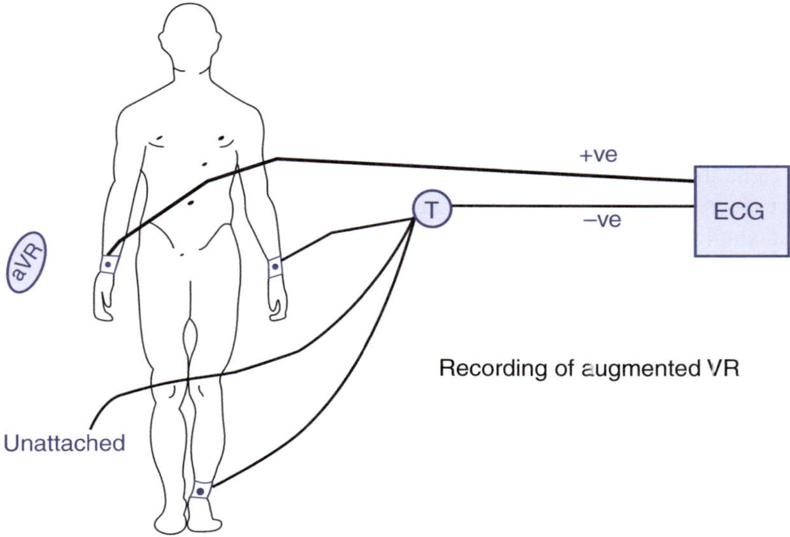

Fig. 16 Recording of augmented VR

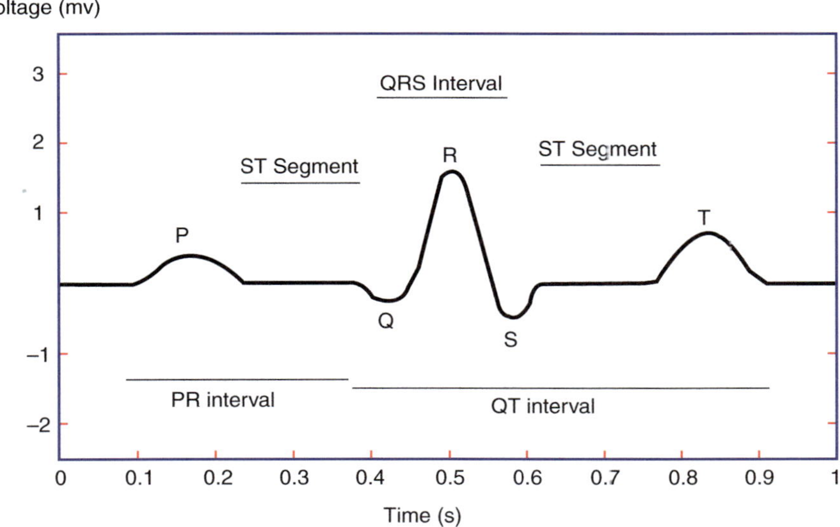

Fig. 17 The normal ECG

As a result of atrial depolarization, a P wave with an amplitude of approximately 0.1 mV and a duration of less than 0.1 s is generated. It is typically positive in all leads except a VR; its initial portion is caused by right atrial activation and its latter portion is caused by left atrial activation.

In hypertrophy of the left atrium, the P waves are enlarged and notched, and their duration increases, because depolarization of the hypertrophied muscle takes longer than usual.

In right atrial hypertrophy, the amplitude and duration of the right portion of the P waves increase and overlap with those of the left, resulting in P waves with nearly normal amplitude and duration and a prominent peak. Additionally, the P waves are inverted in AV nodal rhythm and disappear in atrial fibrillation.

The QRS Complex

This is a representation of the depolarization of the ventricle. This wave has a duration of about 0.06–0.10 s and is formed as a result of ventricular depolarization.

T Wave

This wave is created by the repolarization of the ventricle. Its amplitude is between 0.2 and 0.4 mV, and its duration is between 0.20 and 0.25 s. Its duration is longer than that of the OR complex, as repolarization is slower than depolarization. The last portion of the ventricular muscle to depolarize is the first portion to repolarize, so ventricular repolarization progresses from the myocardial epicardial surface to the endocardial surface, resulting in an upright positive deflection [9].

The P-R Segment

This is a portion of the electrocardiogram that occurs between the termination of the P wave and the beginning of ventricular depolarization [10]. It is characterized by a depolarization that takes place in the conducting system, beginning with the AV node at the very peak of the P wave. However, because the depolarized tissue is not large enough to generate electric changes that are significant enough to reach the body surface, it remains silent and does not contain any waves.

The S-T Segment

This is the line between the S peak and the T peak [10], and its average duration is 0.12 s. During this segment, all ventricular impulses are depolarized, hence its normal isoelectricity suggests myocardial dysfunction or injury.

Cardiac Arrhythmias

The majority of arrhythmias can be categorized as either abnormalities of impulse production or impulse conduction. Abnormalities in impulse generation result in an abnormally rapid firing rate of sinus pacemaker cells or an ectopic pacemaker focus. Impulse conduction abnormalities may occur in delayed or accelerated conduction [11].

1. **Tachycardia: more than 100 per min**

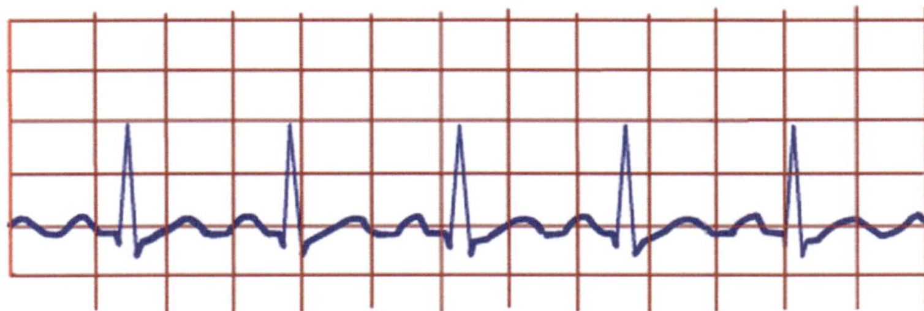

2. **Bradycardia**

Heart rate is less than 60 beats per minute. It may be physiological (most of which are) or pathological.

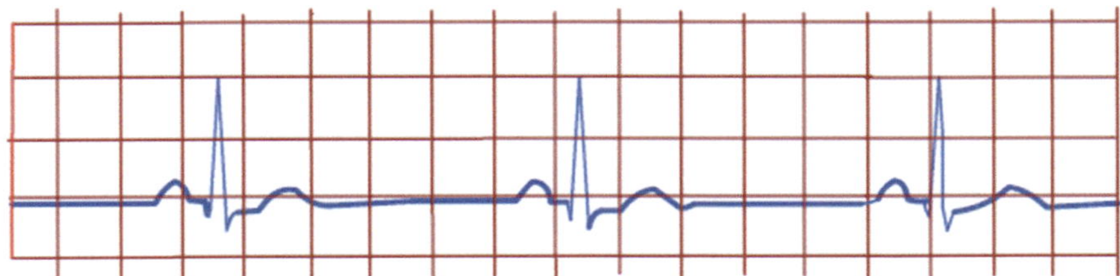

3. **Atrioventricular Block**

Impairment of impulse conduction from atria to ventricle.

- First-degree block (prolonged P-R interval).

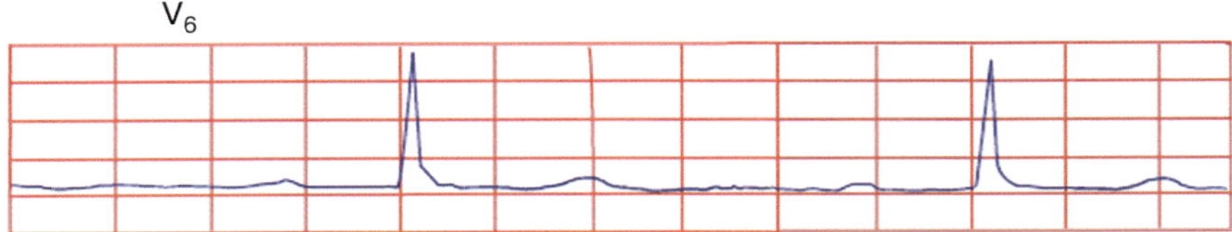

- Second-degree block.

P wave not followed by QRS complex.

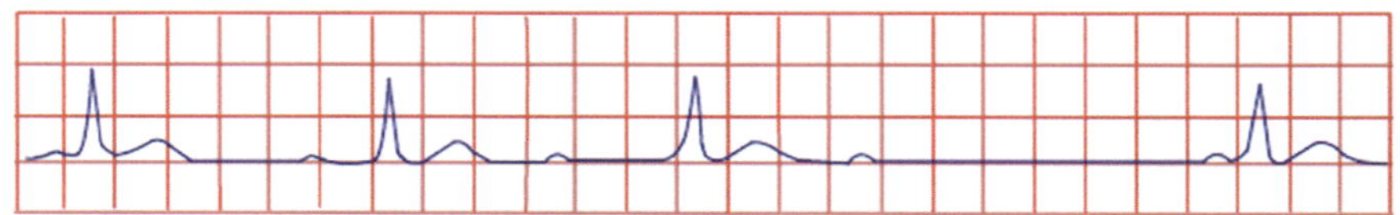

- Complete A-V block (third-degree block).

No impulse moves by the conduction system from part to part [9]. It can be recognized by the dissociation between the P wave and the QRS complex [11].

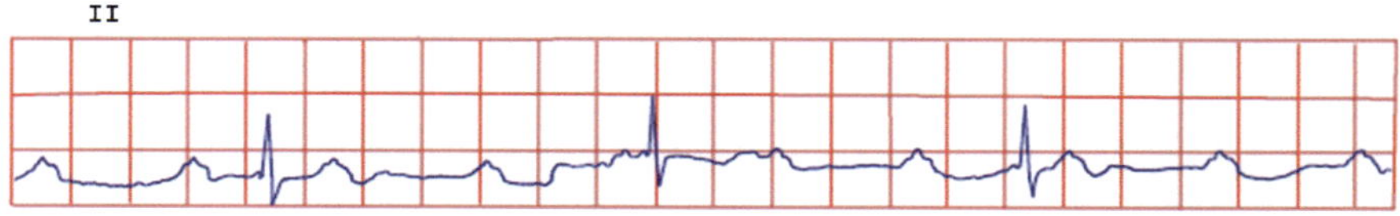

4. Atrial Fibrillation

Irregular tachycardia [11].

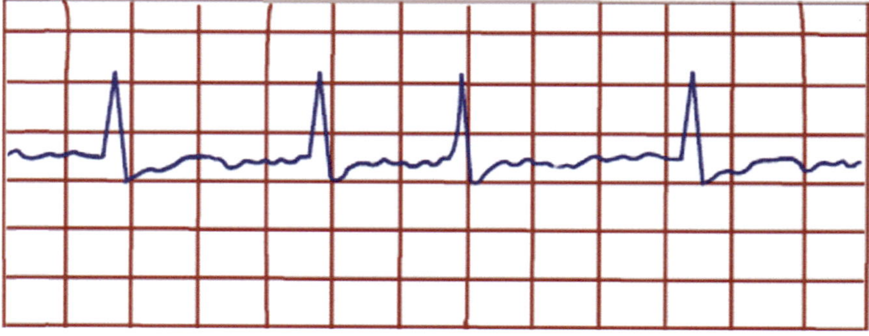

5.   **Ventricular Fibrillation**

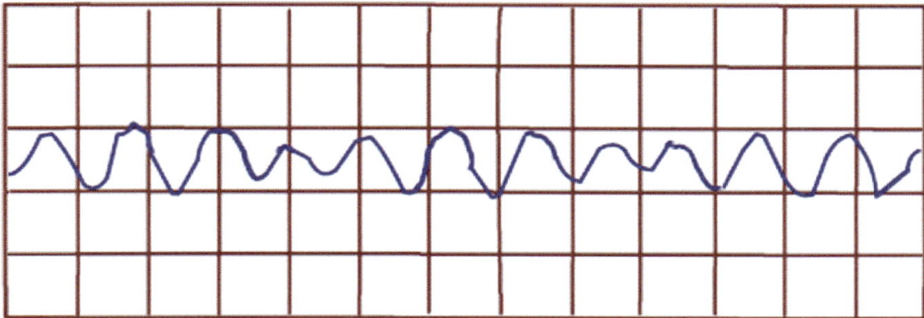

See Figs. 18 and 19.

The Dichotic Notch and Waves

This causes the closure of the semilunar valves, the creation of the second heart sound, and a little oscillation on the downslope of the aortic and pulmonary arterial pressure curves, known as the dichotic notch or incisura. This is caused by blood vibrations when semilunar valves are suddenly closed.

Following the dichotic notch, a wave known as the dichotic wave is recorded as a result of a slight increase in the aortic and pulmonary arterial pressures, which subsequently progressively decline due to blood flow to the peripheral smaller vessels. This wave occupies the diastolic period and is produced as a result of the elastic recoil of the aortic and pulmonary arterial walls. The latter effect is caused by a mechanism known as the windkessel effect, which occurs as a result of the stretching of the aorta and pulmonary artery during the ejection phases and creates potential energy in their walls. During isometric relaxation, this potential energy is converted into kinetic energy, causing these vessels to rebound and recoil. The windkessel effect maintains forward blood movement during ventricular diastoles, making blood flow to tissues continuous throughout both systoles and diastoles and not pulsatile, that is, not intermittent during systoles alone [12] (Fig. 20).

10   Heart Sounds

A sensitive microphone implanted on the chest wall can record heart sounds, a process known as phonocardiography (Fig. 21).

The first sound heard at the beginning of ventricular systole is "lub", while the second sound heard at the beginning of ventricular diastole is "dup". In tachycardia, the diastolic periods are shortened, therefore the pauses are shorter and it becomes

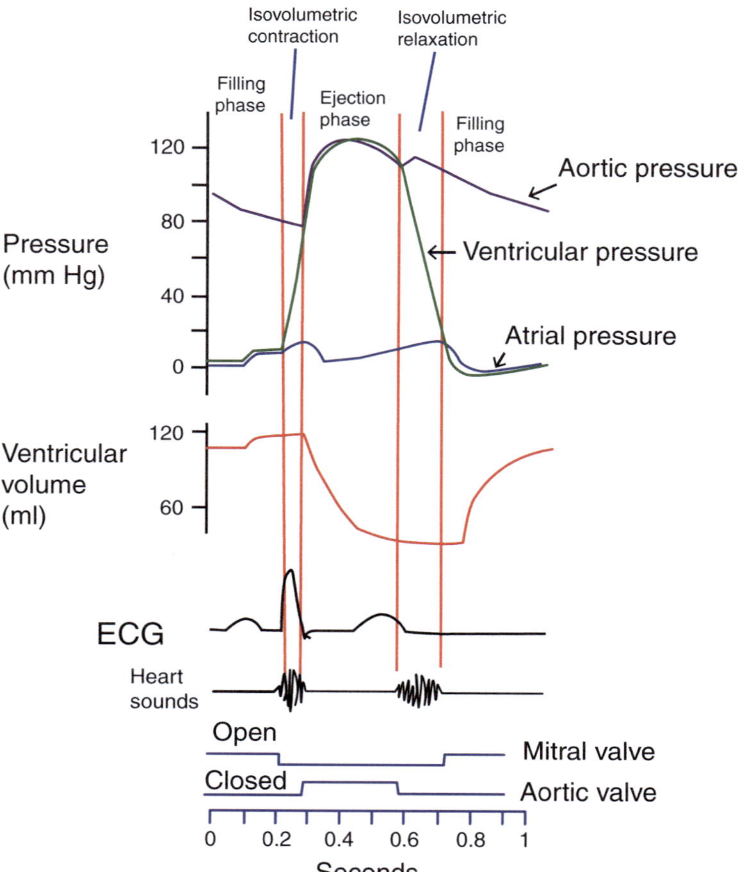

Fig. 18 Cardiac cycle

difficult to distinguish between the two sounds. However, they can still be distinguished by palpating the carotid pulse simultaneously. The first cardiac sound occurs simultaneously with the carotid pulse.

The First Heart Sound

Timing in the cardiac cycle: This sound coincides with the onset of ventricular systole, so it falls mainly during the isometric contraction phase and also extends in the early part of the maximum ejection phase.

Cause: Closure of the AV valves.

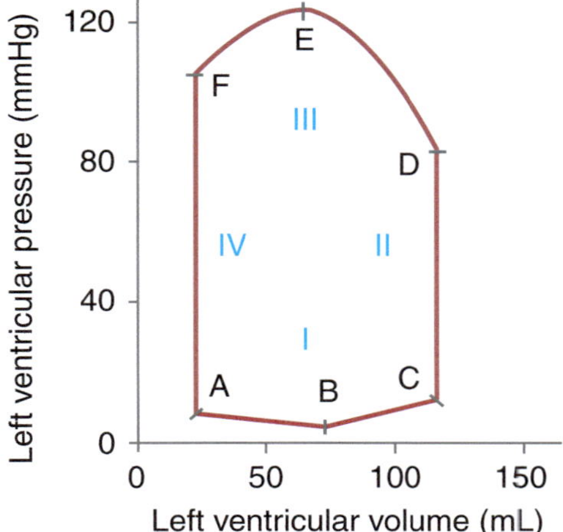

Fig. 19 Left ventricular volume

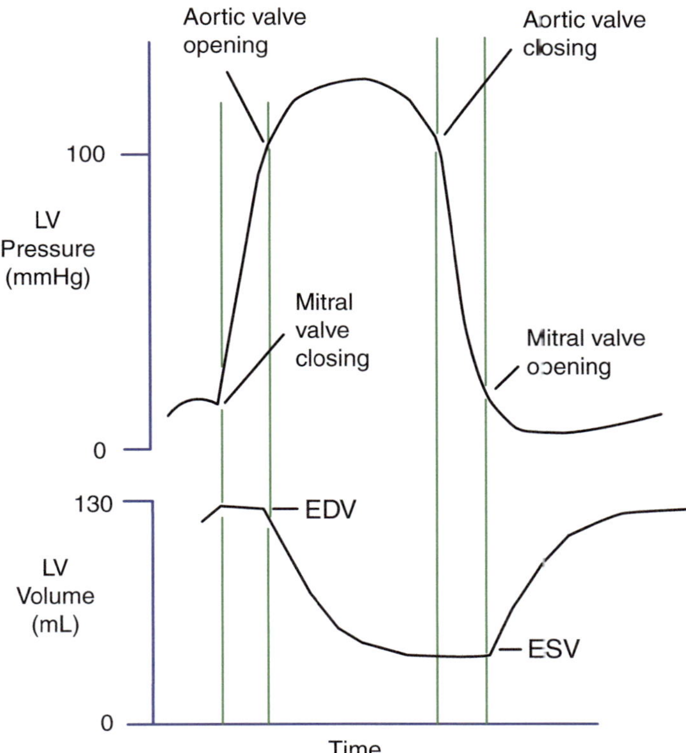

Fig. 20 Movement of valves

Fig. 21 Phonocardiogram

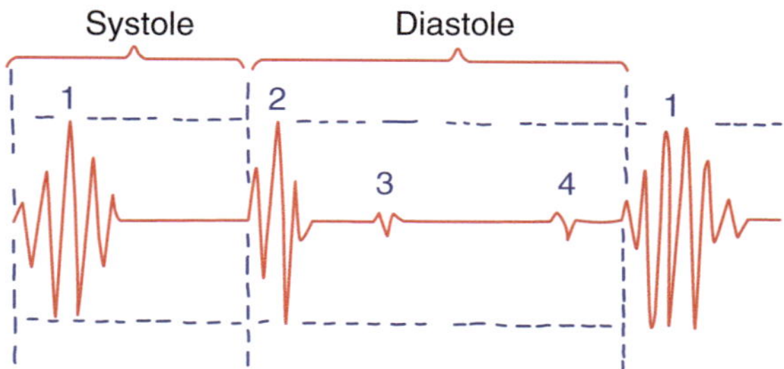

Mechanism: The sound is produced by the vibrations set up in the blood, chordae tendineae, and ventricular wall after closure of the AV valves. It is not the result of snapping shut of the valves (because blood greatly damps the effect of the slapping of the valve leaflets together) [12].

Character: It is a soft low-pitched sound.

Duration: About 0.15 s.

Site of bearing: Closure of the mitral valve is best heard over the apex of the heart at the fifth left intercostal space, 10 cm from the midline, just internal to the midclavicular line. On the other hand, closure of the tricuspid valve is best heard at the lower end of the sternum (Fig. 18).

Splitting of the first heart sound: Normally, the mitral valve closes before the tricuspid valve, and this would produce a splitting of the first sound. However, this is difficult to detect by auscultation (and even by phonocardiography) because the sounds produced by closure of both valves are low pitched and merge into each other.

The Second Heart Sound

Timing in the cardiac cycle: This sound coincides with the onset of ventricular diastole, so it falls during the isometric relaxation phase (Fig. 14).

Cause: Closure of the semilunar valves

Mechanism: The sound is produced by the vibrations set up in the blood, ventricular walls, and walls of the aorta and pulmonary artery after closure of the semilunar valves [7]. It is also not the result of the snapping shut of the valves.

Character: It is sharp and has a higher pitch than that of the first sound.

Duration: About 0.12 s.

Site of hearing: Closure of the aortic valve is heard over the second costal cartilage at the right sternal border, while closure of the pulmonary valve is heard at the second left intercostal space close to the sternum [7].

Physiological splitting of the second heart sound [7].

Normally, the pulmonary valve closes after the aortic valve (because the right ventricle is weaker than the left ventricle, so its systole is longer) leading to splitting of the second sound. Such splitting is more apparent during deep inspiration because this increases the venous return which further delays closure of the pulmonary valve (=physiological splitting) [7]. In addition, splitting of the second sound is characterized by the following:

1. It is easier to hear than the splitting of the first sound (because closure of the semilunar valves produces high pitched sounds).
2. It is heard almost only at the pulmonary area (because closure of the aortic valve is audible in all areas of the precordium [13].
3. It is more easily heard in children and it may be inaudible in older individuals, specially males (due to muscle noise and the thick chest wall).

Paradoxical splitting of the second heart sound:

This is a condition in which the pulmonary valve closes before the aortic valve. It is characteristic of left ventricular failure (due to the slower ejection from the left ventricle than normal which delays closure of the aortic valve). In this case, deep inspiration does not increase the splitting of the second sound but rather decreases it (= paradoxical splitting) [13] (Fig. 22).

The Third Heart Sound

This is a soft low-pitched sound that occurs during the rapid filling phase of the cardiac cycle (Fig. 14).

The Fourth Heart Sound

This is a faint very low-pitched sound that occurs during atrial systole; its mechanism is similar to that producing the third sound. Its duration is 0.03–0.05 s and is normally inaudible (see above).

Gallop Rhythm

In some heart diseases (specially left ventricular failure) and certain other conditions (e.g. severe anemia and thyrotoxicosis), the third or fourth heart sound is augmented and becomes audible. On auscultating the heart in the second itions, more than two sounds will be heard during each cardiac cycle, and these sounds follow each other in a rhythm similar to that produced by a galloping horse (so it is referred to as a gallop rhythm) [6].

Heart Murmurs

In contrast to a gallop, a heart murmur is an abnormal sound, as it is not ordinarily present. It develops when the normal laminar blood flow is replaced by turbulent blood flow, which occurs when the blood velocity exceeds a specified threshold. Blood velocity increases following a region of partial obstruction in a blood vessel, as well as when it passes through stenotic or insufficient heart valves. A stenotic valve is a stiff, narrowing valve that does not open completely, whereas an insufficient valve does not close fully.

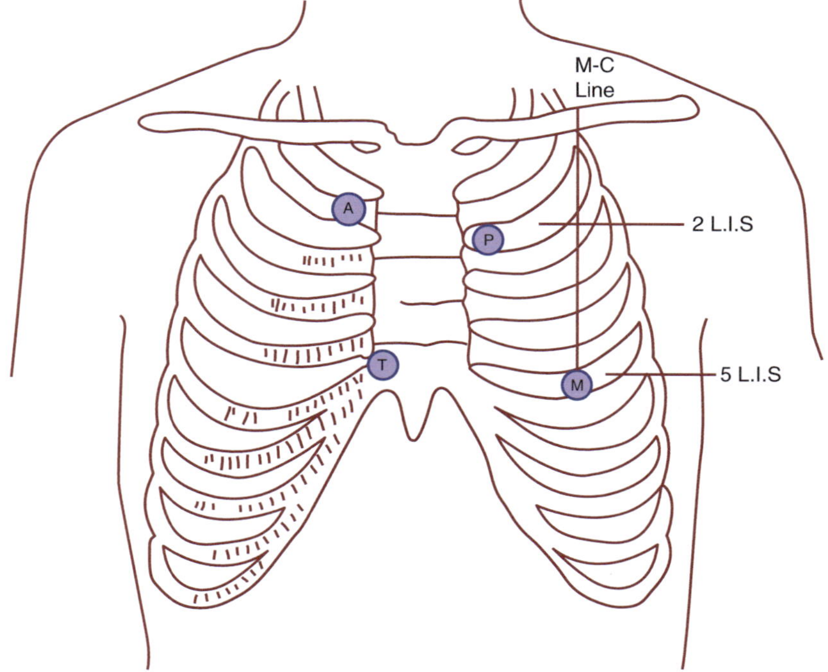

Sites of hearing the heart sounds by the stethoscope.
M,T,A,P= mitral, tricuspid, aortic, pulmonary areas.
L.I.S= left intercostal space.
M . C line = midclavicular line

Fig. 22 Site of hearing heart sounds

Types of Heart Murmurs

(1) Systolic murmurs: These are the murmurs that occur during the ventricular systolic phase (i.e. between the first and second sounds). They can arise in the absence of cardiac illness, as in anemia, fevers, and exertion, or as a result of valvular disorders caused by diseases, such as rheumatic fever or congenital abnormalities. These are the valvular diseases that cause systolic murmurs:

a. Stenosis of a semilunar valve

   (a) Stenosis of one of the semilunar valves
   (b) Incompetence of one of the AV valves may result from scarring of the valve cusps or a problem in the papillary muscle-chordae tendinea system.

During ventricular systole, blood regurgitation toward the atria occurs in these defective valves, producing the abnormal sound.

(c)   Ventricular Septal Defect (VSD).

(2)   Diastolic murmurs: These occur during the ventricular diastolic period (i.e. between the second and subsequent first sounds) as a result of one of the following valve disorders:

(a)   Stenosis of one of the AV valves, as in rheumatic fever.

(b)   Failure of one of the semilunar valves: In aortic incompetence, which can be caused by conditions like syphilis, blood regurgitates frcm the aorta into the left ventricle during ventricular diastole, causing a murmur and a decrease in diastolic pressure. Because the left ventricle will discharge a higher volume of blood than usual, the systolic pressure also rises, as does the pulse pressure (see below) [7].

(3)   Continuous murmurs are those that occur during both systole and diastole. This is typical of patent ductus arteriosus, as aortic blood pressure is always greater than pulmonary arterial blood pressure (Fig. 23).

Clinical Significance of the JVP

(A)   The a-interval, which extends from the beginning cf the "a" wave to the beginning of the "c" wave, is an indicator of conductivity via the A-V node.

(B)   Because jugular venous pressure waves are altered in many heart diseases, recording them can aid in the diagnosis of these conditions [3]. In cases of tricuspid incompetence caused by blood regurgitation from the right ventricle into the right atrium during ventricular systole, large "c" and "y" waves are detected [7].

Fig. 23   JVP wave

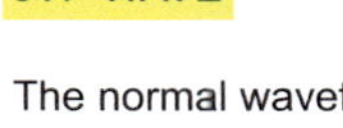

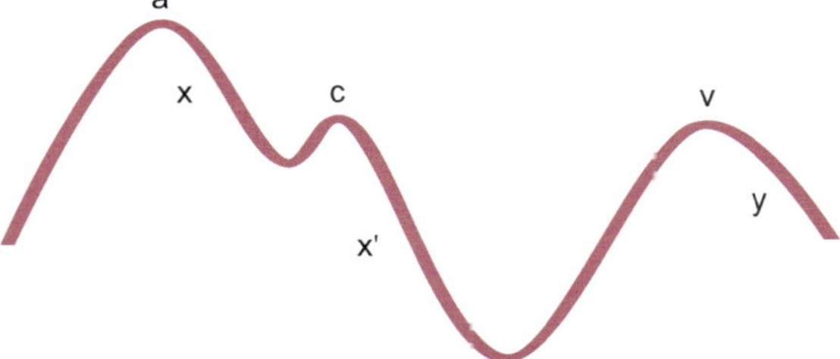

(1) The amplitude of the "a" wave is greatly increased in cases of tricuspid stenosis, pulmonary stenosis, and pulmonary hypertension.

(2) Cannon waves are detected when the right atrium and right ventricle contract at the same time, causing the tricuspid valve to close and causing a significant rise in right atrial pressure. This occurs in A-V dissociation cases, such as total heart block and ventricular tachycardia.

(3) Due to inadequate atrial contraction, the "a" wave disappears in atrial fibrillation. However, the number of "c" and "v" waves is higher than usual in this case, although they are highly irregular [6].

(4) Jugular venous pressure can be used to distinguish between atrial and ventricular extrasystoles because atrial extrasystoles create jugular venous pressure with an "a" wave while ventricular extrasystoles produce jugular venous pressure without an "a" wave.

11 Cardiac Output (CO)

"The cardiac output is the volume of blood pumped each minute by each ventricle; it is also known as the cardiac minute volume" [7, 10, 13].

Normal cardiac output at rest is 5.0–5.5 L per minute, with both ventricles contributing equally

Factors that Affect the End Systolic Volume (ESV)

These are the same factors that affect myocardial contractility.

Diastolic (Relaxation) Properties of the Ventricles

Relaxation of the ventricles is essential for optimal cardiac function, as inadequate relaxation reduces stroke volume and cardiac output due to ventricular filling impairment. The process of ventricular relaxation is determined by both active and passive properties; however, the active relaxation property of the ventricles is responsible for the majority of ventricular filling during early diastole, so the majority of positive inotropic factors increase ventricular filling.

(2) The passive relaxation property of the ventricles refers to a variety of mechanical elements that influence ventricular relaxation passively. These factors, particularly ventricular compliance and stiffness, influence the extent of ventricular filling. The degree of ventricular relaxation is reduced when ventricular compliance is reduced, as in cardiac tamponade, or when ventricular stiffness is increased, as in infarction and hypertrophy (Table 1).

Table 1 Factors that affect the end diastolic volume (EDV)

Atrial pressure	This is the ventricular filling pressure. Its increase is caused by atrial systole, which raises end-diastolic volume, and vice versa
Blood volume	Hypovolemia causes a decrease in the mean circulatory pressure (MCP), venous return (VR), atrial pressure and end-diastolic volume. Hypervolemia has opposite effects
Venous tone	Venoconstriction induced by sympathetic stimulation raises the MCP, leading to an increase in VR, atrial pressure, and end-diastolic volume
Intrapericardial pressure	Its increase in conditions of fluid or blood accumulation decreases the end-diastolic volume
Atrial fibrillation	This weakens atrial contraction, hence decreasing the atria's pumping function and the end-diastolic volume
Intrathoracic pressure	An increase in its negativity, such as during deep inspiration, increases the VR and promotes ventricular relaxation, both of which increase the end-diastolic volume. If its negativity is lost or turns positive, as in pneumothorax, opposite effects occur
Muscle contraction	This increases the VR, atrial pressure, and end-diastolic volume

Methods of Measurement of Cardiac Output

(1) Echocardiography: is a non-invasive technique since it does not require cardiac catheterization or chemical injection [4].

(2) Application of Fick's Principle: This states that the amount of a substance taken up by an organ per minute equals its arterial concentration minus its venous concentration multiplied by the organ's blood flow per minute [10]. This principle can be used to calculate the cardiac output of the right ventricle by determination of the following:

    (a) The total O consumption/minute (normally 250ml/min):

    (b) O content in venous blood (known by analysis of blood obtained from the pulmonary trunk by a cardiac catheter and is normally 140 ml/l).

    (c) O content in arterial blood (known by analysis of blood obtained from an artery by puncture under local anesthesia and is normally 190 ml/l).

(3) Indicator Dilution Method: A known quantity of a drug or radioactive isotope is injected into an arm vein, and its concentration is measured every two seconds in successive arterial blood samples and plotted over time. The dye concentration progressively increases to a maximum, then decreases before rising again. Extrapolation of the curve determines the time of a single circulation of the dye through the heart, the end of which is signaled by a re-rise in its concentration in the arterial blood.

The average concentration of the dye in the arterial blood is determined. Suppose it was 1.6 mg per liter, and if the time of a single circulation of the dye through the heart was 39 s during rest, then the blood flow from the left ventricle in 39 s = 5/1.6 = 3.1 L, and its output per minute = 3.1 × 60/39 = 4.7 L.

Factors that Affect the Cardiac Output

(A)　Effects of Changes in the HR on the CO

>　(1)　As the HR falls below 70 beats per minute, the SV rises because the ventricles have sufficient time to fill to capacity and the cardiac output remains nearly constant.
>　(2)　If the heart rate decreases below 50 beats/minute, the increase in the SV cannot compensate for the slowing of the heart, and the cardiac output is decreased.
>　(3)　As the heart rate increases from 70 to 180–200 beats/minute, the diastolic periods during which ventricular filling occurs are shortened, resulting in a drop in SV. However, the cardiac output remains constant or slightly increases due to the acceleration of the heart.
>　(4)　If the heart rate exceeds 180–200 beats/minute, the diastolic periods become significantly reduced, resulting in a significant fall in SV and a decrease in cardiac output since the decrease in SV is not compensated by cardiac acceleration.

(B)　Factors that Affect the Stroke Volume

(1)　The Cardiac Pumping Power

This is affected by the cardiac inotropic state, preload and afterload, and the myocardial blood supply, in addition to other factors, such as an increase in sympathetic overactivity and ventricular hypertrophy, and a decrease in cases of severe loss of functioning myocardium, such as massive infarction.

(2)　The Venous Return (VR)

The VR is a key factor in determining the SV and cardiac output. It influences the end-diastolic volume via the Frank-Starling law, and its volume is regulated by the following variables.

(a)　The mean circulatory pressure (MCP) or mean systemic filling pressure (MSFP).
(b)　The right atrial pressure (RAP): This is normally about 2 mmHg during recumbency and 0 mmHg in the standing position; the VR is inversely proportional to it.
(c)　The resistance to the VR: Normally, this is about 1.4 mmHg lite of blood flow, and the VR is inversely proportional to it (Table 2).

12　The Central Venous Pressure (CVP)

This is closely related to the right atrial pressure and affects the cardiac output and VR in opposite ways. It typically ranges from about 2 mmHg when standing to 4.6 mmHg when lying down.

Table 2 Factors that affect the venous return (VR)

Venous pressure gradient	This is the difference between the MCP and right atrial pressure, and it is the most important factor in determining the VR. This pressure gradient increases the VR, and vice versa [6]
Skeletal muscle pump	When skeletal muscles contract, the veins within them are compressed. This drives blood towards the heart, while the venous valves inhibit retrograde flow. These effects are likewise exerted, although to a lesser degree, by vascular pulsations
Respiratory pump	During inspiration, the intra-thoracic pressure becomes more negative, causing the thoracic veins to expand and their resistance to blood flow to decrease. Simultaneously, the intra-abdominal pressure rises due to descent of the diaphragm
Venous (venomotor) tone	This is a partial constriction of the venules caused by persistent sympathetic discharge to these veins during rest. It generates an upstream pressure that maintains the VR in opposition to gravity
Cardiac suction forces	During ventricular systole, the downward movement of the A-V ring functions as a suction force to draw blood from the veins into the atria. During early ventricular diastole, the rapid ventricular expansion is also accompanied by a rise in inflow from the filled atria, resulting in a decrease in atrial pressure and venous suction
Blood volume	In cases of bleeding, a decrease in blood volume decreases the MCP, leading to a decrease in the VR, and vice versa
Gravity	This antagonizes the VR in the lower extremities. However, this action is typically antagonized by thoracic and muscular pumps, venomotor tone, and heart suction forces
Arteriolar and capillary diameters	Arteriolar dilatation decreases the resistance to blood flow and increases the VR, and vice versa
Sympathetic stimulation	This increases the VR by increasing venous tone, cardiac suction forces, and arteriolar vascular resistance in skeletal muscles

Regulation (Control) of the Cardiac Output

This occurs through the regulation of the stroke volume and heart rate, which is generated by the two mechanisms:

(1) Extrinsic Regulation

This regulates both the stroke volume and heart rate. Activation of the sympathetic system improves cardiac output by increasing both heart rate and SV, whereas activation of the parasympathetic system decreases cardiac output by opposite effects. Catecholamines and thyroxine hormones also increase cardiac output via positive inotropic and chronotropic effects. Glucagon and insulin exert an inotropic effect as well.

Table 3 Physiological variations of the CO

Sleep	The cardiac output remains almost constant during calm sleep
Posture	By pooling blood in the lower limbs due to the effects of gravity, changing from a recumbent to an upright position tends to reduce the cardiac output by about 30%. However, certain compensatory mechanisms stop the VR from declining and aid in maintaining constant cardiac output and arterial blood pressure
Meals	During the first few hours after meals, the cardiac output is increased due to increase of blood flow in the splanchnic circulation
Temperature	Due to an increase in blood flow to the skin, the cardiac output is increased at temperatures above 30 degrees Celsius
Pregnancy	During pregnancy, particularly in the later months, the cardiac output increases significantly due to the increased uterine blood flow
Emotions	In response to stimulation of the sympathetic-adrenal system, the cardiac output increases by up to 100% during the majority of emotions
Muscular exercise	This produces the highest physiological increase in the cardiac output. It increases up to sevenfold or more in well-trained athletes

(2) Intrinsic Regulation

Including heterometric and homeometric regulation, this only regulates the stroke volume. Homeometric autoregulation, in contrast to heterometric regulation, which is based on the Frank-Starling law, regulates the SV without changing the length of the muscle fibers. While the end-systolic volume decreases less than its normal level due to more vigorous ventricular contraction, the end-diastolic volume increases for a prolonged period of time before decreasing to its normal level. The SV remains high as a result. This effect happens when an afterload develops, such as when the aortic impedance rises as a result of an increase in arterial blood pressure (Table 3).

Multiple Choice Questions

1. **Phase one of cardiac muscle action potential is:**

    A. Depolarization
    B. Initial repolarization
    C. Plateau
    D. Rapid repolarization
    E. Resting membrane potential

Answer: B

2. **The effect of excess potassium ions on heart function is:**

    A. A. Increased heart rate.
    B. B. The heart becomes dilated and flaccid.
    C. C. Spastic contractions.
    D. D. Enhances the heart.

Answer: B

3. **P–R interval is shortened except in:**

   A. A-V nodal rhythm
   B. Sympathetic overactivity
   C. Wolff–Parkinson–White syndrome.
   D. First degree heart block

Answer: D

4. **The electrocardiographic lead for a VR is best described as:**

   (a) Unipolar.
   (b) Bipolar.
   (c) Augmented unipolar.
   (d) Augmented bipolar

Answer: C

5. **Cardiac output is decreased:**

   (a) On standing up.
   (b) During stimulation of sympathetic to the heart.
   (c) By increasing the end-diastolic volume of the heart.
   (d) On cutting the vagal nerve to the heart.

Answer: A. By pooling blood in the lower limbs due to the effects of gravity, changing from a recumbent to an upright position tends to reduce the cardiac output by about 30%. However, certain compensatory mechanisms stop the VR from declining and aid in maintaining constant cardiac output and arterial blood pressure.

6. **Stroke volume is increased by all of the following EXCEPT:**

   (a) Sympathetic stimulation.
   (b) Decreased venous return.
   (c) Digitals.
   (d) d) Stretched cardiac muscle fibers.

Answer: B.

7. **All of the following increases COP, EXCEPT:**

   (a) Increased end-diastolic volume.
   (b) The Valsalva maneuver.
   (c) Increased venous return.
   (d) Moderate tachycardia.

Answer; B

8. **In the heart, parasympathetic stimulation causes all the following effects EXCEPT:**

   (a) Decreased rate of discharge from the S.A.N.
   (b) Coronary V.C.
   (c) Increased ventricular contractility.
   (d) Decreased atrial contractility.

Answer: C

References

1. Dong J-G. The role of heart rate variability in sports physiology. Exp Ther Med. 2016;11(5):1531–6.
2. How Does the Circulatory System Maintain Homeostasis | Biology Dictionary [Internet]. Biology Dictionary. 2022 [cited 30 July 2022]. https://biologydictionary.net/how-does-the-circulatory-system-maintain-homeostasis//.
3. Katz AM, editors. Physiology of the Heart. Lippincott Williams & Wilkins;2010.
4. Opie LH, editors. Heart physiology: from cell to circulation. Lippincott Williams & Wilkins;2004.
5. What to Know About the Endocardium [Internet]. Verywell Health. 2022 [cited 30 July 2022]. https://www.verywellhealth.com/endocardium-definition-5088789.
6. Hall JE, Michael EH. Guyton and hall textbook of medical physiology e-Book. Elsevier Health Sciences;2020.
7. Kibble JD, Halsey CR. Medical physiology: the big picture. Singapore Med J. 2009;50(8):833.
8. Triposkiadis F et al. The sympathetic nervous system in heart failure: physiology, pathophysiology, and clinical implications. J Am Colle Cardiol. 2009;54(19):1747–1762.
9. Vela D. Balance of cardiac and systemic hepcidin and its role in heart physiology and pathology. Lab Invest. 2018;98(3):315–26.
10. Khurana I. Textbook of human physiology for dental students. Elsevier Health Sciences;2012.
11. Adamopoulos S et al. Exercise training in patients with ventricular assist devices: a review of the evidence and practical advice. A position paper from the Committee on Exercise Physiology and Training and the Committee of Advanced Heart Failure of the Heart Failure Association of the European Society of Cardiology. Eur J Hear Fail. 2019;21(1):3–13.
12. Bedzra EKS et al. Mechanical support of superior cavopulmonary (Glenn) physiology to heart transplantation. JTCVS Tech. 2021;6:144–146.
13. DePasquale N, Burch G, Phillips J. The second heart sound. Am Heart J. 1968;76(3):419–31.

Embryology of the Heart

Abbas Mohammad, Adil Alhaideri, and Zanyar Qais

Abstract The human heart is the first organ to evolve functionally. About day 21 or 22, a mere three weeks after fertilization, it starts beating and pumping blood. The process of heart development is called "Carcinogenesis" which includes the formation of the heart and its blood vessels. It starts as a tube that goes into the looping process and septation process progressively, till the final heart is being formed.

Keywords Embryology · Heart tube · Heart field · Cardiac looping · Cardiac separation · Semilunar valves · Germ cells · Cardiogenic cords · Ectoderm · Primitive heart

1 Introduction

The heart is the first organ to develop and function during the embryological life. The process of heart development consists of four main regions including the following:

1. First heart field.
2. Secondary heart field.
3. Cardiac neural Crest.
4. Proepicardial organ.

Each of these are important structures in the development. It is therefore important to understand these embryological sites for further understanding of congenital heart disease. Initially, the simple diffusion is enough to supply the embryo with the nutrients and oxygen but later it becomes inadequate, the heart will then take up this task [1].

A. Mohammad (✉)
College of Medicine, Dhi-qar Qar University, Al-Nasiriyah, Iraq
e-mail: Abbasmohammad199600@gmail.com

A. Alhaideri
College of Medicine, University of Baghdad, Baghdad, Iraq
e-mail: adel.ferras1700b@comed.uobaghdad.edu.iq

Z. Qais
Medical University of Lublin, Lublin, Poland

© The Author(s), under exclusive license to Springer Nature Switzerland AG 2022
H. T. Hashim et al. (eds.), *Heart Transplantation*,
https://doi.org/10.1007/978-3-031-17311-0_3

2 Primary Heart Tube Formation

The heart forms from the germinal mesoderm. The lateral plate of the mesoderm divides into splanchnic and somatic layers. Splanchnic layer of the mesoderm differentiates and gives rise to the first heart field. The first heart field can be further divided into two areas, cranial and caudal. The cranial portion will travel ventrally and caudally to line the newly formed foregut endoderm. Fusion occurs in the position of the anterior intestinal portal and passes in a craniocaudal direction by lengthening of the forgot tube. As a result of this fusion, the endocardial tubes will be recognized as a pair of vascular elements in each limb of the first heart field. The heart tube from each limb will then fuse during folding and give rise to a single tube, the primary heart tube. When the limbs fail to fuse, it results in two tube-like structures instead of one, and this is called Cardia Bifida. The newly formed primary heart tube then undergoes elongation and looping to give rise to atria, ventricles and their endocardium lining. Within the first heart field continuous proliferation will occur and give rise to segments [2].

This mass contains the progenitor cells for the myocardium that aggregate around fused endocardium tubes and result in the formation of the myocardium. The myocardium is separated from the endocardium by the deposition of substances called cardiac jelly which is an acellular matrix. Later the mesoderm will migrate to the outer surface of the myocardium to give rise to the epicardium. The primary heart tube undergoes a series of expansion and contraction resulting in lengthening of the heart tube over the next 5 weeks which contribute to Heart Chambers (Fig. 1).

The second heart field gives rise to the right ventricle and outflow tract, meaning the Aorta and Pulmonary trunk. The outflow tract of both ventricles is subdivided into two parts, Proximal and Distal. The lineage of the cardiac cell within the second heart field remains suspended until the formation of the primary heart tube [3] (Fig. 2).

Later the major arteries that transport the blood to the trunk and head arise from these aortic arch arteries. Initially, the pericardial cavity contains a suspended primary Heart tube by dorsal mesentery of the heart (dorsal mesoderm) which is formed by splanchnic mesoderm [2].

The cells of the second heart field are divided into the following:

1. Cells that are located cranial to the arterial outflow of the heart tube and ventral to developing pharyngeal endoderm give rise to the right ventricle.
2. Cells that are located caudal to arterial outflow give rise to the wall of the proximal and distal outflow tracts.
3. Cells within the outflow end of the heart tube give rise to the atrial wall, atrial septal and sinus venosus.

The proliferation of cells within the second heart field of the arterial pole gives the bulk of the heart tube lengthening (Fig. 3).

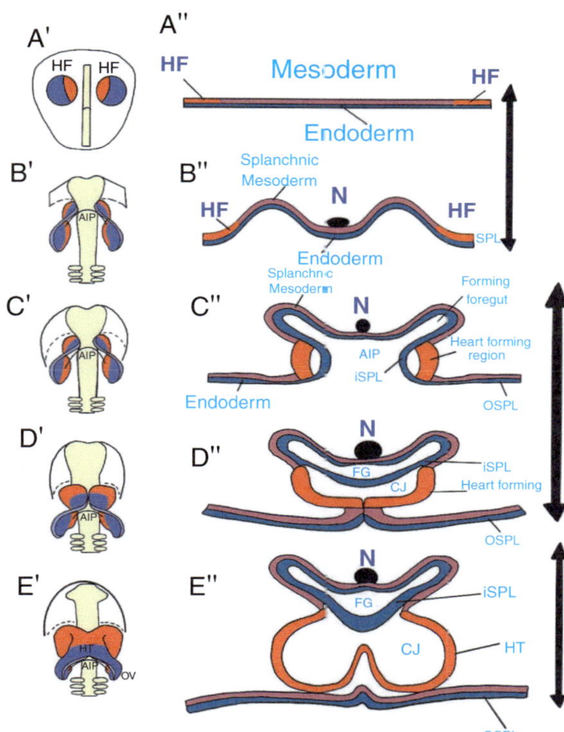

Fig. 1 New hypothesis for foregut and heart tube formation based on differential growth and actomyosin contraction

3   Cardiac Looping

The primary heart tube undergoes elongation and tends to become c-shaped on day 23 of embryonic life. For giving the heart the characteristic shape the tube, needs to bend in different directions at different points. The primitive ventricle (which will give rise to the Left Ventricle) will then turn in the opposite direction to the left. The tube is now shaped like an S. The primitive atrium then displaces cranially and dorsal, making the process of elongation complete on day 28. However, there is continuous remodeling so that the outflow tract becomes aligned with both ventricles. The future heart chambers are now in the correct spatial relationship to each other (Fig. 4). The further development of these chambers now only involves remodeling.

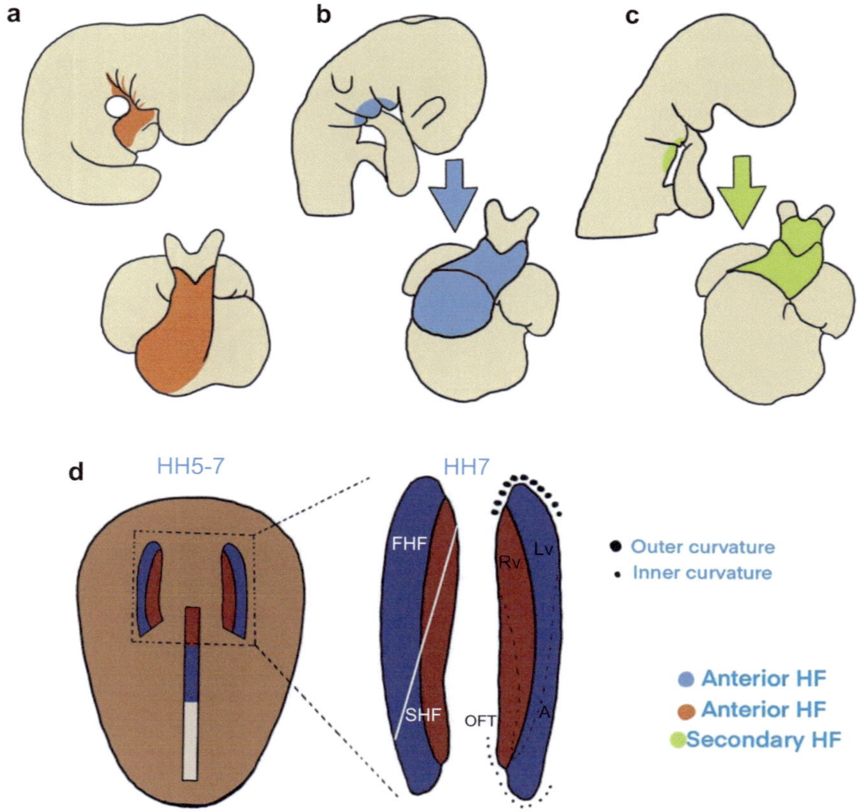

Fig. 2 The role of the secondary heart field in cardiac development

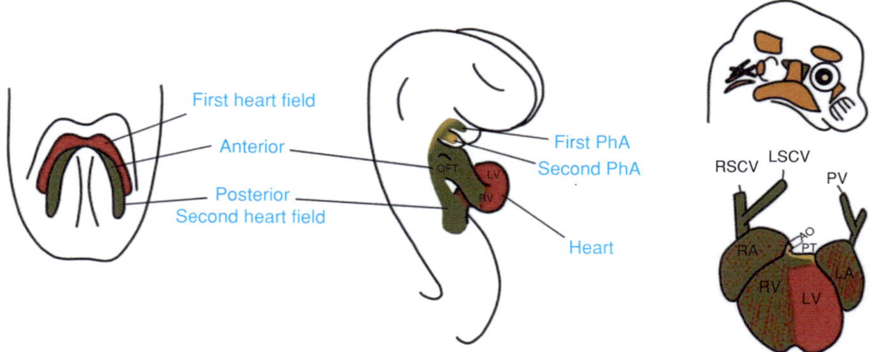

Fig. 3 First and second heart fields and further subdivisions of the myocardial lineage

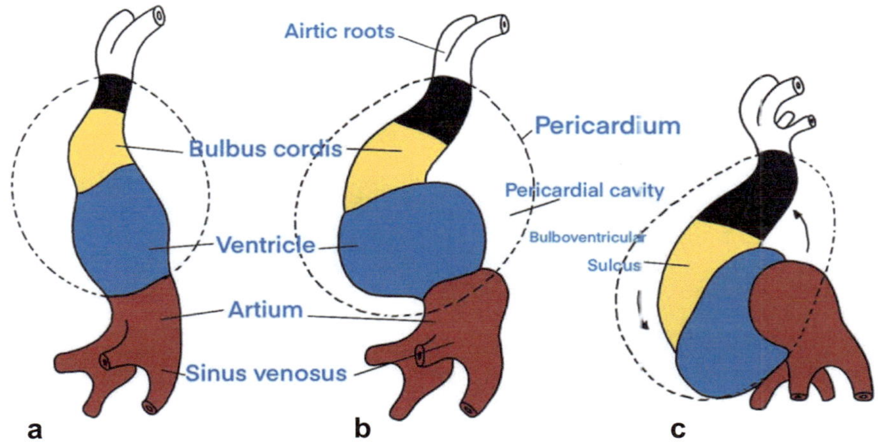

Fig. 4 Cardiac looping

4 Cardiac Separation

Cardiac separation is the process of separation of systemic circulation from pulmonary circulation, which is connected in series in adults. This separation involves the separation of atria, ventricle and outflow tract which we will discuss further below.

4.1 Atrial Separation and Canal Separation

After elongation and looping, the atrium is one large chamber and needs to be separated to form a right and left atrium. The separation of atria is the first to occur in the separation process and it is the last to finish because the Foramen Ovale is still open till after birth. The pulmonary circulation begins to develop in the 6th week by evagination of pulmonary venous confluence into the roof of the embryonic atrium between the two atrial appendages. The primary atrial septum (septum primum) develops distal to this evagination as the muscular septum, crescent shaped. It arises from the dorsal atrial wall toward the atrioventricular canal. It is called septum primum because it is firstly dividing the atria and then becomes a perforator to form Foramen Ovale. Along the rim of the pulmonary vein, the Septum Secundum will develop as a structure called mesenchymal protrusion (also called vestibular spine or spina vestibule or atrial spine). The septum secundum divide the atrioventricular valves to form mitral and tricuspid valves. If there is an extreme defect in the formation of dorsal mesenchymal protrusion, it causes the formation of a common atrioventricular canal. Mild defects cause the formation of Atrial Septal Defect (ASD). While septum secundum defect leads to formation of primum ASD [4] (Fig. 5).

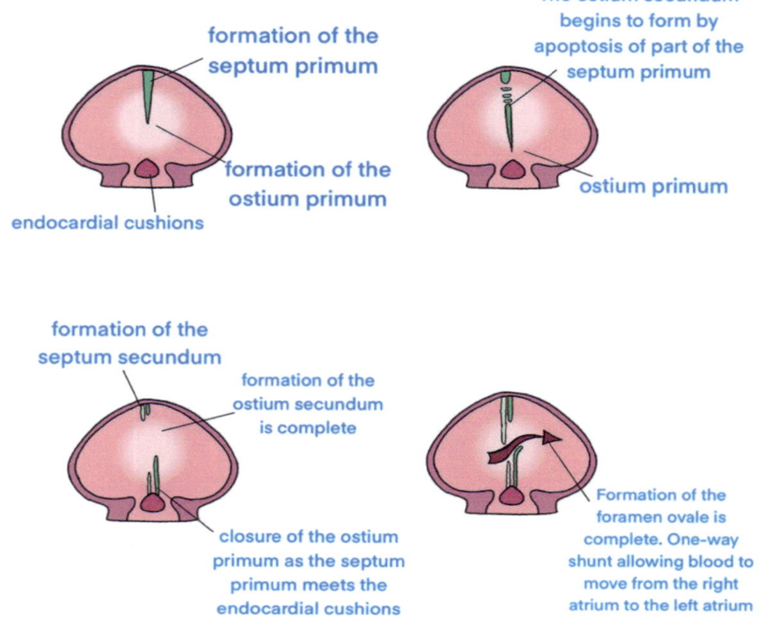

Fig. 5 Atrial separation

4.2 Ventricular Separation

After completion of the cardiac looping process, the primitive left and right ventricles have positions leftward and rightward, respectively. The inflow is directed more toward the right and left ventricles as development progress. At the junction of both ventricles, the ventricular septum arises and grows toward the AV canal which forms the muscular interventricular septum. Any defect in the formation of this septum results in the development of VSD. When the interventricular septum reaches the canal septum between AV valves, the ventricular separation process is completed. If joining between the ventricular septum and cannot septum not occur lead to the development of conoventricular defect (Fig. 6).

4.3 Outflow Tract Separation

The last process of separation we will talk about in this chapter is the separation of the outflow tract, which plays an important role in separating pulmonary circulation from systemic. During the development of the heart, we have cells called the Cardiac neural crest. These cells travel from the dorsal neural tube and aggregate around

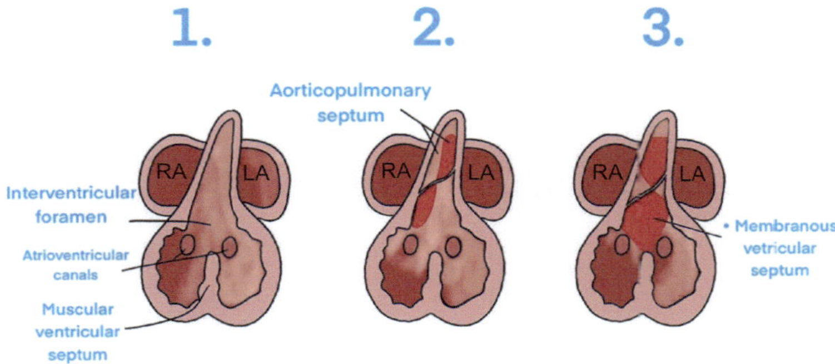

Fig. 6 Ventricular separation

the pharyngeal arch arteries. The sixth and fourth arch arteries are joined together and grow in the truncus. Any interference with the neural crest results in truncus arteriosus, meaning that there is only one large vessel exiting from the heart [4] (Fig. 7).

5   Development of Great Arteries

The vascular system is composed of many arteries which begin to develop in the third week of embryonic life. It arises from a specific type of cell called meso-derm/ectoderm-derived antigenic cells as a result of the combination of pharyngeal mesoderm and ectoderm (which is a part of the neural crest) [5].

These aortic arches pass along the pharyngeal walls in pharyngeal arches. The pharyngeal arch receives pair of branches to form an aortic sac during pharyngeal arch development. The structures that originate from the aortic arch are as follows:

First aortic arch:

"It regresses at time of development of the third pair, except the small part which forms maxillary artery" [5].

Second aortic arch:

also regress accept small part that from the stapedial artery.

Third aortic arch:

It gives rise to the following:

- Common carotid artery.
- Proximal part of internal carotid artery.
- External carotid artery.

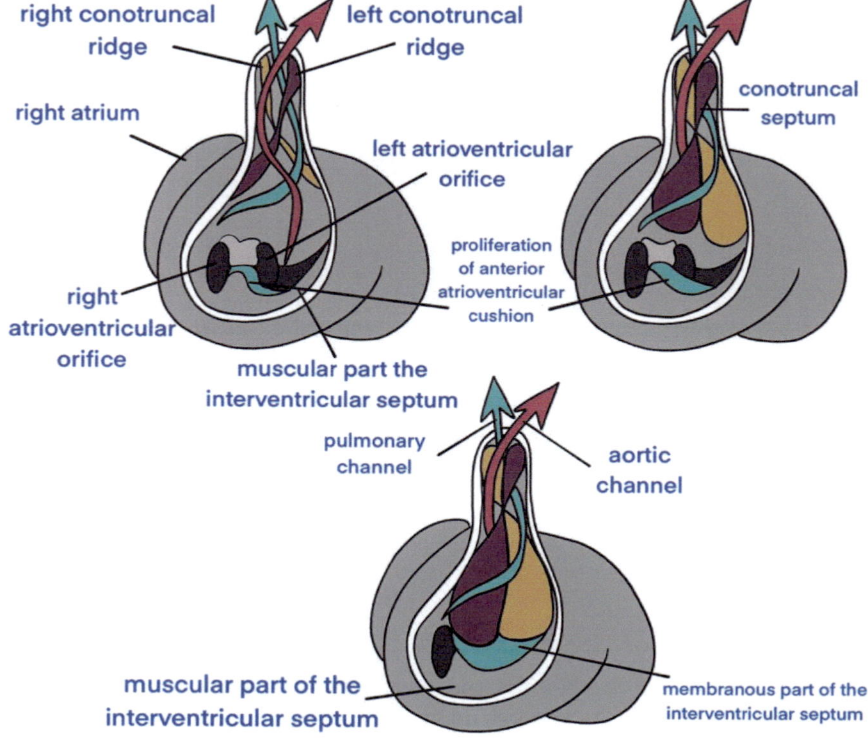

Fig. 7 Outflow tract separation

Right fourth aortic arch:

It gives rise to the proximal part of the right subclavian artery.

Left fourth aortic arch:

It forms the medial part of the aortic arch.

The aortic sac is composed of two horns, the left and right (Fig. 8).

6   Development of the Conductive System of the Heart

The adult conductive system starts in the Sinoatrial node (SAN), which is located at the junction of the right atrium and superior vena cava which generates the electrical impulses (pacemaker). These impulses pass through the atrial muscle to reach the AV node which slows the impulses by about 0.2 s. The AVN is located on the right atrial floor at the apex of the Kock triangle. The impulses then pass from there through right

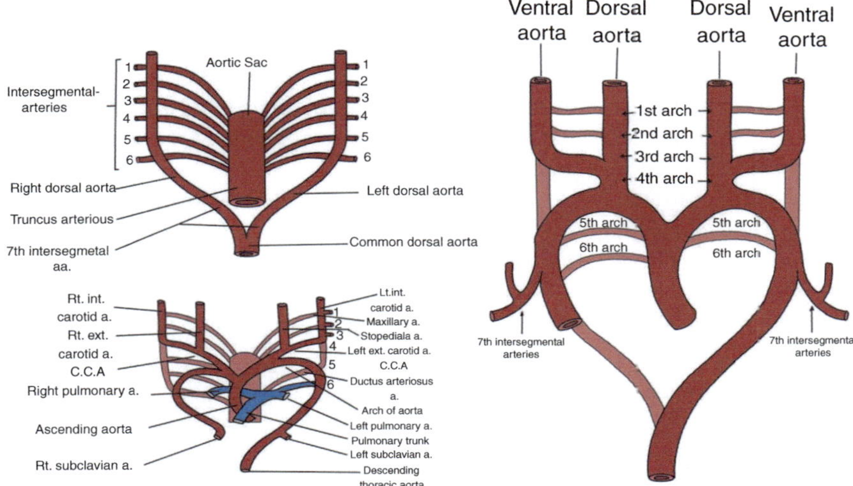

Fig. 8 Development of great vessels

and left bundle branches and finally to Purkinje fiber which stimulates the ventricular myocytes [5].

The origin of cells of the cardiac conductive system is not clearly known. Many studies on chicken's heart show that the cells of the conductive system are multicellular in the form containing myocardial cells of the conductive system and working myocardium. We have other cells which are important for the generation and propagation of the cardiac impulses. These cells are called cardiomyocytes. In embryonic life, the source of electrical impulses of the conduction system is cardiomyocytes because there are no fibroblasts. In the stage of the primitive heart tube, there is no specific conduction system and there is no specific pacemaker. The electrical impulses are generated in myocytes. In lab studies by using a photodiode, it is shown that the primitive pacemaker activity is located in the primitive atrium just before the folding and generation of the heart tube. The proliferation of cells in primitive heart tubes and the development of contractile cells happen, and cells specific to Heart chambers, in this stage, begin to differentiate into two cell types, specialized conduction system myocardium and working myocardium. Also, these cells of the conductive system differentiated into fast conducting and slow conducting myocardium depending on intercellular communication in these cells. In the slow conducting myocytes, the depolarization action potential is transmitted through sparse gap junction which in turn prevents fast conducting myocytes from overwhelming in the pacing node.

The SAN is composed of two parts, the head and tail. It is located in the Crista terminalis at the junction between the venous valve and atrium in the adult. During the development of the SA node from the second heart field along with atria, sinus venosus specifically form the right horn. While the left contains Pitx2c that inhibits the expression of genes responsible for the left side SA node. One of the important genes for the development of the SA node is SHOX2. Deficiency of this gene results in SA node hypoplasia and bradycardia then death. Also, there is another gene expression called PITX2c. The deficiency of this gene results in the formation of the left side SA node. The AV node develops from precursor cells on the dorsal side of the atrioventricular junction [6] (Fig. 9).

AV canal myocardium forms an AV ring bundle which is responsible for the transition from fast conducting gene profile to slow conducting gene profile. Transition between compact node and his bundle. Maturation of fibrous tissue and fibroblast gives rise to the bundle of His. During cardiac chamber formation, the ventricular conduction system arises from the ventricular trabecular myocardium.

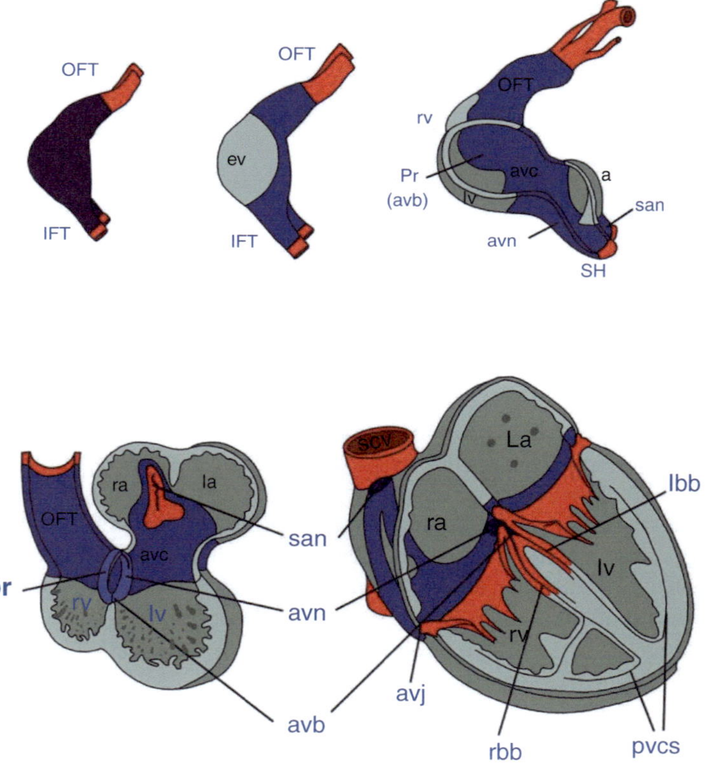

Fig. 9 Development of the conductive system of the heart

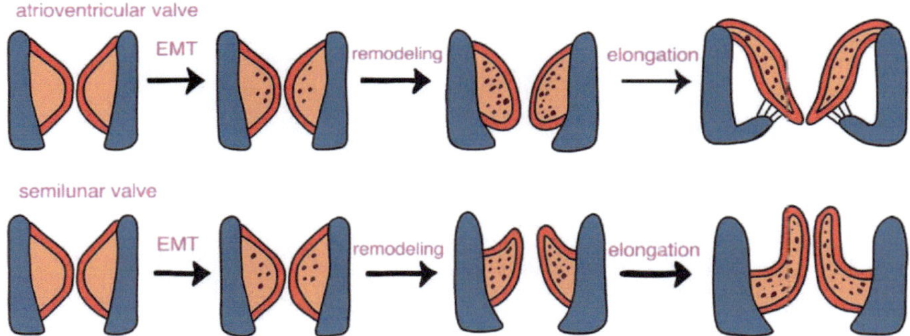

Fig. 10 Development of semilunar valves

7 Development of Semilunar Valves

They arise as cushions in the distal outflow tract during the formation of the outflow tract septum which are called intercalated cushion tissue. A cavity is formed in place of the future pulmonary artery and ascending aorta from the lateral intercalated cushion and the two outflow cushions. From these cavities, the semilunar sinuses and valves will arise. A recent study showed that the semilunar valve arises from the endocardial-derived cushion, along with a contribution from the neural crest. At the 9th week of embryonic life, the development of semilunar valves is completed (Figs. 10, 11 and 12).

8 Development of the Venous System

The primitive venous system is composed of two main components at week 4 as follows:

(1) Dorsal systemic nutritional network.
(2) Double nutritional network.

The dorsal systemic nutritional network itches the main drainage of the embryonic body. It develops from two veins. The posterior and anterior cardinal veins pass to sinus venosus through the common cardinal vein. While the double nutritional network is responsible for drainage of extraembryonic blood. It is composed of two parts as follows:

- Vitelline system:

which carry blood from yolk sac to heart.

- Umbilicoallantoic system:

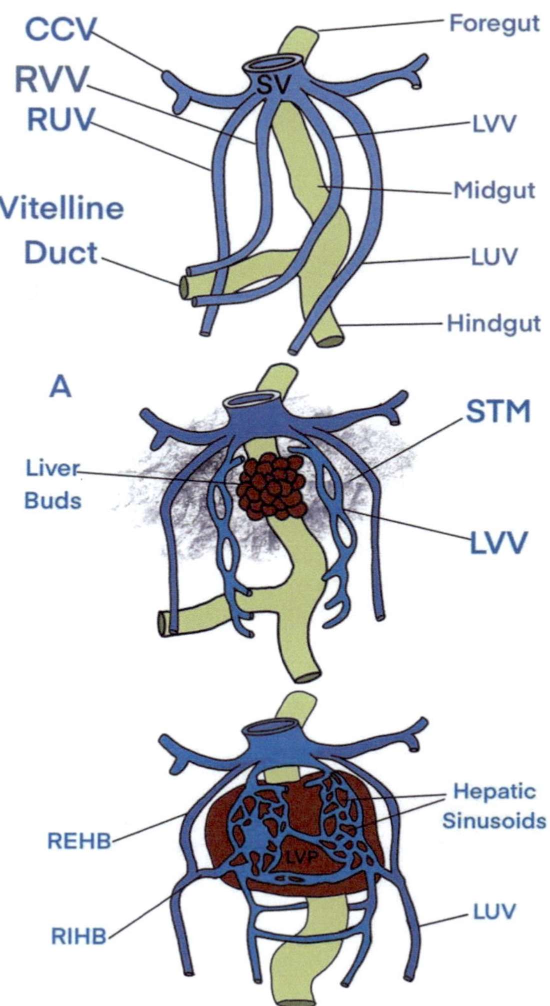

Fig. 11 Development of venous system

which carry the oxygenated blood from placenta toward embryo.

These networks firstly are symmetrical and in pair. They then become series of transverse anastomosis which become one major trunk on the embryonic right side while the vessels on the left side are obliterated.

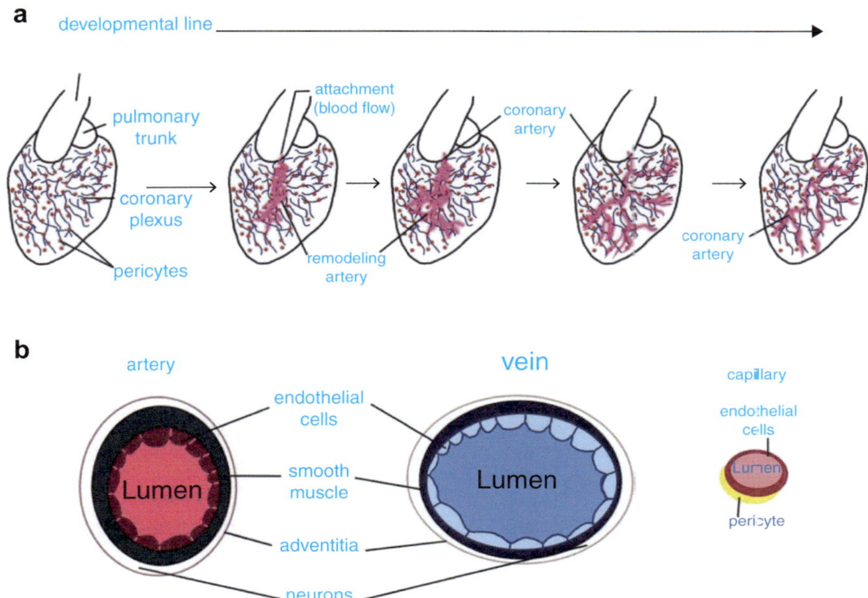

Fig. 12 Development of coronary vessels

9 Development of Superior Venal Cava

A large anastomosis between thyroid and thymic vein drains the blood from superior cardinal vein to the right, which result in formation of the future brachiocephalic Venous trunk. The internal jugular vein arises from anterior cardinal vein above the anastomosis while the external jugular vein arises from anterior vein of mandibular region. The subclavian vein arises from fusion of upper limb venous plexus [7].

9.1 Development of Coronary Arteries

The myocardium initially received nutrition and oxygen by diffusion from common chambers because it is avascularized but when the myocardium became thick it leads to formation of trabeculations to maintain the diffusion. The origin of coronary arteries is aortic sinuses. The aortic sinuses occupying the proximal aortic roof pass beyond the upper border of Cusp to form circumferential, complete, well-defined sinotubular ridges. These ridges are called according to their location as right posterior, left posterior or anterior aortic sinuses [7].

Multiple Choice Questions:

(1) **What are the four main regions in the process of heart development?**

    (A) First Heart Field, Second Heart Field, Third Heart field and Fourth Heart Field.

    (B) First Heart Field, Second Heart Field, Vagal neural crest and Proepicardial Region.

    (C) First Heart Field, Second heart Field, Cardiac neural crest and Proepicardial Region.

    (D) None of the above are main region.

(2) **When does the heart start beating?**

    (A) Second week of pregnancy.

    (B) After 21 days from fertilization.

    (C) Beginning of second trimester (13 week).

    (D) None of the above.

(3) **Cardiac separation means separation of systemic circulation from pulmonary circulation.**

    (A) True.

    (B) False.

(4) **First heart field gives rise to**

    (A) Atria.

    (B) Patent ductus arteriosus.

    (C) Atria and Ventricle.

    (D) Coronary Arteries.

(5) **The heart forms from which of the germ layers**

    (A) Ectoderm.

    (B) Mesoderm.

    (C) Endoderm.

    (D) B + C.

(6) **When does the semilunar valve form?**

    (A) Between week 5 and 9.

    (B) Between week 5 and 8.

    (C) After 3 weeks.

    (D) After 8 weeks.

(7) **When does the atrioventricular valve form?**

    (A) Between week 5 and 9.

    (B) Between week 5 and 8.

    (C) After 3 weeks.

    (D) After 7 weeks.

(8) **During cardiac looping the bending**

(A) Occurs toward the right side which makes the left side of the heart represent the inner curvature.

(B) Occurs toward the right side which makes the left side of the heart represent the outer curvature.

(C) Occurs toward the left side which makes the left side of the heart represent the inner curvature.

(D) Bending does not take place during cardiac looping.

(9) **The septum secundum divides the semilunar valves to form aortic and pulmonary valves.**

(A) True.

(B) False.

(10) **How many pairs of aortic arches is there during development of great arteries?**

(A) 6 pairs.

(B) 6.

(C) 5 pairs.

(D) 5.

(11) **The third aortic arch gives rise to**

(A) Common carotid Artery and External carotid artery.

(B) Proximal part of external carotid artery.

(C) External carotid artery.

(D) Common carotid artery, Proximal part of internal carotid artery and External carotid artery.

(12) **From which arch does the pulmonary artery arise from?**

(A) 4th arch.

(B) 5th arch.

(C) 6th arch.

(D) Does not arise from the aortic arch.

(13) **Deficiency of SHOX2 gene can cause**

(A) Hypolasia of SAN.

(B) Bradycardia.

(C) Right sided SAN.

(D) A + B.

(14) **Which arteries arise from the coronary sinus?**

(A) Right Coronary artery.

(B) Left Coronary Artery.

(C) A + B.

(D)   Right Coronary Artery, Left Coronary Artery, Posterior Coronary Artery.

(15) **The cardiogenic area starts to form from three strands called the cardiogenic cords**.

(A)   True.
(B)   False.

(16) **Second heart field gives rise to**

(A)   Right Ventricle and outflow tract.
(B)   Left Ventricle.
(C)   Atrium.
(D)   All of the above.

(17) **When does the closure of foramen ovale occur?**

(A)   1 week before birth.
(B)   2 weeks before birth.
(C)   After birth.
(D)   It closes when the heart starts beating.

(18) **Of the great arteries the primitive aortic arteries are among the first ones to be developed**.

(A)   True.
(B)   False.

(19) **The external jugular vein arises from**

(A)   Posterior vein of mandibular region.
(B)   Anterior vein of mandibular region.
(C)   Posterior cardinal vein.
(D)   Anterior cardinal vein.

(20) **Neural crest cells are responsible for separation of the outflow tract**.

(A)   True.
(B)   False.

(21) **In embryonic life what type of cell is mainly responsible for conduction?**

(A)   Cardiomyocytes.
(B)   Fibroblast.
(C)   Ganglionic cells.
(D)   None of the above.

Answers

(1)   **C**.
(2)   **B**.
(3)   **A**.
(4)   **C**.

(5) **B.**
(6) **A.**
(7) **B.**
(8) **A.**
(9) **B.**
(10) **A.**
(11) **D.**
(12) **C.**
(13) **D.**
(14) **B.**
(15) **A.**
(16) **C.**
(17) **A.**
(18) **B.**
(19) **A.**
(20) **A.**

References

1. de Groot G, Adriana C, et al. Embryology of the heart and its impact on understanding fetal and neonatal heart disease. Seminars in Fetal and Neonatal Medicine, vol. 18, No. 5. WB Saunders;2013.
2. Clark EB. Cardiac embryology: its relevance to congenital heart disease. Am J Dis Child. 1986;140(1):41–4.
3. Martinsen BJ. Reference guide to the stages of chick heart embryology. Developmental dynamics: an official publication of the American Association of Anatomists. 2005;233(4):1217–37.
4. Abdulla R-i, Blew GA, Holterman MJ. Cardiovascular embryology. Pediatr Cardiol. 2004;25(3):191–200.
5. Foley A, Mercola M. Heart induction: embryology to cardiomyocyte regeneration. Trends Cardiovasc Med. 2004;14(3):121–5.
6. Hiroyuki Y, et al. Molecular embryology for an understanding of congenital heart diseases. Anat Sci Int. 2009;84(3):88–94.
7. Kazuki K, Yamagishi H. A decade of advances in the molecular embryology and genetics underlying congenital heart defects. Circ J. 2011; 1109091402.

The Pathological Changes Seen in Cardiac Diseases Indicated for Transplantation

Ahmed Dheyaa Al-Obaidi, Mohammed Tareq Mutar, Mustafa Majid,
Sara Shihab Ahmad, Rema Yousif Bakose, Mustafa Najah Al-Obaidi,
Hasan Al-Abbasi, Shaymaa Saadi Shaalan, and Mustafa Ismail

Abstract Heart transplantation is the treatment of choice for patients with end-stage heart failure who remain symptomatic despite optimal medical therapy after trying other surgical options. The pathological changes will be described in multiple aspects like morphological, cellular, molecular, structural, and hemodynamic changes.

Keywords Transplantation · Heart · Failure · Pathology · Cellular · Molecular · Hemodynamic · Morphological · Genes · Arrhythmia · Ischemic · Remodeling · Fibrosis · Cardiomyopathy · Dilated · Hypertrophic · Restricted · Congenital · Hypoplastic · Valves

1 Introduction

Heart transplantation is the treatment of choice for patients with end-stage heart failure who remain symptomatic despite optimal medical therapy after trying other surgical options. It's indicated for cardiogenic shock requiring continuous mechanical support or inotropes, in cases of stage III or IV NYHA despite optimal therapy, refractory life-threatening arrhythmia despite all other available options, and end-stage congenital heart disease not amenable to medical or surgical therapy.

In this chapter, the various pathological changes necessitating heart transplantation will be discussed. Pathology will be described in multiple aspects like morphological, cellular, molecular, structural, and hemodynamic changes.

A. D. Al-Obaidi · M. T. Mutar · M. Majid · S. S. Ahmad · R. Y. Bakose · M. N. Al-Obaidi · H. Al-Abbasi · M. Ismail (✉)
College of Medicine, University of Baghdad, Baghdad, Iraq
e-mail: mustafalorance2233@gmail.com

S. S. Shaalan
College of Medicine, Al- Mustansiriyah University, Baghdad, Iraq

© The Author(s), under exclusive license to Springer Nature Switzerland AG 2022
H. T. Hashim et al. (eds.), *Heart Transplantation*,
https://doi.org/10.1007/978-3-031-17311-0_4

2 Morphological Changes of the End-Stage Heart Failure

The heart undergoes various compensatory modifications to accommodate the underlying disease and body demands; these morphological alterations are not disease-specific and can be attributed to the clinical findings of these individuals. As the condition progresses, these changes eventually result in a reduction in cardiac performance as well as end-stage heart failure [1]. All of these changes are progressive.

This remodeling process end result is deleterious, as it becomes a maladaptive process, impairing both systolic and diastolic cardiac function as a result of increased wall tension, interstitial fibrosis, and myocardial apoptosis [2]. Cardiomegaly refers to an enlarged heart, while hypertrophy refers to an increase in weight with respect to normal values [3, 4]. In contrast to concentric hypertrophy, which refers to increased heart weight and wall thickness without cavity dilatation, eccentric hypertrophy refers to increased weight and cavity dilatation; the wall thickness can be reduced, normal, or increased [5]. In both cases, the LV mass index (LVMI) is elevated. Eccentric hypertrophy is associated with chronic volume overload, and individuals with moderate to severe mitral regurgitation may be associated with eccentric hypertrophy. Concentric hypertrophy is less common in individuals with heart failure, and its treatment response is less beneficial in terms of survival than eccentric hypertrophy [6].

Symmetric LV hypertrophy occurs in some cases of heart failure and refers to an equal thickness of the LV and septum, whereas asymmetric LV hypertrophy occurs when the thickness of the LV and septum is not equal and the increased thickness occurs in either the septum or free wall [5]. Asymmetrical hypertrophy may occur in the septal, apical, and mid-ventricular planes or include the right ventricle [7]. Left atrial enlargement arises as a result of chronic overload and is regarded as a risk factor in people with heart disease. Left atrial enlargement can be identified by echocardiography [8]. Heart failure caused by systolic dysfunction is relatively easy to identify with echocardiography, which shows a dilated left ventricle with decreased ejection fraction.

In regards to the morphology of the valves in these cases of heart failure, as vulvar heart disease can cause heart failure and heart failure due to underlying non-vulvar conditions leads to vulvar changes, mostly secondary regurgitation of atrioventricular valves, in which the valves are structurally normal in the early stages in contrast to primary regurgitation, with progression, their pathological changes become more evident worsening ventricular and atrial remodeling [9].

Mitral regurgitation is the most common secondary (functional) change in the case of heart failure, in which it demonstrates severe tenting and poor leaflet cooptation, giving the regurgitant orifice a crescent shape [10, 11].

3 Cellular and Molecular Changes in Heart Failure

In addition to the structural and mechanical changes observed in heart failure patients, the recently developed molecular sciences have revealed a wide spectrum of molecular and cellular changes. These involve changes in genetic profile, metabolism, capillary density, cardiac biomarkers like troponin, cytokine, and catecholamines, and cellular changes like hypertrophy, fibrosis, and necrosis.

3.1 Cardiac Remodeling and Hypertrophy

Pressure or volume stress stimuli are the two main causes of hypertrophy. The effects of these forces are related to genetic activation. The method by which these forces are applied to the extra-cellular matrix and cells being conveyed into the nucleus is variable. One of the well-known methods is through stretch-activated ion protein channels.

These channels could be found in specific cells, including the cardiac muscle cells [12]. Their activation causes calcium ion influx, which in turn activates a cascade of events leading to dephosphorylation of the nuclear factors and activation of the pro-hypertrophic genes [13]. These events could also be induced by adrenergic stimulation [14]. The cellular deformation is also conveyed from the extra-cellular matrix through certain proteins like integrin in association with structural proteins found on the Z disk (muscle lim protein MLP, Costameric protein Melusin, and Filament C) [15, 16]. Mechanical stretch also has an effect through activation of G-protein couple receptors that cause activation of the channels and the same sequence of events [17].

In the case of eccentric remodeling, replication of sarcomeres occurs in series with lengthening of myofibrils leading to thinning of the wall and dilation of cardiac chambers in order to accommodate the increased end-diastolic volume [17], while concentric remodeling occurs due to replication of the sarcomere in parallel with cardiomyocyte thickening and increased LV end-diastolic pressure [17, 18].

3.2 Inflammation and Heart Failure

There is an increased level of pro-inflammatory markers in chronic heart failure, but their level is less than those found in infection (e.g. sepsis) which suggests the chronic nature of inflammation [19, 20].

Directly, the gross evidence of this inflammation is the histopathological detection of numerous T-lymphocytes, natural killer cells, monocytes, CCR2 + (pro-inflammatory) macrophages, and mast cells in patients with ischemic and non-ischemic heart failure. Indirectly, patients with heart failure have persistently elevated levels of troponin suggesting a continuous process of myocardial damage [21–23].

Genetically, it has been proved that the transcription of the DNA related to innate immunity differs significantly between normal people and patients with ischemic or non-ischemic heart failure [24].

However, the role of inflammation is more readily obvious in patients with viral myocarditis or autoimmune diseases affecting the heart [25]. Some autoantibodies can be detected in cases of chronic heart failure. These autoantibodies target some cardiac antigens like cardiac actin, troponin I, Na/K ATPase, M2 muscarinic receptors, and $\beta 1$ receptor. They are found in patients with viral myocarditis, and ischemic or non-Ischemic Cardiomyopathy. These autoantibodies were also found in the absence of any heart disease as well, suggesting their low specificity [22].

Some comorbidities like obesity, especially abdominal obesity, and diabetes mellitus might affect inflammation and the response of the myocardium through their pro-inflammatory role by altering intramyocardial signaling pathways, leading to remodeling and hypertrophic changes [26].

A practical evidence of the damaging effect of inflammation in heart failure is given in the literature: mice with pressure overloaded heart (by using transverse aortic constriction) had increased levels of T-helper cells, macrophages, and increased cytokines parallel with ventricular hypertrophy and dysfunction, while when using lymphocyte blocking agent (CTLA4-Ig) in mice operated with transverse aortic constriction resulted in amelioration of hypertrophy and systolic dysfunction in comparison to the control group which did not receive the agent [27].

3.3 Nitric Oxide in Heart Failure

The pro-inflammatory state in the heart affects coronary micro-vasculature leading to endothelial dysfunction, increased production of reactive oxygen species, and decreased nitric oxide [26]. This will affect intramyocardial signaling like hypophosphorylation of Titin, cyclic GMP, and suppression of phosphatidylinositol 3-kinase (PI3) and mitogen-activated protein, leading to cardiac hypertrophy and stiffness [28]. The vasodilator effect of nitric oxide is also impaired, leading to vasoconstriction with further ischemia. This finding is observed both in cases of ischemic and non-ischemic cardiomyopathy [29].

3.4 Fibrosis in Heart Failure

Fibrosis is a healing process that results in the accumulation of extra-cellular matrix and scar formation. The fibrosis in the myocardium appears in the early stages as an adaptive response, but its persistent activation leads to disrupted tissue structure and function [30]. This process is characterized by increased levels of collagen types I and III as well as activation and differentiation of fibroblasts into myofibroblasts. Three different types of myocardial fibrosis had been identified. These include reactive interstitial fibrosis, replacement fibrosis, and infiltrative interstitial fibrosis [31]. The replacement fibrosis is observed after myocardial necrosis as in myocardial infarction, while the reactive interstitial fibrosis is induced by many stimuli including ischemia, pressure overload, and metabolic derangement without myocardial necrosis. Cells implicated in secreting pro-fibrotic mediators include macrophages, lymphocytes, cardiomyocytes, and vascular cells, which are well known to be present in heart failure states [21]. The myofibroblast is derived from the resident fibroblast in the myocardium and the circulating or resident fibroblast progenitors like epicardial and endocardial cells through their redifferentiation [32].

3.5 Beta Adrenergic Stimulation and Excitation–Contraction Mismatch

In heart failure, there is an increment in the level of catecholamine. This increase is compensatory initially, but with time, it causes dysfunctional signaling, leading to impaired contractility. The detrimental effect of catecholamines appears to affect the metabolism and survival of myocytes by decreasing the density of adrenergic receptors and impairing their association with G-protein coupled receptors (desensitization) [33]. This is mediated by GRK2, GRK5, β-Arrestin, and protein kinase through phosphorylating the adrenergic receptors, leading to an impaired coupling process [34, 35].

Furthermore, the hormonal system, such as the renin–angiotensin–aldosterone system, is a well-known cause of cardiac myocyte death [36].

3.6 T-Tubule Remodeling

Myocardium of the failing hearts shows distorted, dilated, and misdirected T-tubules with decreased density. These changes are collectively called T-tubule remodeling [37]. T-tubule hosts many calcium ion channels, therefore distortion in their structure, arrangement, and density will affect calcium influx and calcium recycling. This effect is subtle initially, but once it exceeds certain thresholds, it appears to significantly impair excitation–contraction coupling and cardiac function [38].

3.7 Capillary Density

Early stages are characterized by compensatory hypertrophy with increased capillary density, while maladaptive hypertrophy causes a decrease in capillary density, inflamed endothelium, and fibrosis [39]. This effect could be additive to the epicardial coronary obstruction which is associated with atherosclerosis, leading to more ischemia and impaired function [39].

3.8 DNA Changes and Genetic Activation of Fetal Genes

Normally, during fetal life, the main source of energy is driven by glycolysis due to the hypoxic environment of fetal development. The fetal genes responsible for metabolism will be reactivated in advanced heart failure, leading to elevated levels of proteins (like GLUTs, PDKs, and HK-1) with their levels similar to those in fetal life and the myocardium will be dependent on glycolysis for energy. Other changes include changes in the compliance and stiffness of the myocardium.

During maturation, the fetal heart, which was more compliant, becomes stiffer. As it progresses into adulthood, these changes get reversed in the diseased heart with activation of fetal genes, regressing the myocardium into a more compliant version. This reprogramming process can also be seen in neurophysiological and neurohormonal models [40].

3.9 Autophagy Role in Heart Failure

Autophagy plays an important role in heart failure, and inadequate autophagy is a key factor in age-related diseases of the human heart [41].

It is described by Bao Li et al.'s study on mice and by Fang Chi et al.'s study on rabbits that decreased autophagy rate was associated with cardiac hypertrophy and subsequent failure. Meanwhile, at later stages in the mice study (dilation and systolic dysfunction), autophagy was shown to be increased when cardiomyocytes apoptosis is being established. This was associated with more oxidative stress and a higher level of modified proteins, which contributed to the decreased contractility, representing the end stage of heart failure [42, 43].

Christiani et al. support this fact by concluding that using autophagy-inducing agents like rapamycin resulted in less heart weight, less progression of hypertrophy, and more maintained contractility in mice which have been exposed to pressure load by transverse aortic constricting surgery compared to those which were not given this pharmacological agent [44].

In addition, Chi RF et al. described that the reduction of myocytes autophagy in healthy regions of the heart after sustaining MI is associated with progressive hypertrophy and progressive LV dysfunction in rabbits [43].

4 Hemodynamic Changes of Heart Failure

Hemodynamic changes of heart failure can be defined as the changes that occur in the intravascular volume, vascular resistance, and venous pressures due to decreased cardiac output. Despite their importance in maintaining many aspects of the human physiology to prevent compromise of the other body organs, these hemodynamic adaptions can worsen the condition of already diseased heart by depressing cardiac output [44]. If they persist, these changes can lead to decompensation due to intensification of their negative impacts, creating a vicious cycle of dramatic worsening of heart function to the extent of developing cardiogenic shock. These compensatory mechanisms can be summarized as follows:

- **Sympathetic nervous system:** This system is activated by baroreceptors and chemoreceptors which send signals to the nervous system. The sympathetic nervous system responds by releasing catecholamines which in turn elicit chronotropic and inotropic effects on the cardiac muscle in a trial of increasing cardiac output. These effects will shorten the diastolic time and increase oxygen demands for the compromised heart muscle. As the coronary arteries are filled with blood during diastole, the blood supply is decreased for the struggling heart, and this will create a further burden on the failing heart. The chronic effects of catecholamines are those related to the down-regulation of the beta receptors in the cardiomyocytes, causing a reduction in the heart rate and abolish the sympathetic effects [45].
- **Renin–Angiotensin–Aldosterone System**: The activation of this system is usually late in heart failure as it is dependent on the decreased renal blood flow. Thus, decreased renal blood flow stimulates the release of renin from the juxtaglomerular cells; these cells include stretch receptors capable of sensitizing the renal perfusion pressure. Renin stimulates the release of angiotensinogen from the liver, which will be converted to angiotensin 1, then angiotensin 2 by renin, and Angiotensin Conversion Enzyme (ACE), respectively. Angiotensin 2 is the enzyme responsible for the effects of this system by exerting actions on many target organs; these actions include efferent renal and systemic arteriolar vasoconstriction and stimulation of aldosterone release from the zona glomerulosa of the adrenal cortex. Aldosterone causes sodium retention, creating an increase in the intravascular volume, with subsequent increases in both preload and afterload [44].
- **Natriuretic peptides:** They are hormones that are released from the atria and the ventricles in response to stretching of the overloaded myocardial cavity. In general, natriuretic peptides mitigate the effects of RAAS by causing vasodilation and natriuresis [46].
- **Other hormonal and non-hormonal mechanisms:** The antidiuretic hormone or the so-called ADH causes fluid retention in low concentration and acts as a peripheral vasoconstrictor in high doses, so it does take place in the pathology of acute, severe, and chronic heart failure. Another vasoconstrictor is endothelin,

which is opposed by Nitric oxide, prostaglandin E2, and I2, or Bradykinin. Non-hormonal factors can be explained by the increase in the force of cardiac muscle contractility to compensate for the increased afterload caused by high aortic elastance. This positive inotropic modification could be weaned or even diminishes in prolonged or decompensated heart failure [47].

5 Pulmonary Capillary Wedge Pressure (PCWP) and Central Venous Pressure (CVP)

The PCWP, which is an estimate of the left atrial pressure, or left ventricular end-diastolic pressure, is typically elevated in left ventricular failure or heart failure due to mitral stenosis. Normal PCWP is in the range 4–12 mmHg. The CVP represents the right atrial pressure, which is mostly seen elevated in right ventricular failure and is used as an assessment tool for patients in intensive care units. The CVP is normally in the range 8–12 mmHg [48, 49].

In summary, increased strength of cardiac contraction, heart rate, vascular resistance, and intravascular volume due to water and sodium retention are the main hemodynamic adaptations to withstand heart failure at the cost of high energy expenditure. Overexpression of biological molecules results in devastating sequelae on vascular compliance, cardiac remodeling, and systemic organs with prolonged disease course, contributing to further disease progression and worsening, resulting in a transition from compensated to decompensated heart failure.

End-stage heart failure necessitating heart transplant can be caused by a variety of diseases. This chapter will discuss the pathology of the most important diseases.

6 Ischemic Cardiomyopathy

Ischemic cardiomyopathy (ICM) is a term that describes heart failure occurring in the setting of ischemic damage caused by coronary artery syndromes (i.e. myocardial infarction), coronary vascular anomalies, and the end stage of other heart diseases that result in myocardial ischemia, such as end-stage hypertrophic and dilated cardiomyopathy. Atherosclerotic coronary diseases are considered to be the most prevalent cause of ischemic cardiomyopathy, which in turn has become, over the last decades, the most prevalent cause of heart failure necessitating heart transplantation [50, 51].

The impedance of cardiomyocytes' blood supply is the initial event in the cascade that will eventually lead to heart failure. Inadequate blood supply that does not meet the myocardial metabolic demands leads to cellular dysfunction and death. This trigger event will result in reversible impairment in contractility and, if prolonged, will turn into irreversible damage, ending in cardiac remodeling. Remodeling is evident by contractile tissue being partially replaced by "non-contractile, dense scar tissue" thus resulting in ventricular wall thinning and myocytic elongation.

Conversely, the non-infracted myocytes undergo hypertrophic changes. Initially, these changes help to maintain cardiac output. The hypertrophic myocyte elongation will change the ventricular shape, rendering it more spherical. This derangement will affect the pumping ability of the heart by making it less effective. Involvement of at least 40% of the left ventricle is considered to be the point at which severe myocardial dysfunction causing heart failure develops. At this stage, the lost contractile ability will not recover even with attempts at revascularization, which makes heart transplantation the best option for these patients [52].

Typically, the morphological features are represented by the presence of numerous discrete focal areas of damaged myocardium in a dilated left ventricle, which are seen as "defined areas of akinesis and thinning of the wall" on imaging techniques such as echocardiography [53]. At a cellular level, there will be an augmentation of the volume of remaining viable myocardium by hyperplasia of fibroblasts, endothelial cells, collagen deposition, and activation of connective tissue and inflammatory cells such as neutrophils. Stimulation of microvascular growth occurs subsequently, but the adaptation of the microcirculation is disproportionate due to the inability of the vascular bed to grow at a similar rate [54, 55]. Chronic insufficient perfusion of the heart leads to a condition known as "hibernating myocardium" in which metabolism is maintained at a lower level in an attempt to conserve energy. This stage is a potentially reversible condition, however, when cellular necrosis occurs, the transition to pathologic irreversible cardiomyopathy is established [53].

The biochemical signature of irreversibility is macromolecular structural alteration. Factors that are involved in this event are toxic lipid metabolite buildup, cellular hyperosmolarity, cytosolic $Ca + 2$ overload, and the release of reactive oxygen species (ROS) [56].

7 Dilated Cardiomyopathy

Dilated cardiomyopathy can strike anyone at any age, however, it is more common in people under the age of 50 [57, 58]. Mutations in genes encoding structural components of the sarcomere and desmosome, genetic mutations in cytoskeletal components, or an autoimmune response to acute viral myocarditis have all been linked to dilated cardiomyopathy [59]. More than 20 viruses can cause dilated cardiomyopathy; coxsackievirus B is the most common in temperate zones. Chagas disease, caused by Trypanosoma cruzi, is the most common infectious disease in Central and South America. Other causes could include endocrine, toxin exposure, neuromuscular, or pregnancy-related, although none of these is likely the cause [59, 60].

It is related to reduced sarcomere contractility which raises ventricular size (Frank–Starling mechanism) to sustain cardiac output, resulting in the thin-walled dilated LV [58]. Valvular changes seen in dilated cardiomyopathy are not typical; they are usually secondary to dilated chambers in the form of valvular regurgitation [61, 62]. Coronary anatomy is usually normal as many cases may have no occlusive atherosclerotic plaques or thrombi, especially in atrial and ventricular appendages [62].

On histological examination, DCM is characterized by widespread fibrosis, myocyte apoptosis, and compensatory enlargement of other myocytes [63]. The most common pattern in DCM is the accumulation of both interstitial and perivascular fibrosis, with various severity degrees. The apoptosis seen in cases of dilated cardiomyopathy mainly involves the subendocardium [62].

The dilation of the ventricular cavity causes a decreased systolic pressure while the diastolic pressure increases. With decreased contractility, cardiac output is decreased. In advanced cases, systemic blood pressure is decreased, which leads to an increased load on the right ventricles with subsequent elevated right ventricular pulmonary systolic pressure and pulmonary hypertension [64].

Several pathways of ventricular dysfunction in DCM have been suggested by genetic mutations. These include the following:

1. The most common cause of DCM **is sarcomere gene mutations (defect in force generation)** [65].
2. **Laminopathies (defects in the nuclear envelope).**
3. **Cytoskeletal cardiomyopathies (defect in force transmission),** which are frequently linked with DCM, are caused by mutations involving protein members of the cytoskeletal apparatus, such as filamins, dystrophin, desmin, d-sarcoglycan, and vinculin [60].
4. **Glycosylation processes cardiomyopathies (defect in protein post-translational modifications):** Dolichol kinase gene mutations [60, 66].
5. **Mitochondrial cardiomyopathies:** These conditions are characterized by abnormalities in oxidative phosphorylation that result in low ATP synthesis [66].
6. **Calcium-cycling abnormalities:** Increased SERCA inhibition with faulty calcium reuptake results from gene mutations will lead to reduced contractility and cardiac dilatation [63, 66].
7. **Disruption of the RAS-MAPK pathway.**

8 Hypertrophic Cardiomyopathy

Dilated cardiomyopathy can strike anyone at any age, however, it is more common in people under the age of 50 [57, 58]. More than 20 viruses can cause dilated cardiomyopathy; coxsackievirus B is the most common in temperate zones. Chagas disease, caused by Trypanosoma cruzi, is the most common infectious disease in Central and South America. Other causes could include endocrine, toxin exposure, neuromuscular, or pregnancy-related, although none of these is likely the cause [59]. It is related to reduced sarcomere contractility which raises ventricular size (Frank–Starling mechanism) to sustain cardiac output, resulting in the thin-walled dilated LV [58]. Valvular changes seen in dilated cardiomyopathy are not typical; they are usually secondary to dilated chambers in the form of valvular regurgitation [61, 62]. Coronary anatomy is usually normal as many cases may have no occlusive atherosclerotic plaques or thrombi, especially in atrial and ventricular appendages [62].

On histological examination, DCM is characterized by widespread fibrosis, myocyte apoptosis, and compensatory enlargement of other myocytes [63]. The most common pattern in DCM is the accumulation of both interstitial and perivascular fibrosis, with various severity degrees. The apoptosis seen in cases of dilated cardiomyopathy mainly involves the subendocardium [62].

The dilation of the ventricular cavity causes a decreased systolic pressure while the diastolic pressure increases. With decreased contractility, cardiac output is decreased. In advanced cases, systemic blood pressure is decreased, which leads to an increased load on the right ventricles with subsequent elevated right ventricular pulmonary systolic pressure and pulmonary hypertension [64].

Several pathways of ventricular dysfunction in DCM have been suggested by genetic mutations. These include.

9 Restrictive Cardiomyopathy

Restrictive cardiomyopathy (RCM) is the rarest type of a collective group of disorders called cardiomyopathies. However, the systolic function is usually maintained. This functional, rather than anatomical alteration, may lead to heart failure if left without treatment [67, 68]. RCM has the worst prognosis and the highest sudden cardiac death records among all cardiomyopathies, with only a 2–5-year survival rate [69].

Using imaging techniques, such as echocardiography, the restricted cardiomyopathic heart has "bilateral atrial dilation and non-hypertrophied, non-dilated ventricles" that cannot be regarded as valvular, ischemic, inflammatory, hypertensive, or infiltrative in origin [70].

RCM is divided into two types: idiopathic (non-infiltrative) and secondary (infiltrative). The idiopathic type refers to the occurrence of hemodynamic disturbances in the absence of apparent histological evidence signifying abnormalities in the myocardium [67]. Myocardial biopsy may show interstitial fibrosis and a variation in the size and shape of myocytic nuclei, but the endocardium remains normal without collagen deposition [71].

On the other hand, secondary RCM is due to infiltration of foreign substances into cardiomyocytes, retention of abnormal metabolic byproducts, or fibrotic injury, as in some diseases like amyloidosis, hemochromatosis, sarcoidosis, Fabry disease, glycogen storage diseases, radiation, and as a result of drugs (i.e. anthracycline and ergotamine) [69].

It can also develop as an end-stage event in hypertrophic and dilated cardiomyopathy. In this type, histological changes can be seen both in the myocardium and the endocardium. They differ among the different types of diseases. For example, depositions can be seen between the myocytes in infiltrative diseases like amyloidosis, while they are within the myocytes in storage diseases like hemochromatosis [67, 72].

These changes may be accompanied by cardiomyocyte death, fibrosis, or compensatory myocardial hypertrophy. Papillary muscle infiltration may also occur, resulting in malfunction of mitral or tricuspid valves thus leading to functional regurgitation. If the infiltration extends to involve the nodal and conduction tissues, different degrees of atrioventricular and sinoatrial block may occur [73].

At a cellular level, assays have shown that cardiac fibroblasts display an impaired relaxation velocity due to deregulation in the components of their extra-cellular matrix and cytokine expression (70).

The primary hemodynamic outcome is diastolic dysfunction, with usually a normal systolic contraction. Ventricular pressure shows immense reductions at diastolic onset followed by a significant increase, demonstrating the "dip-and-plateau" filling pattern typical of RCM [68]. RCM can cause a variety of systolic dysfunctions as the disease progresses. All of these changes contribute to the eventual development of pulmonary venous hypertension and heart failure [67, 73].

RCM's genetic basis has captivated the interest of researchers over the last few decades. Several mutations affecting the genes encoding proteins involved in the formation of the cardiac muscle cytoskeleton and sarcomeres were identified, such as ACTC1, β-MyHC, TNNI3, MYH7, and mutations in the DES gene. These mutations are now used to identify families who may be at risk of developing idiopathic RCM, as the genetic etiology was shown to be the cause of 30% of all reported familial RCM cases [67, 74].

9.1 Lysosomal Storage Diseases

Lysosomal storage diseases (LSDs) represent a group of heterogeneous rare inborn diseases characterized by a deficiency or impaired function of lysosomal enzymes or other proteins related to the lysosomes, resulting in the accumulation of various substrates. These diseases manifest in the myocardium as hypertrophic or less frequently, dilated cardiomyopathy, arrhythmia, coronary involvement, or valvular lesions [75].

Examples of storage diseases include

1. PRKAG2 cardiac syndrome due to mutation in PRKAG2 leading to increased activity of AMPK and accumulation of glycogen, causing abnormal activation of the mTOR pathway.
2. Pompe disease due to mutation in GAA gene causing decreased GAA and accumulation of glycogen.
3. Fabry disease due to mutation in LAMP2 causing glycogen deposit, altered expression of mitochondrial genes, and impaired mitochondrial respiration [76].

10 Fatty Acid Oxidation Disorder

It represents a heterogeneous group of metabolic recessive diseases due to mutations in genes encoding proteins involved in lipid metabolism and transport through the carnitine shuttle pathway in the mitochondria, causing accumulation of their substrate as well as depletion of important intermediates of the tricarboxylic acid cycle.

There are several types of fatty acid disorders classified by the length of the fatty acids or the deficiency of fat transport protein. They are manifested as hypertrophic, dilated cardiomyopathy, or arrhythmia. The development of a dilated heart in those diseases may result from the accumulation of fatty acid metabolism intermediates in the cytoplasm or lysosomes, disruption of myofibril alignment, and impaired contraction, while cardiac hypertrophy results from insufficient energy and inefficient contraction stimulating cardiac hypertrophy. The occurrence of arrhythmias in these diseases may be attributed to lack of energy, impaired inward current of potassium as in ventricular tachycardia, and decreased sodium influx leading to reentry arrhythmias, which may lead to impaired calcium influx or altered gap junction [77].

11 Mitochondrial Disease

Mitochondrial disease represents a group of heterogeneous, rare, inborn diseases associated with systemic manifestation due to mutations in nuclear or mitochondrial DNA. Mitochondrial cardiomyopathy is characterized by abnormal myocardial structure, function, or both due to a genetic mutation affecting the respiratory chain. These diseases are manifested in the form of hypertrophic or dilated cardiomyopathy or arrhythmia.

These mutations affect various structures involved in the respiratory chain. The most common identified abnormalities are deficiencies in NADH-coenzyme Q (CoQ) reductase (complex I) [78, 79].

12 Arrhythmias

The role of heart transplantation in arrhythmia is indicated for fatal arrhythmia like (ventricular tachycardia) refractory to medical treatment. The pathological changes induced by arrhythmia (tachycardia-induced cardiomyopathy) are reversible, and transplantation is indicated for refractory fatal ones [80, 81].

Heart transplantation in arrhythmia is indicated for fatal arrhythmias (i.e. ventricular tachycardia) refractory to medical treatment. The pathological changes induced by arrhythmia (tachycardia-induced cardiomyopathy) are reversible, and transplantation is indicated only for refractory fatal ones [80, 81].

Cardiomyocytes go through a lot of changes during arrhythmia. **These include.**

- gradual depletion of Cardiomyocytes from their contractile material.
- clumps of Z-band material which are Remnants of the sarcomeres.
- accumulation of Glycogen in sarcomere-depleted areas; there was a network of disordered membranes, most likely due to altered sarcoplasmic reticulum profiles.
- Mitochondria have an elongated shape with longitudinally oriented cristae that appear as little doughnut-like features in cross.
- The distribution of nuclear heterochromatin was uniform across the nucleoplasm.

Molecular remodeling in cardiac arrhythmia includes inactivation of sodium channels, changes in calcium and potassium channels, such as decreased L-type $Ca2+$-current, increased inward-rectifier $K+$ current, and modifications in sodium/calcium exchanger function.

Connexins are gap junction proteins that are responsible for cardiomyocyte-to-cardiomyocyte electrical connection. Cardiomyocytes lost many structural proteins, including myosin, tropomyosin, actin, and a-actinin. Only near the cell's perimeter, where the remaining sarcomeres resided, were normal cross-striation patterns still visible [82, 83].

Magnetic resonance T1-weighted images revealed large regions of fibro-fatty infiltration in the left ventricular intramyocardium. The basal inferolateral wall was the most common site of fatty infiltration, with nearly all of the left ventricular inferolateral wall having fatty/fibro-fatty replacement and decreased systolic function. Other parts of the left ventricle, such as the basal anterolateral wall, mid-inferoseptal wall, mid-inferolateral wall, and mid-anterolateral wall, may also have fatty/fibro-fatty replacement [84, 85].

13 Congenital Heart Diseases

Cardiac transplantation is indicated for stage C or D heart failure-associated congenital heart disease (previously repaired or palliated), especially those with a high risk for the irreversible elevation of pulmonary [86].

It should be noted that primary surgical options have significantly reduced the need for heart transplantation in this category.

Three common CHDs that require transplants will be discussed in this scope: Hypoplastic left heart syndrome, pulmonary atresia with an intact interventricular septum, and Ebstein anomaly.

1. *Hypoplastic left heart syndrome:*

HLHS represents 3% of all congenital heart diseases. It could be divided into two categories according to the origin of the insult: (i) outflow obstruction, with aortic stenosis being the commonest cause, and (ii) inflow obstruction, like in mitral valve atresia or restrictive foramen ovale, with the first category being more common [87].

Newborns are totally dependent on the ductus arteriosus for systemic perfusion or interatrial communication. If the patient's ductus closes, or the pulmonary vascular resistance falls, systemic circulation will be depleted, as the left ventricle in those patients is nonfunctional and the neonate will present with signs of shock [87, 88].

Oxygen saturation will be 75 and 85% [89]. Supplemental oxygen should not be given as it may further reduce the pulmonary vascular resistance, worsening the systemic perfusion as discussed above. Intubation may be needed to achieve the goal of keeping $PaCO_2$ at controlled levels.

The main aspects of treatment are heart transplantation, staged palliative surgery, or non-surgical palliative treatment, and fetal operations. The second became the method of choice in the management of this anomaly instead of the primary heart transplant. It provides survival for more than half of the cases for 5 years. The procedure includes a series of three operations: Norwood/Hybrid, Hemi-Fontan/Bidirectional Glenn, and Fontan. These are the only methods for the neonate to survive until the heart transplantation. The operation is only a temporary solution, and eventually heart transplantation will be needed [87, 90]. Although statistics differ, in one study done in 2015, the survival rate for HLHS patients who underwent Fontan operation ranged from 72 to 85% at 10 years [91].

Primary heart transplantation for HLHS is limited to neonates with severe right ventricular dysfunction and/or moderate to severe tricuspid regurgitation [92]. In addition, patients who are labeled as high-risk for palliative surgery may undergo a primary transplantation procedure. Heart transplant success is greater if done in the neonatal period (before 30 days), after which the prognosis is worse, attributing the cause to immunologic factors [87].

2. ***Pulmonary atresia with intact interventricular septum:***

The pathology resides in the membranous or muscular segment obstructing the pulmonary valve, contributing to the right with an absence of interventricular connection. The right ventricle may be hypoplastic, carrying a worse prognosis. The tricuspid valve is rarely intact, and its pathologies range from stenotic to regurgitant [93].

Another pathology in this CHD is the abnormal connection between the right ventricle and the epicardial coronary arteries. In some cases, and especially in hypoplastic right ventricles, parts of the myocardium will be dependent on the right ventricle for perfusion (known as right ventricular dependent coronary circulation, or RVDCC), predisposing them in the long term to ischemia and heart failure associated with systemic hypoperfusion and poor peripheral pulses [94].

Echocardiography and catheterization will be needed to examine for interatrial septum, the size of the tricuspid valve and its annulus, the morphology and size of the right ventricle, the type of right ventricle obstruction (muscular or membranous), and any evidence of the connection between the right ventricle and coronary arteries. These factors will determine the type and outcome of surgery.

The 4 groups classified by Chikkabyrappa et al. [95] include

1. Adequate, functional, tripartite RV shape and size, Z-score of tricuspid valves more than—2.5 and normal coronary arteries anatomy, and membranous atresia with mild to moderate TR: management includes radiofrequency valvotomy or right ventricle outflow obstruction.

2. Borderline hypoplastic RV, which is bipartite, with tricuspid valve Z-scores range from -2.5 to -4.5, moderate to severe TR, absent or small trabecular component, patent infundibulum, small pulmonary valve annulus, subvalvar stenosis or presence of ventriculocoronary connections: management includes radiofrequency valvotomy with PDA stenting or surgical valvotomy/right ventricle outflow obstruction with or without PDA stenting. If future right ventricle growth is affected, bidirectional Glenn or 1.5 ventricular repairs.
3. Severe hypoplastic RV, which is functionally unipartite, with severely hypoplastic tricuspid valve and Z-score of less than -5 and RVDCC: management includes PDA stenting or systemic to pulmonary artery shunt followed by bidirectional Glenn or Fontan completion.
4. Myocardial ischemia and/or coronary ostial atresia: management includes palliative care or cardiac transplant.

Primary heart transplant is indicated in those patients who have coronary atresia or those who develop myocardial ischemia. Patients with a severely hypoplastic right ventricle who developed RDVCC are dealt with an initial palliative surgical therapy followed by a heart transplant.

The 15-year survival of all groups of this treated anomaly ranges from 58 to 87%, but may require re-intervention in the future. The cause of death in adulthood is late-onset arrhythmia [96, 97].

3. *Ebstein anomaly (EA):*

In mild forms of EA, if the pulmonary vascular resistance falls, the right ventricle will be able to pump the blood effectively, thereby reliving the cyanosis. If there is pulmonary valve insufficiency, poor RV function and marked TR with ASD, and intact TR, there will be a circular shunt with severe hemodynamic instability and severe desaturation [98].

The severity of the disease ranges from mild asymptomatic disease to severe disease that is incompatible with the life of the fetus (Hydrops), depending on the degree of leaflet displacement and the severity of regurgitation. There will be hyperactive precordium in severe cases. Imaging will detect evidence of cardiomegaly [99].

Patients with this anomaly associated with anatomic pulmonary atresia, circular shunt, dependency on prostaglandin or mechanical ventilation, worsening cyanosis or heart failure with an inability to tolerate feeds, and generally severe forms as detected by imaging will require surgical intervention during the neonatal period. Intractable arrhythmia is also an indication for surgery [98, 99].

In severe cases, like in severely depressed left ventricular function, options are limited to heart transplantation, and this shows the same outcomes as compared to transplantation in other congenital heart diseases [98].

Multiple choice questions

1. **Regarding the causes of dilated cardiomyopathy: which one is the best answer**

    a. Viral causes, e.g.: cockaxie B virus.
    b. Genetic mutations.
    c. Adverse cardiac remodeling.
    d. All of the above.

2. **The commonest genetic mutation to cause dilated cardiomyopathy is**

    a. Lamin-A/C gene.
    b. Genes encoding filamins, and desmin proteins.
    c. Sarcomere genes, e.g. titin (TTN).
    d. RAF-1 gene.

3. **The type of heart failure in dilated cardiomyopathy is**

    a. Systolic dysfunction.
    b. Diastolic dysfunction.
    c. Systolic then progresses to diastolic dysfunction.
    d. No evidence of heart failure.

4. **Regarding dilated cardiomyopathy, which one is wrong?**

    a. Screening other family members is unhelpful.
    b. Left ventricular or biventricular enlargement.
    c. Catecholamines, TNF, and fibroblasts play a role in pathogenesis.
    d. Alcohol consumption might be a cause.

5. **What is\are the pathophysiological changes seen in dilated cardiomyopathy?**

    a. Reduced sympathetic system activity (RAAS SYSTEM).
    b. The right ventricle is not affected at all.
    c. Myocyte hypertrophy and fibrosis.
    d. Inflammatory cytokines are down-regulated.

6. **The most common morphological variant of HCM is**

    a. Apical.
    b. Right ventricular.
    c. Symmetrical.
    d. Asymmetrical.

7. **Most cases of HCM are due to mutations in**

    a. TNNT2 and TNNI3 genes.
    b. MYH7 and MYBPC3 genes.
    c. MYH7 and MYL2 genes.
    d. MYBPC3 and MYL3 genes.

8. **The predominant histological features of hypertrophic cardiomyopathy include all of the following except**

   a. Cardiac myocyte disarray.
   b. Small-vessel disease.
   c. Fibrosis.
   d. Necrosis.

9. **The primary hemodynamic feature of HCM is**

   a. Systolic dysfunction.
   b. Diastolic dysfunction.
   c. Systolic and diastolic dysfunction.
   d. None of the above.

10. **Regarding systolic dysfunction of HCM, all of the following are true except**

    a. It usually appears late.
    b. It includes both the left and right ventricles.
    c. It's associated with a poor prognosis.
    d. It usually appears before diastolic dysfunction.

11. **Regarding the genetic basis of HCM, all of the following are true except**

    a. Most of the gene mutations associated with HCM are missense.
    b. Mutations in other genes can also cause phenotypes resembling HCM.
    c. HCM primary mode of inheritance is autosomal recessive.
    d. HCM is caused by a mutation in one of the genes encoding for sarcomere proteins.

12. **Restrictive Cardiomyopathy is BEST characterized by**

    a. Systolic dysfunction.
    b. Diastolic under-filling.
    c. A "'dip-and-plateau" filling pattern.
    d. Stiffened non-compliant atrials.

13. **Idiopathic Restrictive Cardiomyopathy differs from its secondary counterpart in that**

    a. It affects the myocardium as well as the endocardium.
    b. It is associated with other systemic diseases.
    c. Myocardial biopsy shows depositions within the myocytes.
    d. It appears normal on histologic examination.

14. **A patient with RCM develops a pan-systolic murmur heard over the mitral area. This can be explained by**

    a. Papillary muscle infiltration leading to functional regurgitation.
    b. Ventricular dilation leading to functional regurgitation.
    c. It is unrelated to the disease process.

    d. The valvular structure is not affected, and it occurs due to the high pressures within the ventricle.

15. **Regarding Ischemic Cardiomyopathy, one of the following changes does NOT occur:**

    a. Ischemic part being replaced by scar tissue.
    b. Ischemic part Akinesis and Dyskinesis.
    c. Non-ischemic part hypertrophy.
    d. Non-ischemic part thinning.

16. **The term "Hibernating myocardium" Implies**

    a. An irreversible event involving myocytic necrosis.
    b. Chronicity of impaired perfusion.
    c. Myocardial metabolism being increased in order to maintain cardiac pumping.
    d. A completely reversible event that will resolve without intervention.

17. **Irreversibility of Myocardial damage is considered to be established when the presence of the following is seen:**

    a. Macromolecular structural alteration.
    b. Foci of cellular necrosis.
    c. Hyperemia surrounding the ischemic part.
    d. a and b.

18. **Regarding structural heart changes during arrhythmia, the most common site for fibro-fatty infiltration is**

    a. Mid-anterolateral wall.
    b. Mid-inferoseptal wall.
    c. Basal anterolateral wall.
    d. Basal inferolateral wall.
    e. Mid-inferolateral wall.

19. **Regarding molecular and cellular remodeling in cardiac arrhythmia**

    a. Ion channel changes include alteration in calcium and potassium channels, such as increased L-type $Ca2 +$ -current.
    b. The distribution of nuclear heterochromatin isn't uniform across the nucleoplasm.
    c. There is an accumulation of Glycogen in sarcomere-depleted areas.
    d. There is a decrease in labeling intensity and redistribution of the gap junction proteins, the most prominent one being connexin 46.
    e. Abrupt depletion of Cardiomyocytes from their contractile material.

20. **Hemodynamic consequences of cardiac arrhythmia:**

    a. It involves reduced cardiac output, reduced stroke volume, and normal or increased arterial pressure.

b. Tachycardia leads to decrease in myocardial oxygen demand.
c. In the case of sinus bradycardia, there may be a massive hemodynamic alteration.
d. Acute tachycardia can eventually lead to systolic heart failure.
e. High rates of contraction lead to decrease in ventricular preload thus reducing stroke volume.

21. **The process of fibrosis in heart failure pathogenesis includes all the following except**

   a. It represents an early adaptive response.
   b. It includes three types, reactive interstitial fibrosis, replacement fibrosis, and infiltrative interstitial fibrosis.
   c. Reactive interstitial fibrosis is mainly seen post-Myocardial Infarction which suggests its reparative role.
   d. The cells involved in secreting pro-fibrotic materials include macrophages, lymphocytes, and cardiomyocyte.

22. **Regarding molecular and cellular remodeling in cardiac arrhythmia**

   a. Ion channel changes include alteration in calcium and potassium channels, such as increased L-type $Ca2+$ -current.
   b. The distribution of nuclear heterochromatin wasn't uniform across the nucleoplasm.
   c. There is an accumulation of Glycogen in sarcomere-depleted areas.
   d. There is decrease in labeling intensity and redistribution of the gap junction proteins, the most prominent one being connexin 46.
   e. Abrupt depletion of Cardiomyocytes from their contractile material.

23. **The most common type of gap junction Proteins involved in structural changes is**

   a. CX43.
   b. CX40.
   c. CX37.
   d. CX46.
   e. CX21.

24. **Regarding Mitochondrial cardiomyopathy, the following is true except**

   a. A group of heterogeneous rare inborn diseases associated with systemic manifestation.
   b. It is caused by mutation affecting only mitochondrial DNA.
   c. These diseases are manifested in the form of hypertrophic or dilated cardiomyopathy or arrhythmia.
   d. The most common identified abnormalities are deficiency in NADH-coenzyme Q (CoQ) reductase.

25. **In chronic heart failure, the following findings can be seen:**

a. Increased anti-inflammatory response in the affected myocardium.
b. Utilization fats as the main source of energy.
c. Reactivation of fetal genes.
d. Decreased catecholamines level in the systemic circulation.

26. **Catecholamines in chronic heart failure is characterized by**

a. Increased levels and increased effects.
b. Increased levels and decreased effects.
c. Decreased levels and increased effects.
d. Decreased levels and decreased effects.
e. Remain unchanged level and effects.

27. **The vascular changes seen in heart failure patients include the following except**

a. Initial increased capillary density as an adaptive response.
b. Decreased capillary numbers and density in long term.
c. Decreased capillary density can be additive to epicardial coronary obstruction.
d. The capillary density decreased as a result of maladaptive hypertrophy.

28. **The top three indications for cardiac transplant in congenital heart disease are all of the following except**

a. Hypoplastic left heart syndrome.
b. Pulmonary atresia with intact interventricular septum.
c. Atrial septal defect.
d. Epstein anomaly.

29. **Epstein anomaly is characterized by**

a. Basal displacement of the leaflets of the mitral valve.
b. Atrialization of the left ventricle.
c. Right to left shunt through patent foramen ovale.
d. Left to right shunt through ventricular septal defect.

30. **Lysosomal storage diseases manifest as structural cardiac**

a. Hypertrophy.
b. Dilation.
c. Non-specific changes involving only the myocardial septum.
d. a and b.

Answers

1. d. Cardiomyopathy is multifactorial and may have a genetic basis, or is caused by environmental exposure to viruses or toxins like alcohol.
2. c. Sarcomere gene mutations are the most commonly found mutations in subjects with dilated cardiomyopathy, but still a number of other mutations can also be found.

3. c. Dilated cardiomyopathy results in heart failure as it is a progressive process of homonymic changes starting as systolic dysfunction with increased cardiac output, and ventricular dilatation then results in diastolic dysfunction as the ventricular walls become thin and fibrosed.
4. a. As dilated cardiomyopathy has a genetic basis, it is much helpful to screen other relatives to detect gene mutation for adequate follow-up and monitoring.
5. c. Myocytes hypertrophy and fibrosis as a result of activation of RAAS system and the inflammatory cytokines along with the remodeling process is noticed in dilated cardiomyopathy pathophysiology, in which the right ventricle will be eventually affected as it is a progressive process.
6. d. Most hypertrophic cardiomyopathies (60–70%) manifest as asymmetrical hypertrophic changes of the interventricular septum.
7. b. Most cases are due to mutations of the MYH7 and MYBPC3 genes.
8. d. The predominant histological features of hypertrophic cardiomyopathy include cardiac myocyte disarray, fibrosis, and small-vessel disease.
9. b. Diastolic dysfunction is a primary hemodynamic feature of HCM and often develops prior to the onset of symptoms.
10. d. Systolic dysfunction generally appears late and is preceded by diastolic dysfunction.
11. c. HCM is inherited in an autosomal dominant pattern.
12. c. RCM is best characterized by the "dip-and-plateau" filling pattern that is considered to be its typical feature. Systolic function is usually not affected and only occurs at late stages. Diastolic under-filling is one of the features of RCM but is not its typical feature. Atrials are usually dilated rather than stiffened.
13. d. Idiopathic RCM usually appears normal on histology examination with no apparent abnormalities hence the name "idiopathic". It usually spares the endocardium. Association with systemic diseases and myocardial biopsy findings are both features of secondary RCM.
14. a. One of the outcomes of RCM is infiltration of different cardiac components such as the papillary muscles, valves, and AV node. Functional regurgitation occurs as a result of papillary muscle infiltration. The ventricles are stiffened and non-compliant rather than dilated. The valvular structure is affected and the "dip-and-plateau" change in the ventricular pressures does not affect the mitral valve in a way as to cause regurgitation.
15. d. Morphological changes occurring in ischemic cardiomyopathy include the ischemic part being replaced by dense scar tissue resulting in its thinning and impairment movement on imaging techniques. On the other hand, the non-ischemic part undergoes hypertrophy which will the ventricular shape leading to ineffective pumping technique.
16. b. Hibernating myocardium is a potentially reversible event. Myocardial metabolism is maintained at low levels in order to conserve energy. Left without treatment, it will turn into irreversible damage.
17. d. Irreversibility is characterized by the presence of macromolecular structural alteration. Foci of cellular necrosis mark the transition between reversible and

irreversible events. Hyperemia means increased blood supply to the affected area which makes it potentially salvageable.

18. d. The basal inferolateral wall is the most common site of fibro-fatty infiltration.
19. c. Accumulation of Glycogen in sarcomere-depleted areas is one of the prominent cellular changes. Other changes include decrease in L-type Ca2+-current, decrease in labeling intensity and redistribution of connexin 43, and gradual depletion of cardiomyocytes from their contractile material.
20. e. High rates of contraction lead to decrease in ventricular filling time (preload), thus stroke volume is reduced together with the cardiac output and blood pressure.
21. c. The replacement fibrosis is observed after myocardial necrosis as in myocardial infarction, while the reactive interstitial fibrosis is induced by many stimuli, like ischemia, pressure overload, and metabolic derangement without myocardial necrosis.
22. c. Accumulation of Glycogen in sarcomere-depleted areas is one of the prominent cellular changes. Other changes include decrease in L-type Ca2+-current, decrease in labeling intensity and redistribution of connexin 43, and gradual depletion of Cardiomyocytes from their contractile material.
23. a. The most common type of gap junction protein involved in structural changes is connexin 43.
24. b. It is due to mutation affecting nuclear or mitochondrial DNA.
25. c. Heart failure is characterized by reactivation of fetal genes that modify the metabolism, wall compliance, and neurohormones.
26. b. In heart failure, there is an increment in the level of catecholamine, with time, it causes dysfunctional signaling leading to impaired contractility (by decreasing the density of adrenergic receptors and impairing their association with G-protein coupled receptor (Desensitization)).
27. b. The initial adaptive response is increased capillary numbers and density, but with advanced maladaptive hypertrophy, their density appears to be reduced.
28. c. Atrial septal defect is rarely indicated for transplantation in congenital heart disease.
29. c. Epstein anomaly is characterized by apical displacement of the posterior and septal leaflets of the tricuspid valve, leading to atrialization of the right ventricle and regurgitation of blood from the right ventricle to the right atrium, enlarging it and elevating its pressure. This will lead to a right to left shunt through patent foremen ovale, leading to the mixing of deoxygenated blood with the systemic circulation, making the anomaly one of cyanotic heart diseases.
30. d. lysosomal storage diseases can manifest as cardiac muscle hypertrophy or dilation and do not have a predilection for specific cardiac structures.

References

1. O'Grady H, Mostafa K, Zafar H, Lohan D, Morris L, Sharif F. Changes in left ventricular shape and morphology in the presence of heart failure: a four-dimensional quantitative and qualitative analysis. Int J Comput Assist Radiol Surg. 2019;14(8):1415–30.
2. Baba H, Wohlschlaeger J. Morphological and molecular changes of the myocardium after left ventricular mechanical support. Curr Cardiol Rev. 2008;4(3):157–69.
3. Sultan F, Saadia S. Patterns of left ventricular hypertrophy and late gadolinium enhancement on cardiac MRI in patients with hypertrophic cardiomyopathy and their prognostic significance—an experience from a South Asian country. J Clin Imaging Sci. 2021;11:14.
4. Markus MR, Freitas HF, Chizzola PR, Silva GT, Lima AC, Mansur AJ. Left ventricular mass in patients with heart failure. Arq Bras Cardiol. 2004;83(3):232–6, 227–31. (English, Portuguese). https://doi.org/10.1590/s0066-782x2004001500006. Epub 13 Sept 2004.
5. Basso C, Michaud K, d'Amati G, et al. Cardiac hypertrophy at autopsy. Virchows Arch. 2021;479(1):79–94. https://doi.org/10.1007/s00428-021-03038-0.
6. Nauta JF, Hummel YM, Tromp J, Ouwerkerk W, van der Meer P, Jin X, Lam CSP, Bax JJ, Metra M, Samani NJ, Ponikowski P, Dickstein K, Anker SD, Lang CC, Ng LL, Zannad F, Filippatos GS, van Veldhuisen DJ, van Melle JP, Voors AA. Concentric vs. eccentric remodelling in heart failure with reduced ejection fraction: clinical characteristics, pathophysiology and response to treatment. Eur J Heart Fail. 2020;22(7):1147–1155. https://doi.org/10.1002/ejhf.1632. Epub 11 Nov 2019.
7. Sultan FAT, Saadia S. Patterns of left ventricular hypertrophy and late gadolinium enhancement on cardiac MRI in Patients with hypertrophic cardiomyopathy and their prognostic significance—an experience from a South Asian country. J Clin Imaging Sci. 2021;11:14. Published 2021 Mar 9. Cuspidi C, Negri F, Sala C, Valerio C, Mancia G. Association of left atrial enlargement with left ventricular hypertrophy and diastolic dysfunction: a tissue Doppler study in echocardiographic practice. Blood Press. 2012;21(1):24–30. https://doi.org/10.3109/08037051.2011.618262. Epub 13 Oct 2011.
8. Savarese G, Lund LH. Global public health burden of heart failure. Card Fail Rev. 2017;3:7–11.
9. Tomaz P, Victoria D, Jeroen JB. Imaging of Valvular heart disease in heart failure. Card Fail Rev J. 2018;4(2):78–86.
10. Noemi P, Robert AL, Philippe P, Alec V, Gregg WS, Georg G. Secondary valve regurgitation in patients with heart failure with preserved ejection fraction, heart failure with mid-range ejection fraction, and heart failure with reduced ejection fraction. Eur Hear J. 2020;41(29):2799–2810. https://doi.org/10.1093/eurheartj/ehaa129.
11. Ennezat PV, Marechaux S, Pibarot P, Le Jemtel TH. Secondary mitral regurgitation in heart failure with reduced or preserved left ventricular ejection fraction. Cardiology. 2013;125:110–7.
12. Peyronnet R, Nerbonne JM, Kohl P. Cardiac Mechano-gated ion channels and arrhythmias. Circ Res. 2016;118(2):311–29. https://doi.org/10.1161/CIRCRESAHA.115.305043.
13. Zhang Y, Su SA, Li W, Ma Y, Shen J, Wang Y, Shen Y, Chen J, Ji Y, Xie Y, Ma H, Xiang M. Piezo1-mediated mechanotransduction promotes cardiac hypertrophy by impairing calcium homeostasis to activate calpain/calcineurin signaling. Hypertension. 2021;78(3):647–60. https://doi.org/10.1161/HYPERTENSIONAHA.121.17177 Epub 2021 Aug 2.
14. Khalilimeybodi A, Daneshmehr A, Sharif KB. Ca2+-dependent calcineurin/NFAT signaling in β-adrenergic-induced cardiac hypertrophy. Gen Physiol Biophys. 2018;37(1):41–56. https://doi.org/10.4149/gpb_2017022.
15. Frank D, Frey N. Cardiac Z-disc signaling network. J Biol Chem. 2011;286(12):9897–904. https://doi.org/10.1074/jbc.R110.17426.
16. Dierck F, Kuhn C, Rohr C, et al. The novel cardiac z-disc protein CEFIP regulates cardiomyocyte hypertrophy by modulating calcineurin signaling. J Biol Chem. 2017;292(37):15180–91. https://doi.org/10.1074/jbc.M117.786764.
17. Sequeira V, Nijenkamp LL, Regan JA, van der Velden J. The physiological role of cardiac cytoskeleton and its alterations in heart failure. Biochim Biophys Acta. 2014;1838(2):700–22. https://doi.org/10.1016/j.bbamem.2013.07.011 Epub 2013 Jul 13.

18. Cluntun AA, Badolia R, Lettlova S, Parnell KM, Shankar TS, Diakos NA, Olson KA, Taleb I, Tatum SM, Berg JA, Cunningham CN, Van Ry T, Bott AJ, Krokidi AT, Fogarty S, Skedros S, Swiatek WI, Yu X, Luo B, Merx S, Navankasattusas S, Cox JE, Ducker GS, Holland WL, McKellar SH, Rutter J, Drakos SG. The pyruvate-lactate axis modulates cardiac hypertrophy and heart failure. Cell Metab. 2021;33(3):629-648.e10. https://dci.org/10.1016/j.cmet.2020.12.003 Epub 2020 Dec 16.

19. Riehle C, Bauersachs J. Key inflammatory mechanisms underlying heart failure. Entzündungsmechanismen bei Herzinsuffizienz Herz. 2019;44(2):96–106. https://doi.org/10.1007/s00059-019-4785-.

20. Matsumoto H, Ogura H, Shimizu K, et al. The clinical importance of a cytokine network in the acute phase of sepsis. Sci Rep. 2018;8:13995. https://doi.org/10.1038/s41598-018-32275-8.

21. Adamo L, Rocha-Resende C, Prabhu SD, Mann DL. Reappraising the role of inflammation in heart failure. Nat Rev Cardiol. 2020;17(5):269–285. https://doi.org/10.1038/s41569-019-0315-x. Epub 2020 Jan 22. Erratum in: Nat Rev Cardiol. 2021;18(10):735. PMID: 31969688.

22. Dick SA, Epelman S. Chronic heart failure and inflammation: what do we really know? Circ Res. 2016;119(1):159–76. https://doi.org/10.1161/CIRCRESAHA.116.308030.

23. Li F, Li Y, Duan Y, Hu CA, Tang Y, Yin Y. Myokines and adipokines: involvement in the crosstalk between skeletal muscle and adipose tissue. Cytokine Growth Factor Rev. 2017;33:73–82. https://doi.org/10.1016/j.cytogfr.2016.10.003 Epub 2016 Oct 13.

24. Mann DL, Topkara VK, Evans S, Barger PM. Innate immunity in the adult mammalian heart: for whom the cell tolls. Trans Am Clin Climatol Assoc. 2010;121:34–50.

25. Rose NR. Viral myocarditis. Curr Opin Rheumatol. 2016;28(4):383–9. https://doi.org/10.1097/BOR.000000000000030.

26. Paulus WJ, Tschöpe C. A novel paradigm for heart failure with preserved ejection fraction: comorbidities drive myocardial dysfunction and remodeling through coronary microvascular endothelial inflammation. J Am Coll Cardiol. 2013;62(4):263–71. https://doi.org/10.1016/j.jacc.2013.02.092 Epub 2013 May 15.

27. Kallikourdis M, Martini E, Carullo P. T cell costimulation blockade blunts pressure overload-induced heart failure. Nat Commun. 2017;8:14680.

28. Alexander EB, Alexander AB, Michael L. Myokines and heart failure: challenging role in adverse cardiac remodeling, myopathy, and clinical outcomes. Dis Markers. 2021;(6644631):17. https://doi.org/10.1155/2021/6644631.

29. Infante T, Costa D, Napoli C. Novel insights regarding nitric oxide and cardiovascular diseases. Angiology. 2021;72(5):411–25. https://doi.org/10.1177/0003319720979243 Epub 2021 Jan 22.

30. Sweeney M, Corden B, Cook SA. Targeting cardiac fibrosis in heart failure with preserved ejection fraction: mirage or miracle? EMBO Mol Med. 2020;12(10): e10865. https://doi.org/10.15252/emmm.20191086.

31. Hinderer S, Schenke-Layland K. Cardiac fibrosis—a short review of causes and therapeutic strategies. Adv Drug Deliv Rev. 2019;146:77–82. https://doi.org/10.1016/j.addr.2019.05.011 Epub 2019 May 31.

32. González A, Schelbert EB, Díez J, Butler J. Myocardial interstitial fibrosis in heart failure: biological and translational perspectives. J Am Coll Cardiol. 2018;71(15):1696–1706. https://doi.org/10.1016/j.jacc.2018.02.021.22; de Lucia C, Eguchi A, Koch WJ. New insights in cardiac β-adrenergic signaling during heart failure and aging. Front Pharmacol. 2018;9:904. https://doi.org/10.3389/fphar.2018.00904. PMID: 30147654;PMCID: PMC6095970.

33. van Gastel J, Hendrickx JO, Leysen H, Santos-Otte P, Luttrell LM, Martin B, Maudsley S. β-arrestin based receptor signaling paradigms: potential therapeutic targets for complex age-related disorders. Front Pharmacol. 2018;28(9):1369. https://doi.org/10.3389/fphar.2018.01369.

34. Najafi A, Sequeira V, Kuster DW, van der Velden J. β-adrenergic receptor signalling and its functional consequences in the diseased heart. Eur J Clin Invest. 2016;46(4):362–74. https://doi.org/10.1111/eci.12598 Epub 2016 Feb 19 PMID: 26842371.

35. Bellinger DL, Lorton D. Autonomic regulation of cellular immune function. Auton Neurosci. 2014;182:15–41.
36. Vitale G, Coppini R, Tesi C, Poggesi C, Sacconi L, Ferrantini C. T-tubule remodeling in human hypertrophic cardiomyopathy. J Muscle Res Cell Motil. 2021;42(2):305–22. https://doi.org/10.1007/s10974-020-09591-6 Epub 2020 Nov 22.
37. Yamakawa S, Wu D, Dasgupta M, Pedamallu H, Gupta B, Modi R, Mufti M, O'Callaghan C, Frisk M, Louch WE, Arora R, Shiferaw Y, Burrell A, Ryan J, Nelson L, Chow M, Shah SJ, Aistrup G, Zhou J, Marszalec W, Wasserstrom JA. Role of t-tubule remodeling on mechanisms of abnormal calcium release during heart failure development in canine ventricle. Am J Physiol Heart Circ Physiol. 2021;320(4):H1658–69. https://doi.org/10.1152/ajpheart.00946.2020 Epub 2021 Feb 26.
38. Guillermo L, Stefanie D. The vasculature: a therapeutic target in heart failure? Cardiovasc Res. 2021;cvab047.
39. Camici PG, Tschöpe C, Di Carli MF, Rimoldi O, Van Linthout S. Coronary microvascular dysfunction in hypertrophy and heart failure. Cardiovasc Res. 2020;116:806–16.
40. Häseli S, Deubel S, Jung T, Grune T, Ott C. Cardiomyocyte contractility and autophagy in a premature senescence model of cardiac aging. Oxidative Med Cell Longev. 2020;2020:1–14.
41. Li B, Chi R-F, Qin F-Z, Guo X-F. Distinct changes of myocyte autophagy during myocardial hypertrophy and heart failure: association with oxidative stress. Exp Physiol. 2016;101:1050–63. https://doi.org/10.1113/EP085586.
42. Chi RF, Wang JP, Wang K, Zhang XL, Zhang YA, Kang YM, Han XB, Li B, Qin FZ, Fan BA. Progressive reduction in myocyte autophagy after myocardial infarction in rabbits: association with oxidative stress and left ventricular remodeling. Cell Physiol Biochem. 2017;44(6):2439–54. https://doi.org/10.1159/000486167 Epub 2017 Dec 18.
43. Ott C, Jung T, Brix S, John C, Betz IR, Foryst-Ludwig A, Deubel S, Kuebler WM, Grune T, Kintscher U, Grune J. Hypertrophy-reduced autophagy causes cardiac dysfunction by directly impacting cardiomyocyte contractility. Cells. 2021;10(4):805. https://doi.org/10.3390/cells10040805.
44. Hála P, Kittnar O. Hemodynamic adaptation of heart failure to percutaneous venoarterial extracorporeal circulatory supports. Physiol Res. 2020;69(5):739–757. https://doi.org/10.33549/physiolres.934332.
45. Miller WL. Fluid volume overload and congestion in heart failure: time to reconsider pathophysiology and how volume is assessed. Circ Heart Fail. 2016;9(8): e002922. https://doi.org/10.1161/CIRCHEARTFAILURE.115.002922.
46. Nishikawa T, Saku K, Uike K, Uemura K, Sunagawa G, Tohyama T, Yoshida K, Kishi T, Sunagawa K, Tsutsui H. Prediction of haemodynamics after interatrial shunt for heart failure using the generalized circulatory equilibrium. ESC Heart Fail. 2020;7(5):3075–85. https://doi.org/10.1002/ehf2.12935.
47. de la Torre JC. Hemodynamic instability in heart failure intensifies age-dependent cognitive decline. J Alzheimer's Dis: JAD. 2020;76(1):63–84. https://doi.org/10.3233/JAD-200296.
48. Nair R, Lamaa N. Pulmonary capillary wedge pressure. In StatPearls: StatPearls Publishing;2021.
49. Shah P, Louis MA. Physiology. StatPearls Publishing: Central Venous Pressure. In StatPearls;2021.
50. Sekulic M, Zacharias M, Medalion B. Ischemic Cardiomyopathy and heart failure. Circ: Hear Fail. 2019;12(6).
51. Felker G, Shaw L, O'Connor C. A standardized definition of ischemic cardiomyopathy for use in clinical research. J Am Coll Cardiol. 2002;39(2):210–8.
52. Mehrani M, Abbasi S, Amin A, Kassaian S, Mahmoudi M. Ischemic cardiomyopathy. Nanomed Ischemic Cardiomyopathy. 2020;1–8.
53. Vlodaver Z, Asinger R, Lesser J. Pathology of ischemic heart disease. Congest Hear Fail Card Transplant. 2017;59–79.
54. Anversa P, Sonnenblick E. Ischemic cardiomyopathy: pathophysiologic mechanisms. Prog Cardiovasc Dis. 33(1):49–70.

55. Severino P, D'Amato A, Pucci M, Infusino F, et al. Ischemic heart disease pathophysiology paradigms overview: from plaque activation to microvascular dysfunction. Int J Mol Sci. 2020;21(21):8118.
56. Zucchi R, Ghelardoni S, Evangelista S. Biochemical basis of ischemic heart injury and of cardioprotective interventions. Curr Med Chem. 2007;14(15):1619–37.
57. Weintraub RG, Semsarian C, Macdonald P. Dilated cardiomyopathy. Lancet. 2017;390(10092):400–14. https://doi.org/10.1016/S0140-6736(16)31713-5.
58. Sarnoff SJ, Berglund E. Ventricular function: I. starling's law of the heart studied by means of simultaneous right and left ventricular function curves in the dog. Circulation. 1954;9(5):706–18.
59. Patel PA, Ali N. An overview of dilated cardiomyopathy. Ann Cardiovasc Dis. 2018;3(1):1022.
60. De Paris V, Biondi F, Stolfo D, et al. Pathophysiology. In: Sinagra G, Merlo M, Pinamonti B, editors. Dilated cardiomyopathy: from genetics to clinical management. Cham (CH): Springer;2019.
61. Lakdawala NK, Winterfield JR, Funke BH. Dilated cardiomyopathy. Circ Arrhythmia Electrophysiol. 2013;6:228–37.
62. Sisakian H. Cardiomyopathies: evolution of pathogenesis concepts and potential for new therapies. World J Cardiol. 2014;6(6):478–94. https://doi.org/10.4330/wjc.v6.i6.478.
63. Araco M, Merlo M, Carr-White G, Sinagra G. Genetic bases of dilated cardiomyopathy. J Cardiovasc Med. 2017;18:123–30.
64. Bozkurt S, Safak KK. Evaluating the hemodynamical response of a cardiovascular system under support of a continuous flow left ventricular assist device via numerical modeling and simulations [published correction appears in Comput Math Methods Med. 2019;2019:2906543]. Comput Math Methods Med. 2013;2013:986430. https://doi.org/10.1155/2013/986430.
65. Hershberger RE, Hedges DJ, Morales A. Dilated cardiomyopathy: the complexity of a diverse genetic architecture. Nat Rev Cardiol. 2013;10:531–47.
66. Japp AG, Gulati A, Cook SA, Cowie MR, Prasad SK. The diagnosis and evaluation of dilated cardiomyopathy. J Am Coll Cardiol. 2016;67:2996–3010.
67. Albakri A. Restrictive cardiomyopathy: a review of literature on clinical status and meta-analysis of diagnosis and clinical management. Pediatr Dimens. 2018;3(2).
68. Nihoyannopoulos P, Dawson D. Restrictive cardiomyopathies. Eur J Echocardiogr 2009;10(8):iii23–iii33.
69. Brown K, Pendela V, Diaz R. Restrictive cardiomyopathy. StatPearls Puplishing. 2019.
70. Tsuru H, Ishida H, Narita J, Ishii R. Cardiac fibroblasts play pathogenic roles in idiopathic restrictive cardiomyopathy. Circ J. 2021;85(5):677–86.
71. Hosenpud J, Niles N. Clinical, hemodynamic and endomyocardial biopsy findings in idiopathic restrictive cardiomyopathy. West J Med. 144(3):303.
72. Brodehl A, Gaertner-Rommel A, Klauke B, Grewe S. The novel αB-crystallin (CRYAB) mutation p.D109G causes restrictive cardiomyopathy. Hum Mutat. 2017;38(8):947–952.
73. Suboc T. Restrictive cardiomyopathy—cardiovascular disorders . MSD Manual Professional Edition. 2021 [cited 10 January 2022]. https://www.msdmanuals.com/professional/cardiovascular-disorders/cardiomyopathies/restrictive-cardiomyopathy#v942573.
74. Harvey P, Leinwand L. Cellular mechanisms of cardiomyopathy. J Cell Biol. 2011;194(3):355–65.
75. Sestito S, Parisi F, Tallarico V, Tarsitano F, Roppa K, Pensabene L, Chimenz R, Ceravolo G, Calabrò MP, De Sarro R, Moricca MT, Bonapace G, Concolino D. Cardiac involvement in Lysosomal Storage Diseases. J Biol Regul Homeost Agents. 2020;34(4 Suppl. 2):107–119. Special issue: Focus on pediatric cardiology.
76. Sacchetto C, Sequeira V, Bertero E, Dudek J, Maack C, Calore M. Metabolic alterations in inherited cardiomyopathies. J Clin Med. 2019;8(12):2195. https://doi.org/10.3390/jcm8122195.
77. Merritt JL 2nd, MacLeod E, Jurecka A, Hainline B. Clinical manifestations and management of fatty acid oxidation disorders. Rev Endocr Metab Disord. 2020;21(4):479–93. https://doi.org/10.1007/s11154-020-09568-.

78. Meyers DE, Basha HI, Koenig MK. Mitochondrial cardiomyopathy: pathophysiology, diagnosis, and management. Tex Heart Inst J. 2013;40(4):385–94.

79. Zhuge R, Zhou R, Ni X. Advances in diagnosis and management of mitochondrial cardiomyopathy. Zhongguo Yi Xue Ke Xue Yuan Xue Bao. 2017;39(2):290–5. https://doi.org/10.3881/j.issn.1000-503X.2017.02.021.

80. Alraies MC, Eckman P. Adult heart transplant: indications and outcomes. J Thorac Dis. 2014;6(8):1120–8. https://doi.org/10.3978/j.issn.2072-1439.2014.06.4.

81. Povolný J. Tachykardií indukovaná kardiomyopatie [Tachycardia-induced cardiomyopathy]. Vnitr Lek. 2015;61(1):56–9. Czech.

82. Nattel S, Harada M. Atrial remodeling and atrial fibrillation. J Am Coll Cardiol. 2014;63(22):2335–45. https://doi.org/10.1016/j.jacc.2014.02.555.

83. Azevedo PS, Polegato BF, Minicucci MF, Paiva SA, Zornoff LA. Cardiac remodeling: concepts, clinical impact, pathophysiological mechanisms and pharmacologic treatment. Arq Bras Cardiol. 2016;106(1):62–9. https://doi.org/10.5935/abc.20160005.

84. Coats CJ, et al. Arrhythmogenic left ventricular cardiomyopathy. Circulation. 2009;120:2613–4. https://doi.org/10.1161/CIRCULATIONAHA.109.874628.

85. Paetsch I, Reith S, Gassler N, Jahnke C. Isolated arrhythmogenic left ventricular cardiomyopathy identified by cardiac magnetic resonance imaging. Eur Heart J. 2011;32:2840. https://doi.org/10.1093/eurheartj/ehr240.

86. Canter CE, Shaddy RE, Bernstein D, et al. Indications for heart transplantation in pediatric heart disease: a scientific statement from the American Heart Association Council on Cardiovascular Disease in the Young; the Councils on Clinical Cardiology, Cardiovascular Nursing, and Cardiovascular Surgery and Anesthesia; and the Quality of Care and Outcomes Research Interdisciplinary Working Group. Circulation. 2007;115:658–76.

87. Kritzmire SM, Cossu AE. Hypoplastic left heart syndrome. [Updated 2021 Jun 9]. In: StatPearls [Internet]. Treasure Island (FL): StatPearls Publishing;2022. https://www.ncbi.nlm.nih.gov/books/NBK554576/.

88. Roeleveld PP, Axelrod DM, Klugman D, Jones MB, Chanani NK, Rossano JW, Costello JM. Hypoplastic left heart syndrome: from fetus to fontan. Cardiol Young. 2018;28(11):1275–88.

89. Mackie SA, Aiyagari R, Zampi JD. Balloon atrial septostomy by a right internal jugular venous approach in a newborn with hypoplastic left heart syndrome with a restrictive atrial septum. Congenit Heart Dis. 2014;9(5):E140–2.

90. Gobergs R, Salputra E, Lubaua I. Hypoplastic left heart syndrome: a review. Acta Med Litu. 2016;23(2):86–98. https://doi.org/10.6001/actamedica.v23i2.3325.

91. Pundi KN, et al. 40-year follow-up after the Fontan operation: long-term outcomes of 1052 patients. J Am Coll Cardiol. 2015;66(15):1700–10.

92. Thrush P, Hoffman T. Pediatric heart transplantation—indications and outcomes in the current era. J Thorac Dis. North America 6 June 2014. https://jtd.amegroups.com/article/view/2685. Accessed: 17 Jan 2022.

93. Zuberbuhler JR, Anderson RH. Morphological variations in pulmonary atresia with intact ventricular septum. Br Heart J. 1979;41:281–8.

94. Akagi T, Benson LN, Williams WG, Trusler GA, Freedom RM. Ventriculo-coronary arterial connections in pulmonary atresia with intact ventricular septum, and their influences on ventricular performance and clinical course. Am J Cardiol. 1993;72:586–90.

95. Chikkabyrappa SM, Loomba RS, Tretter JT. Pulmonary atresia with an intact ventricular septum: preoperative physiology, imaging, and management. Semin Cardiothorac Vasc Anesth. 2018;22(3):245–55.

96. Bui C, Lam W, Franklin W, Ermis P. Long-term follow-up in adult survivors of pulmonary atresia with intact ventricular septum. J Am Coll Cardiol. 2017;69:567.

97. Schneider AW, Blom NA, Bruggemans EF, Hazekamp MG. More than 25 years of experience in managing pulmonary atresia with intact ventricular septum. Ann Thorac Surg. 2014;98:1680–6.

98. Sainathan S, Silva L, Silva J. Ebstein's anomaly: contemporary management strategiesJ Thorac Dis. North America, 12 Mar. 2020. https://jtd.amegroups.com/article/view/37143. Accessed 25 Jan 2022.

99. Singh DP, Mahajan K. Ebstein Anomaly And Malformation. [Updated 2021 May 3]. In: Stat-Pearls [Internet]. Treasure Island (FL): StatPearls Publishing;2022. https://www.ncbi.nlm.nih.gov/books/NBK534824/.

Cardioimmunology and Heart Transplantation

Ali Talib Hashim, Ahed El Abed El Rassoul, Inas Khalifa Sharquie, and Haya Mohammed Abujledan

Abstract A new interest in cardiac immunology is the result of the recent ability to diagnose and obtain unbiased data on heart cells with high cytogenetic resolution. This is rare and is believed to be missing 10 years ago. The adopted immune system focuses on traditional immunosuppression. Increased awareness of innate immunity has many potentials, blocking the response of Toll-like receptors to I/R damage, depleting or blocking NK cell activation, and interfering with complement activation and deposition. Suggests therapeutic goals. Given the remarkable advances in diagnosis and care that have emerged over the last few decades, the essential pathogenic signaling pathways are not well understood and significantly limit the effectiveness of therapeutic treatment. This chapter aims to broaden our knowledge of the factors performed by the immune system in ischemic heart disease, non-ischemic myocarditis, ejection fraction-maintained heart failure, endocarditis, and conduction disorders. increase. Many features of innate and adaptive immune cells are mobilized by ischemic injury, and the function of immunity in myocarditis is still being studied. In addition, the chemokine community regulates the transport of immune cells at specific stages of homeostasis and inflammation, and chemokines, along with some sclerosis, bronchial asthma, AIDS, and even transplants, are inflammatory reactions caused by T cell-related diseases. Rejection mechanisms that may be mentioned in five major titles have been specifically studied. Immunization, immunological memory, cell memory, humoral memory, antibody secretion, opsonization, and supplement cascade activation.

A. T. Hashim (✉)
Golestan University of Medical Sciences, Gorgan, Iran
e-mail: talibhashim42@gmail.com

A. E. A. El Rassoul
Faculty of Medical Sciences, Lebanese University, Hadath, Beirut, Lebanon

I. K. Sharquie
Department of Microbiology and Immunology, College of Medicine, University of Baghdad, Baghdad, Iraq

H. M. Abujledan
Genetic Engineering, Hashemite University, Amman, Jordan

© The Author(s), under exclusive license to Springer Nature Switzerland AG 2022
H. T. Hashim et al. (eds.), *Heart Transplantation*,
https://doi.org/10.1007/978-3-031-17311-0_5

Keywords Cardioimmunology · Heart transplantation · Adaptive immune
system · Natural killer cells · Traditional immunosuppressive medications ·
Antiproliferative agents · Calcineurin inhibitors · Innate immune system

1 Introduction

Heart-specific infectious myocarditis with phenotype inflammatory dilated
cardiomyopathy (iDCM) is not a rare target for histopathological remodeling and
coronary heart failure. Our project explores the mechanical aspects of the improvement and development of viral and autoimmune heart infections that lead to the
abandonment of heart failure. In human and experimental animal models, the phenotype of heart failure after myocarditis is morphologically characterized with the help
of ventricular dilatation and novel tissue fibrosis that impair cardiac function.

Cardiovascular disease (CVD) continues to contribute significantly to morbidity
and mortality in Western countries, as diagnosis and care have improved significantly
over the last few decades. This is because, in most cases, the essential cause is not
well understood, significantly limiting the effectiveness of curative treatment [1].

The effects of immunity and infection on the improvement of atherosclerosis and
associated headaches have been the subject of numerous reviews. In homeostasis and
infectious diseases, the trade in immunotransmission helps infectious marketers, and
a large dedicated circle of chemotactic cytokines from relatives collectively known as
chemokines is against a variety of harmful factors. It shows a tremendous protective
reaction specially managed and customized through borrowing [1].

2 The Population of Immune Cells in the Heart

In 4,444 healthy adult mice, the heart is composed of a complete collection of major
leukocytes, including skeletal muscle 1, neutrophils, B cells, and 10 times more
mononuclear phagocytes than T cells.

This population of cells regenerates itself after birth without the contribution of
monocytes. The smaller number of CCR2+ when compared to adult mice is due to
the diffusion of precursors, probably monocytes. That said, there is sufficient fact
and evidence to deny that a simple depiction of the origin of macrophages is possible.
The yolk sac progeny actually lives longer than adults, but the fact that many adult
macrophages appear later in mid-pregnancy, even in the CCR2 population, is also
true [1, 2]. Some cardiac macrophages such as.

B. Fetal liver precursors can occur prenatally, some immediately after birth 15,
and in some cases from subsequent monocytes. There is a possibility. In addition,
when the expression of various surface markers on the cell is lost or acquired, the
subgroups overlap and the ontogeny line is further weakened.

However, the data support the general conclusion that mouse and human circulating monocytes have little input to cardiac macrophages in healthy heart tissue.

DC18 is found primarily in the aortic valve, but the conduction system contains very high concentrations of macrophages, including the atrioventricular node. The heart is also not isolated. The pericardium, a cavity containing the protective serosa, is surrounded by strongly placed chambers, blood vessels, and valves. The serous fluid contains white blood cells, macrophages, and B cells, which can be a source of white blood cells that infiltrate tissues during provocation, similar to those found in the lungs and liver. White blood cell abundance is rich in white blood cells, and when this space is exposed during myocardial infarction or heart surgery, lymphocytes can be supplied, but white adipose tissue causes mast cell accumulation in the heart after myocardial infarction [3].

The exact way leukocytes fit the heart locally means that leukocytes have a unique experience with non-leukocyte residents.

3 The Immune System's Role in Heart Disease

The inflammatory response is urgent and intense in some situations, and long and mild in other situations, and the role of the immune system is rare or difficult to explain in the rest.

A. *The Myocardial Infarction:*

Ischemic damage to the heart area is the result of an oxygen-rich and occluded coronary artery due to normal blood supply.

Various activities or functions of innate and adaptive immune cells are mobilized by ischemic injury. It is derived from inflammatory cytokines such as 45 and heart growth factors that initiate the production of chemokines and hematopoietic growth factors such as GMCSF31 [3].

Neutrophils and monocytes are actively involved in a series of inflammations after they accumulate in the heart. Their main function is to collect dead substances such as dead cardiomyocytes and dying cardiomyocytes in the first few days. This is an active mechanism involving the tyrosine-protein kinase MER (MERTK), a variety of scavenger receptors [4, 5].

Immune cells also feed on DNA obtained from cardiomyocytes via interferon regulatory factor 3 (IRF3) 55. IL-1, TNF, and IL-5 inflammation further increases inflammation by affecting leukocytes, endothelial cells, and myocardial cells, producing proteolytic enzymes that help digest dying dead people and tissues. It releases sex cytokines. Neutrophils do not survive very long in the infarcted myocardium. After 3 days, their numbers decrease, and after 7 days, they disappear almost completely [1].

B. *Remodeling the Remote Myocardium:*

After a non-perfused myocardial infarction, especially if the myocardium has had its major myocardial infarction removed, a profound remodeling procedure is performed, which can reduce ejection fraction over time and cause heart failure. Part of the heart muscle is necrotic. This is a long process and can take months [1].

C. *Myocarditis:*

The immune system function is further investigated in myocarditis. In mice, the primary model for studying viral myocarditis is myocarditis caused by the Coxsackievirus B3. Coxsackievirus infects the myocardium through its own receptors, causing many innate and adaptive immune responses.

Among the first cells to react are the Mast cells which degranulate and produce inflammatory cytokines including TNF, IL1β, and IL4 within 6 h of infection. By producing additional inflammatory mediators, amassing neutrophils and monocytes further spread the inflammatory cascade.

D. *Endocarditis:*

Most often, it is present in existing endothelial lesions covered with fibrin and platelets. In the acute form, the infection can be fatal because the valve is easily killed by bacteria, leading to acute heart failure.

E. *Conduction Disorders:*

The most common cardiac arrhythmia is atrial fibrillation, which affects 1 in 10 elderly people. In this condition, chaotic behavior that interferes with organized atrial contraction is lost by orderly general atrial depolarization. This has two main implications. Existing treatment options are primarily focused on stroke prevention with anticoagulant therapy [4, 5].

4 Heart Transplant Cardioimmunology

An independent risk factor for ischemic stroke is also higher systemic CXCL10 levels. The immune response to the donor MHC protein is triggered by allogeneic transplant rejection. Recently, we discovered that this reaction could lead to Ag degradation of the recipient's autoimmune tolerance. However, the contribution of this autoimmune response to graft rejection has not yet been determined. Here, we found that the autoimmune response of de novo CD4 + T cells and B cells to cardiac myosin (CM), an important contractile protein of cardiac muscle, is triggered in recipients after allogeneic mouse heart transplantation. Importantly, CM is an autoantigen that induces autoimmune myocarditis, a cardiac autoimmune disease whose histopathological features are similar to those found in rejected heart transplants. In addition, T cell responses were observed in heart-transplanted mice targeting the recognized cardiomyoplasty determinant CM peptide Myhcpha. No response to CM was seen in

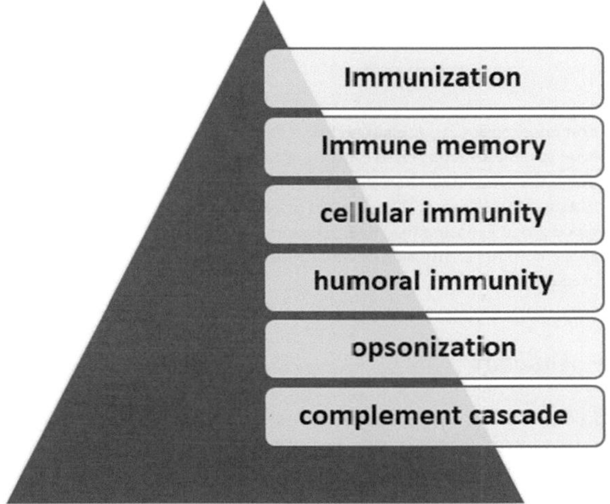

Fig. 1 Immunologic mechanisms of rejection

mice that received allogeneic skin grafts or allogeneic heart transplants, suggesting that this response is tissue-specific and requires an allogeneic response to break CM resistance. Next, we showed that sensitization of CM recipient mice significantly accelerated allogeneic cardiac rejection. Therefore, the autoimmune response to CM after transplantation is important for the rejection phase. We conclude that the autoimmune response to CM caused by transplantation is a new mechanism that may play an important role in heart transplant rejection [1] (Fig. 1).

5 Immunology of Transplant Rejection

- *Immunization*

Exposure to antigens can stimulate the immune system to protect the body against further infection by producing antibodies.

CD4 recognizes foreign peptide in the context of Class II MHC and is crucial in the helper functions (B cell activation and Antibody production and switch) [6].

- *Cellular Immunity*

CD8 recognizes foreign peptides in the context of class IMHC, which is the donor's own peptide. (In living donors, such presentation of self-antigens helped maintain self-tolerance.). And it is associated with cytotoxicity and effector T cell function.

- *Humoral Immunity* [7]

primary exposure: transplant recipient can have specific antibody cross reacting with the donor tissue upon the transplant event, a *secondary exposure*. This is typical of minor blood group exposure (e.g. Kell) following allogenic blood transfusion or trauma during pregnancy

secondary exposure: At secondary exposure, these cross-reactive antibody molecules interact with aspects of innate immunity, soluble immune proteins called complement and innate immune cells called phagocytes, which inflames and destroys the transplanted tissue.

- *Antibody*

B cells can recognize antigens by IgD or monomeric IgM. Together with other related proteins, they form the B cell receptor (BCR).

- *Opsonization*

The ability of antibodies and complement components (and other proteins) to coat dangerous antigens. It is recognized by antibodies or complement receptors on phagocytes.

- *Complement Cascade*

Complement activation is a major cause of tissue damage in patients with antibody-mediated rejection (AMR) of transplanted organs [7].

Multiple Choice Questions:

1. **Considering leukocytes in the heart, all are true except.**

    (a) Are at frequencies in the heart muscle greater than that in the skeletal muscle.
    (b) A network of neutrophils is embedded within cardiomyocytes.
    (c) The heart contains populations of non-cardiomyocyte cells.
    (d) Leukocytes can be found interspersed at various locations in the heart.
    (e) None of the above.

2. **All are found in the heart except.**

    (a) Endothelial cells.
    (b) Fibroblasts.
    (c) Hematopoietic cells.
    (d) Neutrophils.

3. **All are not found within the coronary artery space except.**

    (a) Adipocytes.
    (b) Conducting cells.
    (c) Macrophages.
    (d) All of the above.

4. **Regarding the population of macrophages in the heart.**

   (a) There are at least 5 subsets of macrophages in the heart as by their surface markers expression.
   (b) Macrophages groups vary mainly in their expression of MHC class I.
   (c) The higher population of macrophages is in the population expressing Lys6C11-13.
   (d) CC-chemokine receptor 2 macrophages express MHC class II.

5. **During embryogenesis, CCR2+ and Ly6C+ cardiac macrophages emerge after the definitive hematopoiesis from embryogenic progenitors.**

   (a) True.
   (b) False.

6. **Considering the origin of macrophages in the heart.**

   (a) CCR2+ and Ly6C+ macrophages populate later in embryogenesis.
   (b) Yolk sac progeny doesn't persist into adulthood.
   (c) Fetal liver precursors cardiac macrophages arise before birth.
   (d) Circulating monocytes contribute to a large fraction of cardiac macrophages in healthy tissue heart.

7. **Regarding the dendritic cells population in the heart:**

   (a) Resident dendritic cells comprise about 10% of total cardiac leukocytes.
   (b) Dendritic cells' expression of transcription factors decreases within the heart.
   (c) Classical subsets of CD103+ CD11b+ and CD103−CD11b−.
   (d) Can be found along the aortic valve.

8. **The populations of cardiac macrophages can self-renew after birth without monocyte input.**

   (a) True.
   (b) False.

9. **Regarding leukocyte distribution in the heart, all are true except.**

   (a) Monocytes, neutrophils, and B and T cells can be detected by flow cytometry.
   (b) Different macrophage subsets occupy different niches.
   (c) The homogeneous nature of the heart allows for a standardized leukocyte distribution.
   (d) All are true.

Associate Each Cell With its Corresponding:

Cell	Distribution
10. Fetal monocyte-derived macrophages	(a) Coronary vasculature
11. DCs18	(b) Atrioventricular node
12. Macrophages	(c) Endocardial trabecular
13. Embryonic CCR2 macrophages	(d) Aortic valve

14. **Pericardium:**

    (a) Serosal fluid contains macrophages and T cells.
    (b) A source of tissue-infiltrating leukocytes.
    (c) Pericardial adipose tissue is a source of mast cells.
    (d) All of the above.

15. **Following a myocardial infarction, all are true regarding M2 macrophage action except.**

    (a) Suppress inflammatory responses.
    (b) Facilitate angiogenesis.
    (c) Promotes collagenase activity.
    (d) Vascular remodeling.

16. **Following a myocardial infarction.**

    (a) Mast cell granules facilitate the conversion of fibroblast to myofibroblast.
    (b) Eosinophils activate intrinsic tissue repair cascades.
    (c) Type 2 cytokines serve as biomarkers in determining the severity and prognosis of MI.
    (d) All of the above.

17. **Cytokines responsible for amplifying an inflammatory response:**

    (a) IL-1.
    (b) TNF.
    (c) IL-6.
    (d) All of the above.

18. **Neutrophils in the heart:**

    (a) Persist for 7 days in the infarcted myocardium.
    (b) Enhance cardiac healing through neutrophil gelatinase-associated lipocalin.
    (c) Decrease macrophage activity.
    (d) Increase cardiac fibrosis.

19. **Myocarditis:**

    (a) Irrelevant to leucocytosis.
    (b) Can be due to several infectious and non-infectious causes.
    (c) Causes an acute cardiac function degradation.
    (d) b and c.
    (e) All of the above.

20. **Cardiomyocytes viral infection, which is not true:**

    (a) Cardiomyocyte infection exposes antigens that can have shared epitopes with the virus and cause autoimmunity.
    (b) Initiates exclusively a cascade of innate immune responses.
    (c) Autoantigens and endogenous antigens can lead to chronic myocarditis after viral clearance.
    (d) All are true.

21. **IL-2 deficiency:**

    (a) Improves INF-g through feedback mechanisms.
    (b) Decreases viral replication.
    (c) Restricts TNF and INF-g.
    (d) Improves viral recognition.

22. **Endocarditis:**

    (a) Can be associated with septic embolism.
    (b) Chronic infections are highly fatal.
    (c) Bacterial residence occurs on fibrotic pre-existing endothelial lesions.
    (d) a and b.
    (e) a and c.

23. **Atrial fibrillation is characterized by.**

    (a) Decreased ventricular fill and increased cardiac output.
    (b) Rapid atrial blood flow that dislodges clots and causes thromboses.
    (c) Increased ventricular fill and decreased cardiac output.
    (d) Slow atrial blood flow that forms clots and causes ischemic strokes.

24. **Cardiac myosin in cardiac transplants:**

    (a) Autoantigen that induces autoimmune pericarditis
    (b) Its myocarditogenic determinant induces B cell responses.
    (c) Induces a tissue-specific response.
    (d) All the above.

25. **Immunization mechanism in transplant rejection:**

    (a) Macrophages are the primary antigen-imparting cells (APCs).
    (b) APCs constitute recipient self HLA to primed T cells in lymphoid tissue.

(c) Dendritic cells (DCs) are activated with the aid of using donor DAMPs sample release.

(d) Helper T cells coordinate innate immunity directed on the donor's self-peptides or HLA complicated.

26. **Memory helper T cell, all are true except.**

   (a) TCR receptors recognize antigens presented on MHC class II.
   (b) produce clones that are effector cells that will secrete cytokines.
   (c) Their function is irrespective to that of B cells and antibody production and class switch.
   (d) All are true.

27. **Transplant rejection and self-tolerance:**

   (a) CD4+ and donor MHC class I, CD8+ and recipient MHC class I, respectively.
   (b) CD4+ and donor MHC class II, CD8+ and donor MHC class I, respectively.
   (c) CD4+ and recipient MHC class II, CD8+ and recipient MHC class I, respectively.
   (d) CD4+ and recipient MHC class II, CD8+ and donor MHC class II, respectively.
   (e) None of the above.

28. **Regarding antibodies:**

   (a) The target antigen region comprises the paratope that is a 3d conformation of epitopes.
   (b) Insoluble proteins secreted by activated B cells called plasma cells.
   (c) Basic unit that constitutes 2 Fab regions with tips called the paratope and a single Fc region called epitope.
   (d) None of the above.

29. **Opsonization is the process by which Fc receptors on macrophages in the blood bind to the Fc stem of antibody molecules, thereby enhancing the ability of macrophages to take up antigens in.**

   (a) True.
   (b) False.

30. **Complement cascade, all are wrong except.**

   (a) Is an antibody-mediated acceptation of transplanted tissue.
   (b) Mediated by IgM's Fab region paratope binding to its specific epitope.
   (c) Causes cell rupture and tissue injury of transplanted organs.
   (d) Characterized by the conformational change in the Fab region of IgG.

Answers:

1. Answer: b

 (a) The frequency of all the major groups of white blood cells in the heart is 12 times higher than that of skeletal muscle.
   Bright; a network of macrophages embedded in cardiomyocytes.
 (c) The heart contains a population of non-cardiomyocytes such as endothelial cells, fibroblasts, pericytes, smooth muscle cells, and macrophages.

2. Answer: c
3. Answer: c
4. Answer: d

 (a) Wrong; there are at least 4 subsets of macrophages in the heart as by their surface markers expression; CD4+ , F4/80+ , CD11b+ , CD64+ , and MERTK+.
 (b) Wrong; macrophage groups differ from MHC class II in their expression.
 (c) Wrong; The Ly6C+ macrophage population is the only subgroup expressing Lys6C1113, a small population.

5. Answer: b

 (b) Wrong; detailed cell fate mapping studies show that during embryogenesis, CCR2− and Ly6C+ cardiac macrophages populate the heart, emerging before the start of definitive hematopoiesis from embryonic progenitors.

6. Answer: c

 (a) Wrong; CCR2+ and Ly6C+ macrophages populate the heart before the start of definitive hematopoiesis from embryogenic progenitors.
 (b) Wrong; yolk sac progeny survives into adulthood.
 (d) Wrong; circulating monocytes contribute to a small fraction of cardiac macrophages in healthy tissue heart.

7. Answer: d

 (a) Wrong; resident dendritic cells comprise about 1% of total cardiac leukocytes.
 (b) Wrong; dendritic cells resident in the heart express the transcription factor zinc-finger and BTB domain-containing protein 46 (ZBTB46).
 (c) Wrong; cardiac resident DCs fall into classical subsets of CD103+ CD11b− and CD103−CD11b+.

8. Answer: a
9. Answer: c

 (c) Wrong; The heart is not homogeneous and there is no standardized distribution of leukocytes.

 Associate Each Cell with Its Corresponding:

10. c
11. d
12. b

13. a
14. Answer: b

   (a) Wrong; Serous fluid contains white blood cells such as macrophages and B cells, which can be a source of tissue-infiltrating white blood cells at the time of induction, similar to those found in the lungs and liver.
   (c) Wrong; epithelial adipose tissue is a source of abundant white blood cells that lymphocytes can supply if this space is exposed during myocardial infarction and heart surgery, and white adipose tissue is myocardial infarction. It may be a source of mast cells that later accumulate in the heart.

15. Answer: c

   (c) Correct; M2 macrophages promote the production of collagen, neoangiogenesis, and inflammation resolution, and it facilitates angiogenesis and deposition of collagen, supplying the infected myocardium with benefits.

16. Answer: d
17. Answer: d
18. Answer: b
19. Answer: b
20. Answer: d
21. Answer: c

   (b) Wrong; IL-12 deficiency will increase viral replication and restricts the improvement of TNF and IFNγ, the latter of which regulates viral replication.
   (d) Wrong; IL-2 is a crucial issue among inflammatory mediators, gathering neutrophils and monocytes in addition to unfolding the inflammatory cascade.

22. Answer: e

   (a) Correct; the 'vegetation' of endocarditis (a combination of bacteria, thrombi, and leukocytes) will dislodge the mind, kidneys, and coronary heart and reason septic embolism.
   (b) Wrong; Infection may be deadly in its acute form because the valves are effortlessly killed via way of means of the bacteria, main to acute coronary heart failure.
   (c) Correct; Bacteria circulating withinside the blood, in particular Staphylococcus aureus and streptococci, absorb house in coronary heart valves, regularly on pre-present endothelial lesions protected via way of means of fibrin and platelets.

23. Answer: d

(a) Wrong; downstream ventricles fill much less efficaciously with blood, which can lower cardiac output, in particular in sufferers with coronary heart failure.

(b) Wrong; the sluggish float of blood through the atria results in clots which can byskip to the arteries of the mind inflicting ischemic stroke.

(c) Wrong; downstream ventricles fill much less efficaciously with blood, which can lower cardiac output, in particular in sufferers with coronary heart failure.

24. Answer: c

(a) Wrong; CM is the autoantigen that induces autoimmune myocarditis, an autoimmune coronary heart ailment whose histopathological functions are just like the ones visible in cardiac transplants which have been rejected.

(b) Wrong; T molecular responses had been discovered in coronary heart-transplanted mice directed at CM peptide myhcpha, an identified myocarditogenic determinant.

(c) Correct; in mice that had acquired allogeneic pores and skin graft or a syngeneic coronary heart transplant, no responses to CM had been discovered, suggesting that this reaction is tissue-unique and that allogeneic reaction is wanted to interrupt CM tolerance.

25. Answer: c

(a) Wrong; the primary antigen-presenting cells (APCs), dendritic cells (DCs), are activated and release related molecular patterns (DAMPS) after damage to the innate immune system.

(b) Wrong; Donor APC migrates to the recipient's lymphatic system and presents foreign HLA to primed T cells (CD4, CD8).

26. Answer: c

(a) Wrong; When the CD4 receptor on memory helper T cells binds to the MHC class II molecule expressed on the surface of the target cell of the transplanted tissue, the T cell receptor (TCR) on the memory helper T cell is the presented target antigen. The MHC class II molecule.

27. Answer: e
    CD4 recognizes foreign (donor) peptides in the context of class II MHC.
    CD8 recognizes self (receiver) peptides in the context of class I MHC.

28. Answer: d

29. Answer: b

(a) Wrong; The Fc region of IgG also allows phagocytic opsonization. This is because of Fc receptors on phagocytic cells.

30. Answer: c

(a) Wrong; Complement activation is a major cause of tissue damage in patients with antibody-mediated rejection (AMR) of transplanted organs.

(c) That's right. The initiation of the complement cascade ends by puncturing the cell membrane. When so many holes are drilled, the liquid will flow into the cell and tear it apart.

(d) Wrong Answer; The conformational change in the Fc region is short enough for the complement protein to correspond to.

References

1. Swirski FK, Nahrendorf M. Cardioimmunology: the immune system in cardiac homeostasis and disease. Nat Rev Immunol. 2018;18(12):733–44.
2. Baritussio A, et al. Predictors of death, heart transplantation and relapse in clinically suspected and biopsy-proven myocarditis in the pre-immunosuppression era. Eur Hear J.2020; **41**(Supplement_2):ehaa946–2059.
3. Pietro Enea L, Murray Hamilton R, Boutjdir M. Cardioimmunology: inflammation and immunity in cardiovascular disease. Front Cardiovasc Med. **6**; 2019:181.
4. Madan S, Mehra MR. The heart–gut microbiome axis in advanced heart failure. J Heart Lung Transplant. 2020;39(9):891–3.
5. Nasrin P, et al. TNF-α and IL-10 gene polymorphisms versus cardioimmunological responses in sudden infant death. Fetal Pediatr Pathol.2008; **27**(3):149–65.
6. Schaenman J, Goldwater D. The aging transplant population and immunobiology: any therapeutic implication? Curr Opin Organ Transplant. 2020;25(3):255–60.
7. Roberts, Luke B, et al. An update on the roles of immune system-derived microRNAs in cardiovascular diseases. Cardiovasc Res. 2021.

Heart Failure Outcomes and Management

Ibad Ur Rehman, Khadija Iqbal, Vanya Ibrahim, Alaa bakhtyar, and Belan Mikael

Abstract "Hear Failure is defined as failure of the heart to contract efficiently and to meet the body's demand of output". An ejection fraction of under 40% is a risk. In the initial stages, regular exercise and avoidance of smoking and alcohol can prevent the worsening of the condition. Keeping a healthy weight and avoiding stress can be a good prognosis.

Keywords Heart failure · Ejection fraction · Heart transplant · Outcomes · Congestive heart failure

1 Introduction

Over the last few decades, many researchers have defined heart failure; some definitions have focused more on the clinical aspect, while some have kept research and other fundamentals as the priority [1–4]. These different definitions proposed by different well-established heart associations and societies have led to ambiguity and have caused confusion [5–7]. Cardiologists spread across over 14 nations organized the following document in Table 1.

As explained by the definitions, there are varying criteria for diagnosis of heart failure. Most of these are centered around blood tests like chloride test, natriuretic peptide tests and radiological tests [8, 9].

I. U. Rehman
Shifa College of Medicine, Shifa Tamer E Millat University, Islamabad, Pakistan

K. Iqbal
Al Nafees Medical College, Isra University, Islamabad, Pakistan

V. Ibrahim (✉) · A. bakhtyar · B. Mikael
College of Medicine, University of Sulaimani, Sulaymaniyah, Iraq
e-mail: vanyaibra-him98@gmail.com

© The Author(s), under exclusive license to Springer Nature Switzerland AG 2022
H. T. Hashim et al. (eds.), *Heart Transplantation*,
https://doi.org/10.1007/978-3-031-17311-0_6

Table 1 Universally proposed definition in comparison with older definitions

Universal definition, [3]	"HF as a clinical syndrome with symptoms and/or signs caused by a structural and/or functional cardiac abnormality and corroborated by elevated natriuretic peptide levels and/or objective evidence of pulmonary or systemic congestion"
JCS/JHFSS [5]	"HF is a clinical syndrome consisting of dyspnea, malaise, swelling and/or decreased exercise capacity due to the loss of compensation for cardiac pumping function due to structural and/or functional abnormalities of the heart"
ESC [6]	"HF is a clinical syndrome characterized by typical symptoms (e.g., breathlessness, ankle swelling and fatigue) that may be accompanied by signs (e.g., elevated jugular venous pressure, pulmonary crackles and peripheral edema) caused by a structural and/or functional cardiac abnormality, resulting in a reduced cardiac output and/or elevated intracardiac pressures at rest or during stress"
ACCF/AHA [7]	"HF is a complex clinical syndrome that results from any structural or functional impairment of ventricular filling or ejection of blood. The cardinal manifestations of HF are dyspnea and fatigue, which may limit exercise tolerance, and fluid retention, which may lead to pulmonary and/or splanchnic congestion and/or peripheral edema. Some patients have exercise intolerance but little evidence of fluid retention, whereas others complain primarily of edema, dyspnea, or fatigue"

2 Outcomes and Controlling the Outcomes

Patient outcome depends and varies in different situations for different patients. Factors like patient's condition at the time of admission, facilities available and patients' demographics are a few of those. Various studies report variable outcomes; in one study, ten percent of patients died in the hospital, while 72% of patients were discharged after symptomatic improvement. They were prescribed commonly used drugs furosemide, aspirin and spironolactone. Mechanical ventilation using NO_2 was used in 85% of patients [8].

Management

The management of the patient depends upon the condition of the heart and the patient. The biggest issue in management is suspected, but unconfirmed, heart failure and amounts to a large number in Western countries. In the past, many studies have shown that a multidisciplinary approach may reduce admission rates in emergencies and may improve compliance of the patient. The impact of admissions in hospitals is not only on the patient and his family but also on the entire healthcare system. The main aim of management should be to delay the progression of the disease and make the patent live an active life [9–11].

One of the best lines of management for HF is heart transplantation which has a lot of compilations and risks. It takes a lot to get a donor, and there a lot of conditions for suitability and matching.

Children have to wait much longer for a suitable match. Unfortunately, this is not the ultimate treatment, and may end the life of patients due to rejection or infection. Cardiac allograft vasculopathy is also a major risk for the failure. This leads to the endothelial damage characterized by intimal thickening of the proximal arteries followed by fibrofatty plaque which leads to circulatory failure.

Estimation of antibodies pre- and post-op may minimize the risks of rejection. Desensitization techniques which lower the circulating antibodies can be an alternative to reduce the failure of transplantation.

Skin malignancies and lymphomas are the most commonly reported cancers in patients 10 years following heart transplant. Bacterial pneumonias also occur frequently in transplanted patients. Aortic dissection and thromboembolism are also reported [11–13].

End-Stage Heart Failure:

When heart failure develops, the body starts to compensate the failure of the heart by many mechanisms to keep the heart pumping the required quantity of blood consistently. When the compensation mechanisms fails, it is called the end stage of heart failure [14].

This stage of heart failure has a lot of symptoms that are progressing over time such as dyspnea, tightness of the chest, weight loss, severe swelling and finally renal and liver failure (organ failure) [14].

The complications of this stage are ranging from organ failure to death, and arrhythmia is a well-known complication as well.

Management of this stage focuses mainly on palliating the symptoms like fluid retention and arrhythmia. There is also device therapy including left ventricular assist device. But the final treatment is the surgery with a new heart transplant, because the progressing heart failure cannot be controlled anymore and some of the cases may become resistant to pharmacological treatment.

Heart Transplantation End-Stage Heart Failure:

One of the indications for heart transplantation is when the ejection fraction is less than 20–25% as in the case of heart failure (severe cases) [15].

While the patients are on the waiting list for a new heart, many other options are available to be used to maintain their failing heart till the new heart is available. Those options include the assisted device, intra-aortic balloon and many other pharmacological medications and mechanical support.

Prognosis in Heart Failure

Age of the patient and ejection fraction are important for the prognosis. An ejection fraction of under 40% is a risk. In the initial stages, regular exercise and avoidance of smoking and alcohol can prevent the worsening of the condition. Keeping a healthy weight and avoiding stress can be a good prognosis. One episode of heart failure lessens the lifespan by 10 years. Patients who do not qualify for a heart transplant may be prescribed a left ventricular assist device (LVAD) or an artificial heart [12, 16].

References

1. Wagner S, Cohn K. Heart failure. A proposed definition and classification. Arch Intern Med. 1977 [cited 2022 Mar 29]; 137(5):675–8. https://pubmed.ncbi.nlm.nih.gov/856090/
2. Denolin H, Kuhn H, Krayenbuehl H, Loogen F, Reale A. The defintion of heart failure. Eur Heart J. 1983;**4**(7):445–8. https://www.zora.uzh.ch/id/eprint/154420/1/ZORA_NL_154420.pdf
3. Bozkurt B, Coats AJ, Tsutsui H, Abdelhamid M, Adamopoulos S, Albert N, et al. Universal definition and classification of heart failure: a report of the heart failure society of America, heart failure association of the European society of cardiology, Japanese heart failure society and writing committee of the universal definition of heart failure. J Card Fail. 2021 [cited 2022 Mar 29]. https://pubmed.ncbi.nlm.nih.gov/33663906/
4. Universal definition and classification of heart failure: a step in the right direction from failure to function. American College of Cardiology [cited 2022 Mar 29]. https://www.acc.org/latest-in-cardiology/articles/2021/07/12/12/31/universal-definition-and-classification-of-heart-failure
5. Tsutsui H, Isobe M, Ito H, Ito H, Okumura K, Ono M, et al. JCS 2017/JHFS 2017 guideline on diagnosis and treatment of acute and chronic heart failure—digest version. Circ J. 2019 [cited 2022 Mar 29];**83**(10):2084–184. https://pubmed.ncbi.nlm.nih.gov/31511439/
6. Ponikowski P, Voors AA, Anker SD, Bueno H, Cleland JGF, Coats AJS, et al. 2016 ESC guidelines for the diagnosis and treatment of acute and chronic heart failure: the task force for the diagnosis and treatment of acute and chronic heart failure of the European Society of Cardiology (ESC). Developed with the special contribution of the Heart Failure Association (HFA) of the ESC. Eur J Heart Fail. 2016 [cited 2022 Mar 29];**18**(8):891–975. https://pubmed.ncbi.nlm.nih.gov/27207191/
7. Yancy CW, Jessup M, Bozkurt B, Butler J, Casey DE Jr, et al. 2013 ACCF/AHA guideline for the management of heart failure: a report of the American College of Cardiology Foundation/American Heart Association Task Force on practice guidelines: a report of the American college of cardiology foundation/American heart association task force on practice guidelines. Circulation. 2013 [cited 2022 Mar 29];**128**(16):e240–327. https://pubmed.ncbi.nlm.nih.gov/23741058/
8. Congestive heart failure: pathophysiology, diagnosis, and comprehensive approach to management—University of Missouri Libraries. Missouri.edu. [cited 2022 Mar 29]. http://link.library.missouri.edu/portal/Congestive-heart-failure--pathophysiology/g5JArSjQyY8/
9. Hosenpud JD, Greenberg BH. Congestive heart failure: pathophysiology, diagnosis, and comprehensive approach to management. 1994th Hosenpud JD, Greenberg BH (eds.). New York, NY: Springer;2013. https://books.google.at/books?id=zI--BwAAQBAJ
10. Palliative care consultation and the transition to hospice for patients with end-stage CVD. American College of Cardiology [cited 2022 Mar 29]. https://www.acc.org/Latest-in-Cardiology/Articles/2022/01/21/13/11/Palliative-Care-Consultation-and-the-Transition-to-Hospice
11. Lund LH, Edwards LB, Dipchand AI, Goldfarb S, Kucheryavaya AY, Levvey BJ, et al. The registry of the international society for heart and lung transplantation: thirty-third adult heart transplantation report—2016; focus theme: primary diagnostic indications for transplant. J Heart Lung Transplant. 2016 [cited 2022 Mar 29];**35**(10):1158–69. https://pubmed.ncbi.nlm.nih.gov/27772668/
12. Deng MC. Cardiac transplantation. Heart. 2002;**87**(2):177–84. https://heart.bmj.com/content/heartjnl/87/2/177.full.pdf
13. Deng MC, De Meester JM, Smits JM, Heinecke J, Scheld HH. Effect of receiving a heart transplant: analysis of a national cohort entered on to a waiting list, stratified by heart failure severity. Comparative Outcome and Clinical Profiles in Transplantation (COCPIT) study group. BMJ. 2000;**321**(7260):540–5. https://www.bmj.com/content/bmj/321/7260/540.full.pdf
14. Friedrich EB, Böhm M. Management of end stage heart failure. Heart. 2007;93(5):626–31.

15. Boilson, Barry A, et al. Device therapy and cardiac transplantation for end-stage heart failure. Curr Probl Cardiol. 2010;**35**(1):8–64
16. Shah P, Bristow MR, Port JD. MicroRNAs in heart failure, cardiac transplantation, and myocardial recovery: biomarkers with therapeutic potential. Curr Heart Fail Rep. 2017;14:454–64.

Donor Management and Organ Procurement

Annalisa Bernabei, Ilaria Tropea, Giuseppe Faggian, and Francesco Onorati

Abstract Heart transplantation remains the gold standard treatment for end-stage heart failure refractory to medical therapy. Donation after circulatory death (DCD) is gaining much attention from the international transplant community. It is estimated that the DCD technique carries the potential to increase heart transplant activity by up to 20%. Although only recent studies with DCD donors are available, preliminary results are promising. In addition to seeking new types of donations, meticulous management of the donor at the procurement site is crucial. A proper harvesting technique must be employed to avoid damaging critical structures leading to donor organ discard. Moreover, accurate coordination and timely and constant communication among all the surgeons involved are crucial for successful heart transplantation. Special attention is deserved for preservation and transportation to the implantation hospital. Although the standard static cold storage preservation with the three-bag technique is still the most employed worldwide, new technologies are under investigation. The Paragonix SherpaPak cardiac transport system has been recently developed to avoid temperature fluctuation and freeze myocardial injury. This new device functions as a small and portable cardiopulmonary bypass machine that aims to minimize ischemic damage during transportation, and it allows for the evaluation of marginal donors before implantation. Its use is auspicious, primarily when combined with donation after circulatory death. This chapter will cover all the aforementioned topics, focusing on the new technologies pushing heart transplantation in a new and exciting era.

Keywords Heart transplantation · Heart Procurement · DBD · DCD · Bicaval Technique · Biatrial Technique · Cold Ischemic Storage · TransMedics OCS · Paragonix SherpaPak · Ex-vivo heart perfusion

Heart transplantation (HT) is the best line of management for patients with end-stage heart failure that cannot be fixed with medications [1]. However, this population with end-stage HF is continuously increasing, whereas the number of donor organs

A. Bernabei · I. Tropea · G. Faggian · F. Onorati (✉)
Division of Cardiac Surgery, University Hospital of Verona, Verona, Italy
e-mail: Francesco.onorati@univr.it

© The Author(s), under exclusive license to Springer Nature Switzerland AG 2022
H. T. Hashim et al. (eds.), *Heart Transplantation*,
https://doi.org/10.1007/978-3-031-17311-0_7

remains constant and an unavoidable limiting factor in HT. Indeed, death on the waiting list is unfortunately common nowadays, accounting for more than one-third of the HT candidates [2]. This chapter will discuss the types of donors and their clinical assessment for successful transplantation, the surgical technique for heart procurement, and current approaches in retrieval and heart preservation.

1 Types of Donors for Heart Transplantation

Christiaan Barnard performed the first successful human heart transplantation at Groote Schuur Hospital in Cape Town, South Africa, on December 3rd, 1967 [3]. Since then, more than 100 heart transplants have been performed worldwide in less than a year [4]. However, no legal definition for organ donors had been defined at that time yet. [5]. Since then, all heart transplant donors have had to meet the DBD criteria. However, with the increased need and concomitant global shortage of suitable donor hearts, extending the acceptability criteria for heart donation became necessary. Thus, the heart transplant community started seeking other potential donors, including donations after circulatory death (DCD).

Historically, this type of donation was not new to the scientific world. Christiaan Barnard's first HT occurred, in fact, after circulatory death. The donor was a female who sustained severe brain damage after being hit by a drunk driver in a motor vehicle accident. The medical team deemed her recovery not possible [3]. Brain stem testing was not available; thus, heart procurement after withdrawal from life support (WLST) was the only viable option.

DCD donors may be classified into four categories based on the Modified Maastricht Classification (Table 1) [6]. Heart donation from DCD donors is performed only in planned withdrawal of life-sustaining treatment (Category III). Exclusion criteria for heart transplantation after circulatory death are previous cardiac surgery or midline sternotomy, known cardiovascular risk factors, high vasopressor requirement, malignancy with increased metastatic potential, or infective diseases such as tuberculosis or HIV positivity [7].

A schematic representation of the difference between DBD and DCD heart donation is shown in Fig. 1.

In both scenarios, the donor suffered from an irreversible brain injury. However, DCD donors are not characterized by complete loss of brain function, even though there is no hope for recovery. Thus, withdrawal of life-sustaining therapy is necessary for death pronunciation. This condition of myocardial hypoperfusion without patient cooling persists until coronary arteries are reperfused. With the onset of cardiac asystole, the "no-touch period" begins. Each country with an active DCD program has legally defined the duration for this stand-off time. In the member states of the Council of Europe, the "no-touch" period ranges from 5 (most of the countries) up to 20 (Italy) or 30 min (Russia) [8]. Only after the end of the "no-touch" time, the donor is declared dead, and the procurement team is allowed to proceed with heart retrieval.

Table 1 The modified Maastricht classification of DCD

CATEGORY I Uncontrolled	Not witnessed CA Ia. Out-of-Hospital Ib. In-hospital	Sudden unexpected CA without any attempt of resuscitation by a medical team
CATEGORY II Uncontrolled	Witnessed CA IIa. Out-of-Hospital IIb. In-hospital	Sudden unexpected CA with unsuccessful resuscitation life-by a medical team
CATEGORY III Controlled	Withdrawal of life-sustaining therapy	Planned withdrawal of life-sustaining therapy; expected CA
CATEGORY IV Uncontrolled/controlled	CA while life-brain dead	Sudden CA after brain death diagnosis during donor life-management but before planned organ recovery

CA = cardiac arrest

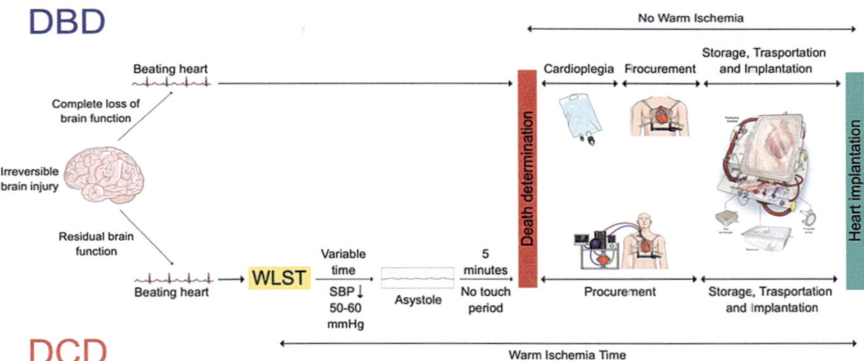

Fig. 1 Graphical representation of the different timelines between DBD and DCD donation. WLST = withdrawal of life-sustaining therapy; SBP = systolic blood pressure

Compared to DBD donors, in which organ hypoxia is minimized due to continuous systemic perfusion maintained by the beating heart, donation after circulatory death is strongly limited by WIT duration. Exceeding 30 min of WIT would increase the risk of irreversible damage due to hypoxia and myocardial ischemia, possibly leading to primary graft failure or delayed graft function [9, 10]. Moreover, assessing the donor's heart function is easier when a "standard" DBD donation is performed.

To reduce WIT, antemortem interventions, such as reducing the "no-touch" period and performing VA ECMO cannulation before death declaration, have been successfully described in the literature [11–13].

Therefore, more effort has been recently put into improving heart retrieval techniques for donation after circulatory death to avoid breaking ethical rules. Four different heart retrieval protocols have been described; however, only three of them are currently in use worldwide.

In 2008, Boucek and colleagues presented the first-ever small case series of 3 pediatric patients who underwent HT from DCD donors in Denver, Colorado [11]. Their *direct procurement followed by static cold storage (DP-SCS)* technique required co-location of patients and donors at the same hospital. In addition, antemortem heparinization and cannulation were used to reduce WIT, and the "no-touch" time was limited to 75 s.

No antemortem interventions are allowed with this protocol. This protocol carries the same issues related to direct procurement mentioned earlier in this paragraph. Yet, this method is still used in Australia [14], UK [15, 16], Austria [17], and USA [18, 19].

The heart is then stopped through cardioplegia infusion, removed from the donor's mediastinum, and normothermic blood-based perfusion is provided during transportation to the recipient hospital through OCS. This protocol recreates a condition that resembles the normal human physiology and allows for the donor's heart visual direct examination [17, 20].

In Belgium, a variation of the protocol just mentioned above has been studied [12]. However, after cardioplegia infusion and removal from the mediastinum, the donor's heart is transported to the implantation hospital through cold storage. Although less expensive than the NRP-NMP protocol, the NRP-SCS technique is not allowed in most countries where antemortem interventions are prohibited. At Papworth Hospital, a single case of NRP-SCS has been performed so far. The donor was already supported by a Veno-Venous ECMO before proceeding to WLST [21]. Another small case series of four patients has been described by the NYU Langone Health team (USA) [22].

It is estimated that DCD donation carries the potential to increase heart transplant activity by up to 20% as well as to reduce the death rate on the waiting list by 40% [23, 24]. Although heart donation after circulatory death is opening a fascinating path to overcome organ shortage worldwide, many programs across Europe and USA have not published their results yet. However, older programs such as St Vincent's in Australia [14] and Papworth in the UK [16, 17].

2 Assessment of the Donor Prior to Heart Procurement

Heart procurement is part of a multi-phased process involving several teams from different hospitals. Accurate coordination and timely and constant communication among surgeons are crucial for successful heart transplantation, both at the donor's procurement site and between the procurement and implant teams (Fig. 2). However, heart donor procurement and preservation procedures have not been internationally standardized yet. Vast differences exist between geographical regions within the same country and even among procurement teams within the same hospital [25].

Donor evaluation begins hours (if not days) before the surgical procedure. If the donor is deemed "increased risk", the recipient must be informed, and separate consent must be duly obtained. A donor–recipient BMI ratio >0.8 is considered

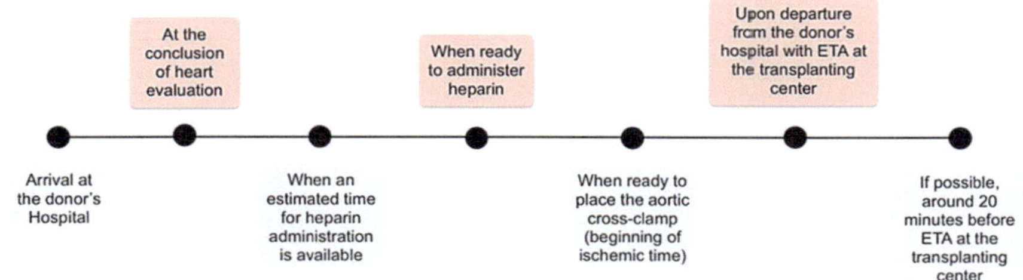

Fig. 2 A suggested standard protocol of communication between procurement and implantation teams. ETA = estimated time of arrival

acceptable [26]. Male and larger donors are preferred for recipients suffering from pulmonary hypertension or who have undergone other cardiac operations before HT. Moreover, in the case of a gender mismatch between the donor and recipient, male donors may be considered appropriate for female recipients, whereas the opposite should be avoided [27]. If no other option is available, a larger size of 10% in height and weight would be acceptable when a female donor is chosen for a male recipient [25]. Donor's age is a recognized factor with a significant impact on heart transplant outcomes [26, 28]. Poorer long-term survival has been associated with donors from 30 years old onwards [27].

However, failure to meet the above criteria is not an absolute contraindication to heart donations. Each case should be evaluated based on a combination of clinical and center experience and the clinical conditions of the recipient. The final decision should result from a careful analysis of the procurement team in conjunction with the transplanting team.

Before the departure, the procurement team is responsible for checking all the supplies necessary for the explant operation. Sternal saw and its batteries, surgical equipment, bags and buckets for organs, *cardioplegia with its* cannula, *tubing* and pressure bag, preservation solutions, ice, saline, and transport devices must be meticulously inspected.

Upon arrival at the procurement center, consent for donation, ABO compatibility to the recipient, serology, verification of brain death that complies with local legislation (if a DBD donor), and any new documentation available since the acceptance must be reviewed carefully. [29]. Maintaining a target central venous pressure (CVP) of 6–10 mmHg and mean arterial pressure (MAP) >60 mmHg is advisable [25]. However, two main physiopathologic events happen after brain dead. Increased intracranial cerebral pressure and progressive brainstem ischemia lead to a sympathetic storm, which is responsible for initial hypertension and raised systemic vascular resistance. This phenomenon is followed by abrupt loss of the sympathetic tone that causes peripheral vasodilation, also known as neurogenic vasoplegia [30–32]. However, aggressive fluid repletion may negatively affect the right ventricular function. If fluid resuscitation is insufficient to keep the MAP >60 mmHg, vasopressor or inotropic support should be started. [33, 34]. Epinephrine and norepinephrine are

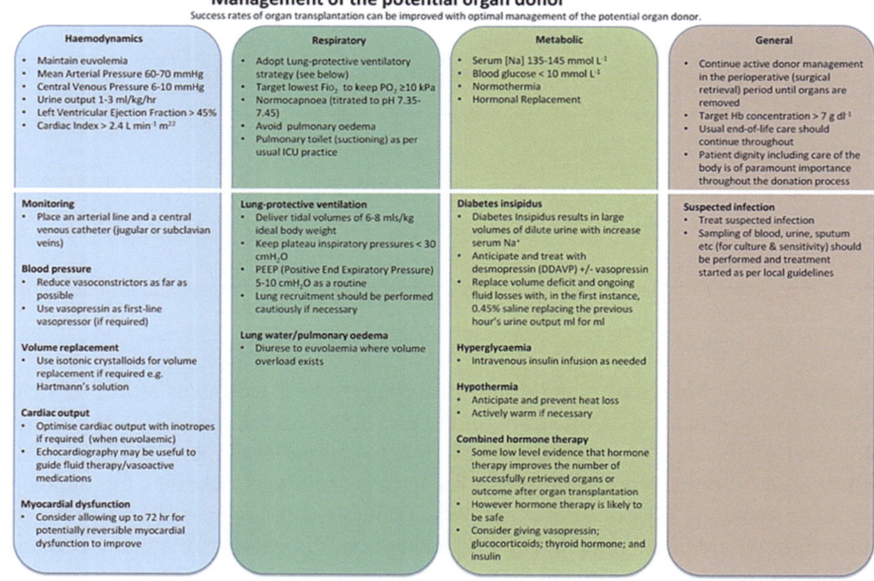

Fig. 3 Reproduced from Conrick-Martin I. et al. Intensive Care Society of Ireland—guidelines for the management of the potential organ donor (2nd edition). Ir J Med Sci 2019; 188: pp. 1111–1118

extensively used in everyday practice for resuscitation support in brain death donors. Their use has been associated with impaired contractility post-transplantation due to down-regulation of β-receptors [35, 36].

Figure 3 summarizes the main strategies for donor management during organ procurement from the hemodynamic, respiratory, and metabolic standpoint.

3 Current Approaches in Retrieval and Heart Preservation

3.1 Cold Ischemic Storage

It is well known that heart retrieval and preservation play a fundamental role in the overall outcome of heart transplantation. Despite significant progress in multiple aspects of heart transplantation, such as donor management, post-operative care, and immunosuppressive therapy, static cold storage at 4 °C remains the preferred technique for preserving the retrieved heart [37]. Moreover, hypothermia does not entirely stop anaerobic metabolism, which continues at low levels in the background. This activity leads to the depletion of adenosine triphosphate (ATP) and increases detrimental myocardial acidosis [38–41]. Later, the two types of solutions showed comparable outcomes [41, 42]. Nowadays, the UW solution is the preferred preservation solution in heart transplantation [42]. However, no consensus about the best preservation solutions commercially available has been reached yet, and many centers still rely on institutionally derived products.

Independently from the preservation solution used, the gold standard for transportation after procurement is still SCS of the heart using the three-bag technique (described earlier in this chapter). To avoid potential complications such as temperature fluctuation and freeze myocardial injury, a new device has been recently developed and approved for clinical usage. "The Paragonix SherpaPak (SherpaPak-CTS; Paragonix Technologies, Braintree Mass) cardiac transport system has been used for the first time in clinical practice in 2018, and it has been approved by both US Food and Drug Administration and CE marked" [43]. "SherpaPak-CTS is a single-use, power source-free, disposable device designed for static hypothermic donor heart preservation" [43, 44]. Moreover, it requires a short learning curve for the procurement team, and it is cheaper than the ex-vivo perfusion system. Despite promising results [45–49], larger studies are needed to validate this new technology better.

3.2 Ex-Vivo Normothermic Preservation

Although universally adopted, static cold ischemic storage is known to be far from perfection. Thus, new approaches have been explored. The only platform that has been CE marked and commercially approved by the Food and Drug Administration is the TransMedics Organ Care System (OCS), commonly known as "heart-in-a-box" (TransMedics, Inc, Andover, MA). The OCS comprises a portable console with a heart console and a perfusion module through which a "maintenance" solution is added to the donor's blood and pumped into the circuit connected to the heart [50]. It allows preserving the beating donor's heart with warm, oxygenated, and nutrient-enriched donor blood. OCS functions as a small and portable cardiopulmonary bypass machine that pumps blood into the aorta, perfusing the coronary arteries during transportation. A diaphragmatic pump generates pulsatile flow. The "maintenance" solution adds insulin, antibiotics, corticosteroids, sodium bicarbonate, and nutrients to the donor's blood.

When ex-vivo heart perfusion is planned, the donor's SVC is cannulated at the level of the azygous vein for donor blood collection. The donor's blood is used to prime the OCS circuit. After stopping the donor's heart through the infusion of cold cardioplegia, the atrial cuff and pulmonary veins are harvested if the heart is taken alone. Pulmonary veins are tied off when the heart is removed from the mediastinum (Fig. 4A). In the case of heart–lung procurement, a transverse incision of the left atrium is made, leaving the defect alone. The blood coming off the defect during OCS perfusion will be collected into the reservoir and returned to the circuit (Fig. 4B). The aorta is then trimmed below the insertion point of the cardioplegia cannula to avoid leakage, and an appropriate-sized aortic tip cannula is inserted into the aorta and secured in place with a cable. The pulmonary artery (PA) is also cannulated,

                                                                      A. Bernabei et al.

and the cannula is secured with a 4–0 polypropylene purse-string suture. The SVC is tied. Now the donor's heart is ready to be positioned into the OCS "box". The donor's heart is placed with the posterior face above. The heart is aligned, and the aorta is connected to the port on the top of the heart chamber. Simultaneously, the aorta is filled with primed blood to avoid any air entrapment in the tip. PA cannula is de-aired through heart massage and connected to the PA connector.

An LV vent is placed through an opening in the left atrium, and the IVC is closed with a 4–0 poly polypropylene pro running suture. Pacing wires are placed, and

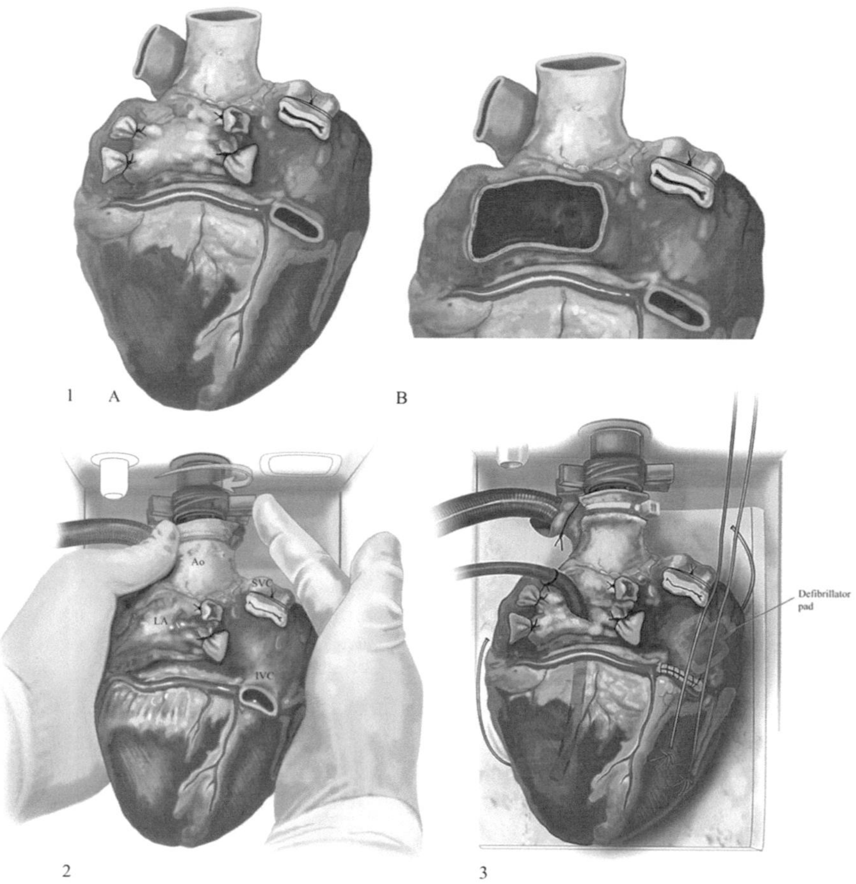

Fig. 4 **a** Donor's heart is harvested, and pulmonary veins and SVC are tied. **b** (1) In the case of heart–lung procurement, the atrial cuff is incised, and the defect is left open. (2) The donor's heart is placed facing down in the OCS chamber. Aorta and PA are connected to the circuit. (3) Final setting of the "heart in a box". A vent is placed into the left ventricle through the left atrium. Pacing wires and defibrillation electrode pads are positioned. Reprinted with permission of Elsevier [51]

defibrillation electrode pads are positioned on the right atrium and left ventricle [51].

A threshold of 5 mmol/L of lactate within the perfusate is set as a limit for contraindication to implantation [50]. Because the "heart-in-a-box" is not placed in an anatomical position facing downwards, direct visual inspection of the kinetics of the right ventricle is not feasible during transportation. However, when angiography at the procurement hospital is not available, the platform allows coronary catheterization [52, 53].

The prospective, open-label, multicenter, randomized non-inferiority PROCEED II trial demonstrated that OCS was safe and effective in human heart transplantation, with short-term results similar to HT after cold ischemic storage [54]. Other trials are still ongoing [55]. The high cost and personnel demanding to adopt the Trans-Medics Organ Care System are currently limiting this technology to high-volume heart transplant programs. However, its use is auspicious, especially with donation after circulatory death. A new era in the heart transplantation field has officially begun by expanding the donor pool to marginal donors.

References

1. McDonagh TA, Metra M, Adamo M, Gardner RS, Baumbach A, Böhm M et al. ESC scientific document group. 2021 ESC guidelines for the diagnosis and treatment of acute and chronic heart failure. Eur Heart J. 2021;42(36):3599–726
2. Bakhtiyar SS, Godfrey EL, Ahmed S, Lamba H, Morgan J, Loor G, et al. Survival on the heart transplant waiting list. JAMA Cardiol. 2020;5(11):1227–35.
3. Barnard CN. The operation. A human cardiac transplant: an interim report of a successful operation performed at Groote Schuur Hospital, Cape Town. S Afr Med J. 1967;41(48):1271–4
4. Stolf NAG. History of heart transplantation: a hard and glorious journey. Braz J Cardiovasc Surg. 2017;32(5):423–7.
5. A definition of irreversible coma. Report of the Ad Hoc Committee of the Harvard Medical School to examine the definition of brain death. JAMA. 1968;205(6):337–40
6. Thuong M, Ruiz A, Evrard P, Kuiper M, Boffa C, Akhtar MZ, et al. New classification of donation after circulatory death donors definitions and terminology. Transpl Int. 2016;29(7):749–59.
7. Messer S, Page A, Axell R, Berman M, Hernández-Sánchez J, Colah S, et al. Outcome after heart transplantation from donation after circulatory-determined death donors. J Heart Lung Transplant. 2017;36(12):1311–8.
8. Lomero M, Gardiner D, Coll E, Haase-Kromwijk B, Procaccio F, Immer F, et al. European Committee on Organ Transplantation of the Council of Europe (CD-P-TO). Donation after circulatory death today: an updated overview of the European landscape. Transpl Int. 2020;33(1):76–88
9. Manara AR, Murphy PG, O'Callaghan G. Donation after circulatory death. Br J Anaesth. 2012;108(Suppl 1):i108-21.
10. Quader M, Toldo S, Chen Q, Hundley G, Kasirajan V. Heart transplantation from donation after circulatory death donors: present and future. J Card Surg. 2020;35(4):875–85.
11. Boucek MM, Mashburn C, Dunn SM, Frizell R, Edwards L, Pietra B, Campbell D. Denver children's pediatric heart transplant team. Pediatric heart transplantation after declaration of cardiocirculatory death. N Engl J Med. 2008;359(7):709–14

12. Tchana-Sato V, Ledoux D, Detry O, Hans G, Ancion A, D'Orio V, et al. Successful clinical transplantation of hearts donated after circulatory death using normothermic regional perfusion. J Heart Lung Transplant. 2019;38(6):593–8.
13. Robertson JA. The dead donor rule. Hastings Cent Rep. 1999;29(6):6–14
14. Chew HC, Iyer A, Connellan M, et al. Outcomes of donation after circulatory death heart transplantation in Australia. J Am Coll Cardiol. 2019;73:1447–59.
15. Messer S, Abu-Omar Y, Large SR, et al. Combined heart-lung transplantation from a donation after circulatory death donor. J Heart Lung Transplant. 2020;39:1366–71.
16. Messer S, Cernic S, Page A, et al. A 5-year single-center early experience of heart transplantation from donation after circulatory—determined death donors. J Heart Lung Transplant. 2020;39:1463–75.
17. Scheuer SE, Jansz PC, Macdonald PS. Heart transplantation following donation after circulatory death: expanding the donor pool. J Heart Lung Transplant. 2021;40(9):882–9.
18. Shudo Y, Benjamin-Addy R, Koyano TK, Hiesinger W, MacArthur JW, Woo YJ. Donors after circulatory death heart trial. Future Cardiol. 2021;17:11–7.
19. Messer S, Large S. Resuscitating heart transplantation: the donation after circulatory determined death donor. Eur J Cardiothorac Surg. 2016;49(1):1–4.
20. Messer SJ, Axell RG, Colah S, et al. Functional assessment and transplantation of the donor heart after circulatory death. J Heart Lung Transplant. 2016;35(12):1443–52.
21. Messer S, Page A, Colah S, Axell R, Parizkova B, Tsui S, Large S. Human heart transplantation from donation after circulatory-determined death donors using normothermic regional perfusion and cold storage. J Heart Lung Transplant. 2018;37(7):865–9.
22. Ngai J, Masuno K, Moazami N. Anesthetic considerations during heart transplantation using donation after circulatory death. J Cardio—Thorac Vasc Anesth. 2020;34:3073–7.
23. Suarez-Pierre A, Iguidbashian J, Stuart C, King RW, Cotton J, Carroll AM, Cleveland JC, Fullerton DA, Pal JD. Appraisal of donation after circulatory death: how far could we expand the heart donor pool? Ann Thorac Surg. 2022;S0003–4975(22):00197–207.
24. Noterdaeme T, Detry O, Hans MF, Nellessen E, Ledoux D, Joris J, Meurisse M, Defraigne JO. What is the potential increase in the heart graft pool by cardiac donation after circulatory death? Transpl Int. 2013;26(1):61–6.
25. Copeland H, Hayanga JWA, Neyrinck A, MacDonald P, Dellgren G, Bertolotti A, et al. Donor heart and lung procurement: a consensus statement. J Heart Lung Transplant. 2020;39(6):501–17.
26. Khush KK, Potena L, Cherikh WS, Chambers DC, Harhay MO, Hayes Jr D, et al. International society for heart and lung transplantation. The International Thoracic Organ Transplant Registry of the International Society for Heart and Lung Transplantation: 37th Adult Heart Transplantation Report-2020; focus on deceased donor characteristics. J Hear Lung Transpl. 2020;39(10):1003–15
27. Sathianathan S, Bhat G. Heart transplant donor selection guidelines: review and recommendations. Curr Cardiol Rep. 2022;24(2):119–30.
28. Weber DJ, Wang IW, Gracon AS, Hellman YM, Hormuth DA, Wozniak TC, et al. Impact of donor age on survival after heart transplantation: an analysis of the United Network for Organ Sharing (UNOS) registry. J Card Surg. 2014;29(5):723–8.
29. Wheeldon DR, Potter CD, Oduro A, Wallwork J, Large SR. Transforming the "unacceptable" donor: outcomes from the adoption of a standardized donor management technique. J Heart Lung Transplant. 1995;14(4):734–42
30. Lazzeri C, Bonizzoli M, Guetti C, Fulceri GE, Peris A. Hemodynamic management in brain dead donors. World J Transplant. 2021;11(10):410–20
31. Essien EO, Fioretti K, Scalea TM, Stein DM. Physiologic features of brain death. Am Surg. 2017;83(8):850–4
32. Kotloff RM, Blosser S, Fulda GJ, Malinoski D, Ahya VN, Angel L, et al. Society of Critical Care Medicine/American College of Chest Physicians/Association of Organ Procurement Organizations Donor Management Task Force. Management of the potential organ donor in the ICU: Society of Critical Care Medicine/American College of Chest Physicians/Association of Organ Procurement Organizations Consensus Statement. Crit Care Med. 2015;43(6):1291–325

33. Venkateswaran RV, et al. The hemodynamic effects of adjunctive hormone therapy in potential heart donors: a prospective randomized double-blind factorially designed controlled trial. Eur Heart J. 2009;30(14):1771–80.

34. Rosendale JD, Kauffman HM, McBride MA, Chabalewski FL, Zaroff JG, Garrity ER, Delmonico FL, Rosengard BR. Hormonal resuscitation yields more transplanted hearts, with improved early function. Transplantation. 2003;75:1336–41.

35. D'Amico TA, et al. Desensitization of myocardial beta-adrenergic receptors and deterioration of left ventricular function after brain death. J Thorac Cardiovasc Surg. 1995;110(3):746–51.

36. Angleitner P, Kaider A, Gökler J, Moayedifar R, Osorio-Jaramillo E, Zuckermann A, Laufer G, Aliabadi-Zuckermann A. High-dose catecholamine donor support and outcomes after heart transplantation. J Heart Lung Transplant. 2018;37(5):596–603.

37. Lund LH, Khush KK, Cherikh WS, Goldfarb S, Kucheryavaya AY, Levvey BJ, et al. The Registry of the International Society for Heart and Lung Transplantation: thirty-fourth adult heart transplantation report. Focus theme: allograft ischemic time. J Heart Lung Transplant. 2017;36:1037–46

38. Buckburg GD, Brazier JR, Nelson RL, et al. Studies of the effects of hypothermia on regional myocardial flow and metabolism during cardiopulmonary bypass. I. The adequately perfused beating, fibrillating, and arrested heart. J Thorac Cardiovasc Surg 1997;73:87

39. Demmy TL, Biddle JS, Bennett LE, et al. Organ preservation solutions in heart transplantation-patterns of usage and related survival. Transplantation. 1997;63:262–9.

40. Mühlbacher F, Langer F, Mittermayer C. Preservation solutions for transplantation. Transplant Proc. 1999;31:2069–70.

41. Nils AH, Henri GDL, Rutger JP. New solutions in organ preservation. Transplant Rev. 2002;16(3):131–41

42. Latchana N, Peck JR, Whitson B, Black SM. Preservation solutions for cardiac and pulmonary donor grafts: a review of the current literature. J Thorac Dis. 2014.6(8):1143–9.

43. Naito N, Funamoto M, Pierson RN, D'Alessandro DA. First clinical use of a novel hypothermic storage system for a long-distance donor heart procurement. J Thorac Cardiovasc Surg. 2020;159(2):e121-3.

44. Michel SG, LaMuraglia Ii GM, Madariaga ML, Anderson LM. Innovative cold storage of donor organs using the Paragonix Sherpa Pak™ devices. Heart Lung Vessel. 2015;7(3):246–55.

45. Radakovic D, Karimli S, Penov K, Schade I, Hamouda K, Bening C, Leyh RG, Aleksic I. First clinical experience with the novel cold storage SherpaPak™ system for donor heart transportation. J Thorac Dis. 2020;12(12):7227–35.

46. Mohite PN, Sef D, Umakumar K, Maunz O, Smail H, Stock U. Utilization of Paragonix SherpaPak for human donor heart preservation. Multimed Man Cardiothorac Surg. 2021;2021

47. Schmiady MO, Graf T, Ouda A, Aser R, Flammer AJ, Vogt PR, Wilhelm MJ. An innovative cold storage system for donor heart transportation-lessons learned from the first experience in Switzerland. J Thorac Dis. 2021;13(12):6790–9.

48. Bitargil M, Haddad O, Pham SM, Goswami RM, Patel PC, Jacob S, El-Sayed Ahmed MM, Leoni Moreno JC, Yip DS, Landolfo K, Sareyyupoglu B. Controlled temperatures in cold preservation provides safe heart transplantation results. J Card Surg. 2022;37(4):732–8.

49. Iyengar A, Atluri P. Commentary: keeping your cool: donor heart preservation using the SherpaPak cardiac transport system. J Thorac Cardiovasc Surg. 2020;159(2):e125-6.

50. Monteagudo Vela M, García Sáez D, Simon AR. Current approaches in retrieval and heart preservation. Ann Cardiothorac Surg. 2018;7(1):67–74.

51. Tsukashita M, Naka Y. Organ care system for heart procurement and strategies to reduce primary graft failure after heart transplant. Oper Tech Thorac Cardiovasc Surg. 2015;20(3):322–34.

52. Ghodsizad A, Bordel V, Ungerer M, Karck M, Bekeredjian R, Ruhparwar A. Ex vivo coronary angiography of a donor heart in the organ care system. Heart Surg Forum. 2012;15:E161-3.

53. Bryner BS, Schroder JN, Milano CA. Heart transplant advances: ex vivo organ-preservation systems. JTCVS Open. 2021;8:123–7.

54. Ardehali A, Esmailian F, Deng M, Soltesz E, Hsich E, Naka Y, et al. PROCEED II trial investigators. Ex-vivo perfusion of donor hearts for human heart transplantation (PROCEED II): a prospective, open-label, multicentre, randomised non-inferiority trial. Lancet. 2015;385(9987):2577–84
55. Messer S, Ardehali A, Tsui S. Normothermic donor heart perfusion: current clinical experience and the future. Transpl Int. 2015;28(6):634–42.

Heart Transplantation Procedure

Abbas Mohammad

Abstract Heart transplantation is the key treatment of heart failure in the end stage when the other options are not useful such as medical treatment, mechanical or electrical devices. The limit of this option for the treatment of heart failure is that impossible to provide this option to all patients due to lacking donors. The prognosis after heart transplantation is good in comparison with medical treatment particularly when there is restricted following of instructions to optimize the selection and management of patients and donors and perioperative management. The limits of good prognosis are graft rejection and complications of immunosuppressive drugs used after transplantation like severe infections, malignant disease, and renal failure.

Keywords Cardiac surgery · Cardiac transplantation · Immunosuppressive drugs · Cardiopulmonary bypass

1 Introduction

The first cardiac transplantation was done in 1950. Which made a leap in the survival of many congenital heart diseases and increase the survival of adulthood. Although cardiac surgery for many types of congenital heart disease have good outcomes and accepted improvement in life pattern for many patients when is done early. The other group of patients with congenital heart disease has poor life patterns even when surgery is done because this surgery is palliative surgery due to more complexity and more complicated congenital heart disease that ends with hemodynamic problems with age progressing. Many adults with congenital heart disease can live longer but they have a shorter mean age of death. The mean age of death in 2007 is about 57 years, the cause of death was mainly cardiovascular events including heart failure which is the most common cause of death that represents about 26% of total death in patients with congenital heart disease according to a recent study. The heart failure caused by congenital heart disease is progressively becoming resistant to medical

A. Mohammad (✉)
College of Medicine, Qar University, Al-Nasiriyah, Iraq
e-mail: abbasmoham-mad199600@gmail.com

therapy and requires either heart transplantation alone or heart–lung transplantation to improve the life quality and survival rate.

2 Epidemiology

According to collected data, about 2000 operations of heart transplantation are done annually in the US. Due to lacking of heart donors, the heart transplantation rate remains constant. According to statistics, the most common indication for heart transplantation is heart failure due to coronary heart disease and cardiomyopathy. Once the immunosuppressive drugs emerged, the survival rate is largely improved which was about 9 years according to a study done on about 43,906 heart transplant patients. The heart transplantation survival rate decreases after 20 years to about 10%. The 7 years survival rate is about 59% between 1994–1998 and about 62% between 1995–2000 and about 65% between 2000–2007. According to other studies on infants, the survival rate in infants during the first post transplantation year is about 74% (which is a poor survival rate). While in other age groups, it is more than 85% with better long-term prognosis in surviving infants compared to the survival of other age groups. In patients who are 65 years old or more, the survival rate begins to decrease more rapidly 8 years post transplantation. Today, heart transplantation is done widely in the world. According to data of international society of heart and lung transplantation reported about 111,068 heart transplantation worldwide in June of 2012, and the mean survival rate also improved to more than 11 years.

3 Indication for Heart Transplantation

Generally, patients with advanced heart failure who are resistant to medical therapy and resynchronization are mostly indicated for heart transplantation according to the American College of Cardiology and American Heart Association (ACC/ AHA) guideline. In case if heart failure has a reversible underlying cause or an underlying cause that can be corrected surgically, then it should be addressed before transplantation so that heart transplantation could be done for more needed patients. Heart failure severity is classified into four categories by New York Heart Association (NYHA classification):

- Category I: the patient develops a symptom (shortness of breathing) only during heavy activities
- Category II: the patient develops a symptom during ordinary activities
- Category III: the patient develops a symptom during minimal exercise
- Category IV: the patient develops a symptom at rest

Also, there is another system for classification of heart failure severity by the American College of Cardiology and American Heart Association (ACC/AHA) which classifies the severity of heart failure into four categories:

- Stage A: patients have high risk for development of heart failure as hypertension but there is no structural heart disease and no symptoms of heart failure
- Stage B: there is structural heart disease but there are no signs or symptoms of heart failure
- Stage C: there is structural heart disease with signs and symptoms of heart failure
- Stage D: patients have advanced heart failure that requires hospital-based support or heart transplantation or palliative care (refractory heart failure)

The patient with stage D heart failure cannot be discharged from the hospital safely. They require specific intervention such as heart transplantation, long-term treatment with inotropic drugs, experimental therapy, permanent medical circulatory support or end-of-life care. The most common cause of heart failure which is indicated for heart transplantation is dilated cardiomyopathy, which represents about 53%, and the second most common cause is coronary artery disease, which represents about 38% [1].

Other causes include valvular heart disease, which represents about 3%, re transportationrepresents about 3%, and other rare indications represent about 10%.

The indications of heart transplantation that are considered by ACC/AHA are:

1. Patients with cardiogenic shock which are refractory and require a left ventricular assisted device or intraoartic balloon pump counterpulsation, continuous intravenous inotropic drugs such as milrinone or dobutamine
2. Patients who have peak VO2 of less than 10 ml/kg/minute
3. Advanced NYHA classes (class III or class IV) which are resistant to maximum medical therapy or resynchronization therapy
4. Patients who experienced recurrent ventricular dysrhythmia who are resistant to catheter-based ablation or ant—arrhythmic drugs or implantable cardiac defibrillator
5. Patients who have end-stage heart failure without pulmonary hypertension
6. Patients with resistant angina without surgical or medical therapeutic options

Before cardiac transplantation, there are many features considered by the European Society of Cardiology that should be met including structural, functional, and symptomatic parameters. These features include:

(1) Attacks of fluid retention inform of vascular congestion (pulmonary or systemic) and peripheral edema or episodes of low cardiac output in the form of peripheral hypoperfusion
(2) Severe ventricular dysfunction in the form of one of the following:

    A. low left ventricular ejection fraction of less than 30%.
    B. Right and/or left ventricular filling pressure is a highly impaired functional capacity which is represented by one of the followings:

Table 8.1 ACC/AHA guideline indications for heart transplantation

• **Absolute indications**	• **Relative indications**	• **Insufficient indications**
1. Heart failure induced hemodynamic instability 2. Refractory cardiogenic shock 3. Patients with Heart failure who completely depend on inotropics to maintain adequate cardiac output 4. Peak VO2 less than 10 ml/kg/min associated with anaerobic metabolism 5. Severely symptomatic ischemia that interferes with routine activities which unsuitable for coronary intervention 6. Recurrent symptomatic ventricular dysrhythmia that does not respond to all therapeutic measures	1. Peak VO2 is 11–14 ml/kg/min for 55% predicted that largely interfere with routine activities of the patient 2. Recurrent unstable angina unsuitable for coronary intervention 3. Recurrent fluid imbalance or renal function abnormality in patients who complained of medical therapy	(1) Low left ventricular ejection fraction (2) Heart failure of NYHA class III or IV (3) Peak VO2 of more than 15 ml/kg/min and more than 55% were predicted in absence of other indications

- exercise intolerance.
- 6 min walking distance less than 30 min or less in elderly (equal or more than 75 years old) or female.
- Maximum oxygen intake less than 12–14 ml/kg /minute

C.   Restrictive or pseudo normal mitral outflow on Doppler echocardiography

(3)   One or more hospital admissions due to heart failure in the last 6 months (Table 8.1)

4   Contraindication for Heart Transplantation

The relative and absolute contraindications for heart transplantation are listed in Table. We will discuss some of these contraindications as follows:

- Irreversible pulmonary hypertension or raised pulmonary vascular resistance:

When the heart transplantation is done in patients with pulmonary hypertension or raised pulmonary vascular resistance, it ends with post transplantation acute right-side heart failure because the pulmonary hypertension is poorly tolerated by the donor heart and may result in perioperative recipient death. So, for any patient who needs transplantation, a mandatory right ventricular catheterization should be done as a preoperative evaluation for heart transplantation candidate selection among optimally treated patients with vasodilators. The use of vasodilators should be considered in patients who have systolic pulmonary pressure of 50 mmHg or more and either pulmonary vascular resistance (PVR) of more than 3 wood units or transpulmonary gradient of 15 mmHg or more. The vasodilators include nitroglycerin, prostaglandin, nitroprusside, nitric oxide, and milrinone. The post transplantation high risk of heart failure or mortality rate should be considered in the following conditions:

a. Transpulmonary gradient more than 16–20 mmHgor pulmonary vascular resistance more than 5 wood units or PVRI more than 6 mmHg
b. If the pulmonary vascular resistance is amenable to reduce to less than 2.5 wood units with using of vasodilators only at cost to lowering of arterial systolic blood pressure to less than 85 mmHg
c. If the pulmonary arterial pressure is more than 60 mmHg in presence of pulmonary vascular resistance of more than 5 wood units or transpulmonary gradient more than 16–20 mmHg or PVRI more than 6 mmHg

- Active systemic infection

When the heart transplantation is done in patients with active systemic infection, this gives rise to serious complications due to the use of immunosuppressive therapy post transplantation at least for the short term because of lacking long-term data. Also, in patients with HIV infection, who are already immunosuppressed, it may cause life-threatening infection.

- Active malignancy or history of malignancy with a high risk of recurrence

Heart transplantation is an absolute contraindication in patients with active malignancy except for skin malignancy because the patients with active malignancy have a low survival rate (skin malignancy is low malignant and can be completely curable). Also, patients with a history of malignancy are contraindicated for heart transplantation when the risk of recurrence is high but can be done if the risk of recurrence is low. In general, patients with malignancy can undergo heart transplantation depending on grading, staging of the tumor, and response to therapy [2].

- Inability to comply with the complex medical regimen

When there is evidence of non-adherence life-long medical therapy, regular follow up or lifestyle changes, the long–term outcomes of cardiac transplantation are poor. These factors can be listed in the following forms:

1. Suboptimal use of immunosuppressive therapy which results in acute rejection 6 months or more after cardiac transplantation. Also, it can result in chronic rejection due to cardiac allograft vasculopathy
2. Lifestyle changes: the most important lifestyle effect is substance abuse as creative drugs or alcohol and smoking, because these substances are potential factors for non-compliance. Also, smoking has an adverse effect on the cardiovascular system and a wide range of malignancies development which can result in death. So, the most avoidable cause of death after cardiac transplantation is smoking cessation. Some studies show that the patients who continue smoking

after transplantation developed malignancy or coronary artery allograft disease which results in a decrease in the survival rate. Also, the patients who were smoking actively in the last 6 months of pre-transplantation have poor outcomes after transplantation, so it's a relative contraindication for heart transplantation. Psychological assessment to evaluate compliance with drugs should be done as a part of pre-transplantation evaluation.

- Severe peripheral vascular disease or cerebrovascular diseases

It's a major comorbidity that can affect the eligibility for heart transplantation because it contributes to poor outcomes after transplantation and affect the life quality due to non–cardiac effects. Some studies suggest that vascular disease will progress rapidly after transplantation, especially in patients who have ischemic heart disease as the indication of the heart transplantation [3].

- Another irreversible organ failure

The most organ failure that influences the decision of heart transplantation is a renal failure because it increases the post transplantation mortality rate, so when the GFR less than 40 ml/minute is considered relative contraindication for heart transplantation because the renal function will deteriorate post–transplantation due to nephrotoxic effect of immunosuppressive therapy. In patients with GFR less than 29 ml/minute, the 5-years survival rate after heart transplantation is 7–21%. Also, some patients with renal failure may require renal replacement therapy in the form of renal transplantation or dialysis after heart transplantation. In this circumstance, using of heart and kidney from the same donor reduces organ donation limitations. Other organ dysfunctions that should be considered are pancreatic endocrine dysfunction including diabetes mellitus and obesity which is considered as an absolute contraindication for heart transplantation by all centers in the first years, but recently, a large study was done on heart transplantation recipients which showed that the patients with non-complicated diabetes mellitus have the same prognosis as for non-diabetic patients, but when there are microvascular complications (nephropathy) or microvascular complications (cerebrovascular accidents, peripheral vascular disease) or sever obesity have poor prognosis and low survival rate after heart transplantation. Now with the development of experience, the non-complicated diabetes mellitus is considered as a relative contraindication for heart transplantation. Regarding obesity, it also has worse effects on patients after heart transplantation. A study shows that the 5-years mortality rate after heart transplantation in obese patients is twice as higher than non-obese patients (in obese patients with BMI > 30, the 5-years mortality rate is about 53%, while in non- obese patients with normal BMI is about 27%). So, one of the important parts of the list for transplantation in obese patients is reducing the BMI to less than 30 [5] (Table 8.2).

Table 8.2 Contraindications for heart transplantation

Age	Patients more than 70 years old are relatively contraindicated for heart transplantation depending on associated health problems
Diabetes mellitus	DM is absolute contraindication when it is uncontrolled or associated with complications
Malignancy	Active malignancy, except for skin malignancy (nonmelanoma), is an absolute contraindication for heart transplantation but then the malignancy is low grade or curable, the transplantation can be done after consultation with an oncologist
Pulmonary hypertension	The pulmonary vascular resistance that cannot be brought lower than 2.5 with inotropic or vasodilators, is contraindicated. those patients can be treated with long-term ventricular assisted device
Rental failure	It may be an absolute contraindication if it is caused by DM
Infection	Absolute contraindication for heart transplantation is hepatitis C and HIV infections
Peripheral vascular disease	Peripheral vascular disease is an absolute contraindications when are unsuitable for revascularization
Substance abuse	Patients who want to undergo heart transplantation, should stops the substance abuse for at least 6 months. Also, the psychologist consultation is important
Psychological problems	Absolute psychological contraindications are dementia and noncompliance

5 Donor Selection

One of the important limitations in heart transplantation is the shrinkage by number and quality, especially in the pediatric age group. A study done between July 2000 to December 2008 shows that only 65.7% of the donor's heart was transplanted due to many causes including the usage of high doses of inotropic agents, prolonged use of CPR, prolonged ischemic time, and trauma to the chest wall. But in general, the studies on heart transplantation are lacking, especially in pediatrics. As a result, the doctors depend on adult data or experience. the heart transplantation should be done on the after confirmed diagnosis of Brain Death depending on the specific criteria for diagnosis of Brain Death. Also, there are other criteria depending on age groups. the diagnosis of brain death should be confirmed on two occasions of 12 - 48 h interval. The donor factors that should be considered for donation are gender, age, body mass index (Height and weight), evaluation of the patients for blunt chest trauma, review of the use of inotropic agents, and evaluation of hemodynamic status. Using of CPR, evaluation of ischemia time because it is poor prognostic factor for survival especially in those of age of 11 to 17 years, but there is no impact on infants of less than 1-year old. The functional and structural disorders should be excluded by echocardiography because an ejection fraction of less than 50% is a large barrier to transplantation and make heart using precluded. Also, pericardial effusion resulting from blunt chest trauma should be detected. Take in mind that some valvular diseases are normal after brain death. As tricuspid or mitral regurgitation. The ECG should be done but generally record nonspecific ischemic changes due to hemodynamic changes caused by brain death. Serum tripping, I also it is recommended because it is a prognostic factor for heart transplantation, but a news show there is no significant effect on outcomes.

Also, the matching of size between recipient and donor is an important factor, which is evaluated by the measurement of the donor–recipient ratio. A ratio of less than 0.6 is considered undersized, which is a poor prognostic factor, and some centers avoid a ratio of less than 0.75, while the oversized ratio can be done safely up to 3. in old children can receive adult heart. A study shows that 25% of all children received adult heart especially in patients with cardiomyopathy because the cardiomyopathy makes a large cavity that harbors the large donor heart (Table 8.3).

Also, routine serological screening should be done for many viruses including HIV, Epstein Barr virus, Cytomegalovirus, Hepatitis, Human T-cell lymphocytic virus (HTLV), and Toxoplasma gonadii. Any donor with positive screening for Hepatitis, HIV, or HTLV is considered a contraindication for donation, while the donors who are positive for Epstein Barr virus, Cytomegalovirus, or Toxoplasma gondii are not a contraindication for donation but require management post transplantation. The donors also should be closely monitored with adequate support to avoid the metabolic changes that increase Demand on hard. Especially catecholamine surge which results in vasoconstriction and increased afterload and Demand on the heart. Blood gas analysis should be done and preserved within normal values. Central venous pressure also should be normal. The donor should receive hormonal support such as insulin, thyroxine or corticosteroids as needed. Also, circulatory support should be done if it is needed (Table 8.4).

Table 8.3 Criteria of the brain death

• **Etiology**	• **Clinical examination**
• Established irreversible CNS injury (hypoxia, ischemia, trauma)	• Deep coma unresponsive to stimuli
• Exclusion of reversible causes as drug intoxication	• No motor response to painful stimuli
• Exclusion of other medical problems (hypoglycemia, severe acid–base balance or electrolytes disturbance)	• No pupillary light reflex
• **Clinical conditions**	• No cough reflex by tracheal catheterization
• No hypotension (systolic BP 90 mmHg or more)	• No gag reflexes
• No hypothermia (body temperature 36.5 C° or more)	• No corneal reflex
• No neuromuscular disabilities	• No caloric response (no oculovestibular reflex)
• No sedation	• **Testing of apnea**
	• No pulmonary response (PaCO2 more than 60 mmHg or 20 mmHg more than baseline

Table 8.4 Donor heart selection criteria

(1) Donor age < 55 years
(2) No history of heart disease or chest trauma
(3) No prolonged hypoxia or hypotension
(4) Acceptable hemodynamic state including central venous pressure 8–12 mmHg and mean arterial pressure more than 60 mmHg
(5) Inotropic used (dopamine or dobutamine less than 10 mcg/kg/min
(6) Normal ECG and echocardiography
(7) Normal coronary artery angiography
(8) Negative viral serology (Hepatitis B and C, HIV)

6 Recipient Preparation

Preparation of the recipient for heart transplantation should be done earlier than other heart surgeries (e.g., valve repair, CABG, valve replacement), so the physician should plan for each step in transplantation process. Upon confirming the donor's availability, the recipient should be admitted to the hospital for routine medical history, physical examination, and routine investigations including blood group, cross matching and coagulation profile, and correction of any abnormality as blood products transfusion. Also, the patient should be given antibiotics. A CT or chest x-ray should be performed to assess the recipient's pericardial space to avoid mismatching of size between donor's heart and recipient's pericardial space, especially in patients who have recently implanted mechanical ventricular assist device, as there is not enough time for the heart to dilate, so should compare the ratio between the donor heart size and recipient chest dimensions and measurement and comparison of the height of both and recipient and donor [4] (Table 8.5).

7 Donor Preparation

The important factors that should be considered in a donor are age, sex, size, and ischemic time:

- Donor age: the donor age which is accepted for donation is variable from the earlier experience of heart transplantation until now. In 1985, the accepted mean age was 23 years, and in 2006–2013, the accepted mean age was increased to 35 years because an increased mean age will decrease the survival rate after transplantation. When the patient has ischemia time more than 4 h and ages more than 50 years, the 1-year and 2-year mortality rate will be high, so it is a poor outcome. A recent study was done to know the effect of interaction between ischemic time and donor age on survival rate. The study shows that the ischemia time above 240 min results in decreased 1-year survival rate to 16.7%, and when aged above 50 years, the 1-year and 2-year survival rate decreased to 50%. Another

Table 8.5 Routine pre-transplantation evaluation

– **History and physical examination**
- Age, BMI (weight and weight), surface area of the body
- Past medical history
- Drug history and allergies
- Immunization stat
  – **Laboratory information**
- Renal function test, urinalysis, GFR
- Liver function test
- Coagulation profile (PT, PTT)
- Complete blood count and differential
- Purified protein derivative (PPD)
- Viral serology (Hepatitis B and C, HIV, Cytomegalovirus, Epstein Barr virus, Toxoplasmosis gondii, Syphilis
- Panel reactivity antibody
- ABO blood type
  – **Consultation reviewing**
- Cardiopulmonary information
- Results of cardiac catheterization
- Echocardiography and ECG
- Chest X-ray
- Pulmonary function test
- Peak VO2
- Endomyocardial biopsy
- Radionucleotide angiography
  – **Psychological information**
- Substance abuse
- Long-term supportive care
- Possible relocation
- Evidence of abuse or neglecting

study shows that there are differences between survival rate and ischemic time suggesting that the younger donors tolerate more ischemic time than older donors because of old age related comorbidities. With a longer duration of comorbidities also the endothelial changes of coronary arteries began after the age of 35 years old, so results in poor outcomes after transplantation. In general, in patients who are candidates for transplantation, the risk of mortality of transplantation from an older donor is lower than the risk of mortality of non-transplanted candidate.

- Donor sex: sex is another important prognostic factor for heart transplantation because recipient–donor sex mismatching increases the risk of mortality due to episodes of rejection. also increased mortality rate after 1-year from transplantation. many studies show that the female donor is associated with mortality rate than male donor and the male recipients who receive heart transplant from female donor have increase mortality rate about 10% and male-recipients who receives heart transplant from male donor have higher 5 years survival rate than female, while female donor to female recipient increase survival rate about 10%. According to Khush and colleagues, there is no difference between sex-match and sex-mismatch when compare in cases of acute rejection. Another single center study shows that sex has no impact on the survival of male and female recipients of age less than 45 years while female donor decreases the survival rate in male recipients of age 45 years old or more. In general, the sex-mismatch is not potential barrier for heart transplantation.

- Donor size: The acceptable donor–recipients ratio for heart transplantation is 0.8–1.2. The donor–recipient ratio is a significant prognostic factor for 5 years survival rate according to a report by the international Society of heart and lung transplantation in 2007. In those with a ratio of less than 0.8, the 30-day mortality rate was highest according to to a study done between 1999–2007 by Patel and colleagues evaluate the United network for Oregon sharing/ organ procurement and transplantation network Registry. The study also evaluated the low ratio in those with pulmonary vascular resistance of more than 4 wood units. Another study uses weight-based matching and found that there are no significant differences in the survival rates between overweight, underweight, and normal weight. Another study uses the left ventricular mass and found that the differences of more than 10 to 15% result in decreased survival rate in some centers paint with pulmonary hypertension are transplanted oversized heart.
- Ischemic time: the ischemic time impact on survival rate and outcomes is unclear but generally the optional ischemic time is less than 240 min. The impact of ischemic time on the outcome is mainly related to donor age because there is no significant impact of ischemic time when the age is less than 20 years, while the ischemic time of 210–375 min in the age of 20 to 33 years and ischemic time of 210–330 min of the age of more than 30 years old decrease the survival rate. As a result of ischemic time of greater impact with increasing age.

Minimizing of ischemic time

Ischemic time can be minimized by the followings:

- Early transplantation of the heart as soon as the heart reaches the hospital.
- A new system was developed to reduce the ischemic time by pumping blood carrying oxygen and nutrients to the heart as early as possible after harvesting. This system is called " The Trans medics Organ Care System ".
- Aorta, pulmonary artery, and left atrium anastomosis are followed by removal of cross clamp to reperfuse of heart then the other anastomoses carried out on reperfused heart when the heart is retrieved immediately and anastomosis of great vessels to connectors that attached to the machine of this system. The system keeps the heart beating in optimal condition by pumping of nutrients, oxygenated blood, afterload, preload, and positive inotropic. Then the heart transplanted to transplanting Hospital under monitoring. The study shows that the system can reduce the ischemic time to 60 min with 100% 30 – days survival rate in 200 transplant patients.

8 Donor Risk Score

This score was used to evaluate short-term mortality and organ acceptance by using about 20 risk factors. It is created or Euro transplant Registry, Smits and colleagues. This score can predict 3–years survival rate. Another scoring system developed by Weiss and colleagues which include blood urea nitrogen/creatinine ratio, donor age, ischemic time, and race mismatching. The total score is 15 points. The 1-year mortality rate increased 9–13% for each one point increasing in scoring system. There is another scoring system named IMPACT, which mainly depends on recipient risk factors. Between 1984–2006, Segovia and colleagues studied about 621 heart transplantation depending on 6 predictors including age 30 years or more, diabetes mellitus, right atrial pressure 110 MmHg or more, inotropic dependence, and ischemic time 240 min or more. Out of 621, about 56 heart transplants developed primary graft failure. According to this study, Segovia and colleagues developed a risk scoring system which is a PADIAL risk calculator. Each one predicting Factor gate 1-point score and the total scoring points are 6 points. increasing of scoring system mean increase the risk of primary graft failure. the risk of primary organ failure increases about 5–folds when the scoring system 4–6 points.

9 Waiting List

The heart transplantation should be done as early as possible because later transplantation may result in some problems such as death before the availability of donor's heart or result in further organ failure of the recipient as renal failure or pulmonary hypertension or worsening of these already coexisting problems. A study showed that individuals who wait for the transplantation of the heart have more mortality rate than those who wait for other solid organ transplantation. The poorest prognostic factor for transplantation is patients who require for hemodynamic support and extracorporeal membrane oxygenation. followed by mechanical ventilation and using of inotropics. Other poor prognostic factors are dialysis, non-white ethnicity, and pretransplantation congenital anomalies of the heart. In September 1988, there were about 929 patients who were waiting for their transplantation. About 22% of those were waiting for 6–12 months and 10% were waiting for more than one year and about 55% died while waiting for heart Transplantation. Later, here are some techniques developed to make waiting time as long as possible by using artificial hearts which make many patients awaiting longer until the availability of a suitable heart. About 60 Artificial hearts were used in 1986. A study in one Hospital shows that the patients who are longer waiting for donor heart are became resistant to medical treatment and most of them require hospital admission. a survey in 18 Hospital show that about 17 of these hospitals reported that the waiting time in 1987 was longer than in 1985. In 1987, The International Society for heart transplantation reported many negative effects of donor shortage on survival rate and noted that some recipients died within 30-days post implantation. Society suggests that the cause of death was due to flexibility of acceptance of heart donor criterion. In 1987, a survey showed that the number of waiting donors was 1000 to 26,000 and suggests that in future the number will increase. This survey reported that about 82% of the population was ready to give permission for organ donation for their loved people, 61% were ready to donate their child's organs, and 48% wanted to donate their organs [5].

10   Selection of Operation Time

The donor heart should be preserved as soon as possible. In some studies, it is reported that the donor heart can be preserved for 4–6 h, but in some conditions should be preserved within 6 h as in marginal donor criteria or when there is pulmonary hypertension or size mismatching because of these conditions the early reperfusion of the heart improve the survival rate by the maintenance of function of the right ventricle. This shortening of the preservation time can be done by the coordination of recipient and donor operation time.

11   Anesthesia

Assessment of recipient for anesthesia.

Anesthetic assessment for heart transplantation is similar to other types of surgeries depending on history, physical examination, laboratory investigation, and imaging. Also, there are some issues should get a specific focusing at night of survey including:

- presence of extra cardiac device as automated implantable cardioverter-defibrillator should be turned off before surgery also pacemaker because these devices can Implicate placement of Central venous Line during anesthesia.
- airways scoring and examination of dental status.
- fasting time assessment; as some patients reach without fasting which requires rapid induction of anesthesia.
- reviewing the latest laboratory investigation such as blood group, hemoglobin, and complete blood count.
- preparing the blood and blood products.
- discussion of the risk and any procedure done before and during operation as risk of the placement of vascular lines, transesophageal echocardiography
- patients with ventricular assist device and planed for resternotomy should be done CT scan to assess the location of ventricular assisted device and its proximity to sternum to avoid damage of device during resternotomy.

- immunosuppressive drugs are given before the beginning of anesthesia, also giving IV short-acting benzodiazepines such as midazolam is preferable to oral sedation. Another premedication for the recipient is unnecessary

12   Monitoring of the Recipient

- Peripheral oxygen saturation.
- ECG monitoring: at least w leads (lead II and lead V5).
- Monitoring of arterial blood pressure in patients who have ventricular assisted device with no pulsation, catheterization done through a radial artery or brachial artery, and monitoring of the volume status and right ventricular infection through monitoring of the central venous pressure and evaluation of the cardiac output, pulmonary hemodynamics status, left arterial filling pressure, mixed venous oxygen saturation, and systemic vascular resistance. This can be done through the insertion of a pulmonary artery catheter following the removal of cardiopulmonary bypass.
- Left arterial pressure line for direct measurement of the left atrial pressure which can also measure ventricular diastolic pressure directly and monitoring of the body temperature, especially for those with moderate hypothermia and those on cardiopulmonary bypass.
- Transesophageal echocardiography for the evaluation of the volume status, right ventricle and left ventricular function, and valve function status.

13   Induction of Anesthesia

As heart transplant recipient is immunocompromised, intense aseptic conditions should be included to avoid the risk of infections, especially through vascular lines. insertion of peripheral line which also following induction of anesthesia. pulmonary artery catheter should be inserted. It is advisable to preoxygenate to avoid hypoxic attacks which occurred immediately after induction of anesthesia. The anesthesia should be titrating the speed of anesthesia to conscious level of the patient who have fluid overload, using of fast-flowing drip line is preferable for induction of anesthesia to give faster induction with low doses of anesthetics. after induction, the flow rate should be reduced to avoid accidental fluid overload. regarding choosing of an aesthetic for induction of anesthesia, all an aesthetic agent can be used safely with careful attention, but generally related to individual preference. Also, the ansthescian can use high dose of narcotics [6].

14 Coagulation Management

Because heart transplantation is a bloody operation, using anti-fibrinolytic agent before sternotomy is recommended by some heart transplantation centers. The most anti-fibrinolytic agents used are tranexamic acid and aprotinin. These agents have an adverse effect on organ function but waiting against the effect of transfusion of blood and blood products on organ function which is significant and cannot be ignored. A supplementary factor should be given post-operatively to patient on warfarin inform of Factor concentrate or fresh frozen plasma. the ISHLT recently recommended INR less than 1.5 in patients on Warfarin, also can use single dose of vitamin K to reverse the effect of warfarin in hospitalized patients using of thromboelastnografy to monitor platelet and factor replacement.

15 Maintenance of Anesthesia

After induction of anesthesia, the patient should be strictly monitored for pulmonary artery pressure, central venous pressure, cardiac output estimation, and trans-esophageal echocardiography to diagnose and deal with hemodynamic deception that occur during the period following induction of anesthesia. In patients with heart transplantation, the anesthesia maintenance can be done safely by remifentanil and propofol, vapor-based inhalation anesthesia. Usually, a combination of these agents is used.

16 Donor Heart Retrieval

Donors usually give permission for the donation of more than one organ. So, heart retrieval surgery is usually a part of multi-organ donation surgery. The donor should receive at least 300 unit/kg of heparin intravenously followed by the insertion of cardioplegia needle into ascending aorta to induce hypothermic cardiac arrest. The first step is ligation of the superior vena cava by using two silk ties for cessation of venous return followed by the opening of the inferior vena cava and ventilation of the left atrium to prevent distension of the left ventricle. Subsequently, cross clamping of the ascending aorta followed by rapid retrieval of the heart, which is then preserved in cardioplegia and kept in cold storage.

17 Cold Ischemic Time

Cold ischemic time represents the period of hypothermic cardiac arrest, which is induced by rapid flushing and cooling of the heart with a crystalloid fluid that protects the heart by many mechanisms:

- Reduce the cell Death caused by hypothermia
- Buffering of intracellular acidosis
- Prevent oxygen free radical induced injury
- Optimize their oncotic pressure which prevents expansion of the extracellular compartment
- Prevent reperfusion injury induced by ATP store depletion.

During the first years of heart transplantation, the cold ischemic storage was at 4 °C, but with an increase in the number of heart transplantation and doing of many studies, this technique is found to be a significant limitation because it was one of the significant risk factors for primary organ dysfunction and death and was the most common cause of 30-days mortality. The ischemic time has been studied by ISHLT registry 2012 heart statistic and Banner Et Al that found that the ischemic time more than 180 min has incremental and significant increase in a primary graft dysfunction. As a result, there are many confrontations emerging to sacrifice some steps of the survey to reduce the ischemic time. Also, there is a limiting donor pool due to the difficulty in the transport of organs to large distances. Studies and investigations are carried out for about 20 years but all failed due to an increase in the ischemic time for suitable donor heart beyond 240 min. There is an alternative technique for the preservation of heart, which includes the preservation of heart in a beating normothermic perfused state. Also, preservation and transporting of heart by OCS device which has similar short-term outcomes to cold ischemic storage but reduces the cold ischemic time which can help increase the donor heart pool and wide heart assessment. Other techniques include CO–treatment and remote pre-conditioning; but these techniques are under experimentation till now [7].

18 Recipient Cardiectomy

The incision for cardiectomy is median sternotomy followed by the dissection and isolation of the great vessels including pulmonary artery, aorta, superior vena cava, and inferior vena cava from adjacent structures, then insertion of tape snares around inferior vena cava and superior vena cava. After heparinization, cannulation of superior vena cava, inferior vena cava, and aorta just proximal to the innominate artery for cardiopulmonary bypass by dissection of the native heart is enough for cannulation. If needed further incision, it is done on cardiopulmonary bypass. If there is a previous sternotomy, preferable cannulation of inferior vena cava through the femoral vein which allows more area for anastomosis of inferior vena cava during implantation. Cross-clamping of the recipient's aorta was done after starting cardiopulmonary bypass and tightening of the snares around superior vena cava and inferior vena cava. For those with the left ventricular assisted device, the device should be turned off and the device outflow should be clamped before starting cardiopulmonary bypass. division of pulmonary artery and aorta just above semilunar valves. Excision of the right atrium completely by transection of the superior vena cava then inferior vena cava adjacent to their junction with the main body of the right atrium. Removal and the preservation of the Swan Ganz catheter on opening of superior vena cava. if there are any pacing leads should be placed on tension followed by the division of them. exposure of the lift atrium dome by retraction of the heart inferiorly. once the left atrium dome is exposed, it is opened and extension of incision to mitral valve annulus circumferentially. Then removal of the heart followed by removal of the left atrial appendage and trimming of the left atrial cuff. Trimming of superior vena cava, inferior vena cava, pulmonary artery and aorta individually. If there is left ventricular assisted device should be removed. Dissection, mobilization and division of the driveline from the thoracic cavity and at the end of the procedure, the remaining of the driveline should be removed because the exist site of driveline is contaminated. now, the donor heart enters the warm ischemic time after removal from the procurement container. before implantation, the donor heart should be inspected for any missed defects as congenital anomalies, valvular heart disease or patent foramen ovale. If the left ventricular appendage used for ventilation during procurement, the incision should be closed.

19 Implantation

The order of anastomosis procedure is left atrium, pulmonary artery, aorta anastomosis then the inferior vena cava and superior vena cava anastomosis. if necessary making of the heart is early reperfused by immediate removal of cross-clamping of the aorta after aortic and left atrial anastomosis but commonly the cross-clamping of aorta is removed after first 3 anastomoses.

- Left atrial anastomosis:

It is done by long double-armed running 3–0 polypropylene suture. The first stitch is placed at the level of the left superior pulmonary vein across the atrial cuff of the recipient. Then to the atrial cuff of the donor,i.e., at the left atrial appendage. The donor's heart is parachuted down inside the recipient's thorax after 3–4 stitch swings toward the left superior pulmonary vein for insulation of the donor's heart against warming from adjacent thoracic structures. The donor's heart should be wrapped with ice for cooling. The remaining stitches are placed at the level of the right inferior pulmonary vein and right superior pulmonary vein of the septum. The suture line is tied after continuation around inferior and superior left at atrial borders. application of excessive tissue If them is donor–recipient discrepancy. during constructing the suture line of the left atrium. It is impatient to sense the position of the donor and recipient superior vena cava and inferior vena cava. During implantation, the warming of the donor heart is caused by the accumulation of the pulmonary venous return by insertion of the left ventricular vent through the right superior pulmonary vein for airing [8].

- Pulmonary artery anastomosis:

Before the anastomosis of the pulmonary artery, it is firstly trimmed and should be fitted to the appropriate anastomosis length. The anastomosis was done by using a double-armed 4–0 polypropylene suture which began on the arterial back wall. It is important to remove the rudimentary issue at the ends pulmonary artery by trimming to avoid arterial kinking. after continuation of the suture line on the front wall, the suture is tied at the anterolateral aspect of the pulmonary artery using of everting suture technique if possible.

- Aortic artery anastomosis:

The aortic artery anastomosis is done in the same maneuver of the pulmonary artery anastomosis and also by using of double armed 4 -0 polypropylene suture and by using two-layer Technic anastomosis. the outer layer informs running suture pattern while the inner layer with horizontal suture pattern. The only difference Between the pulmonary artery anastomosis and aortic artery anastomosis is that the rudimentary tissue in arterial end is important for aortic artery anastomosis to allow seeming of the posterior suture line of the aorta and suture line of pulmonary artery and left atrium if there is a bleeding after removal of cross–clamping of the aorta. Also, to reduce the tension at the anastomosis site. after completing of anastomosis of the aorta, the patient should be Trendelenburg position and administration of steroid (500 mg of methylprednisolone) followed by releasing of cross–clamping. sometimes the aortic artery anastomosis is reinforced by strip of Teflon or natural pericardium as bovine pericardium. Then the vent of aortic roof can be placed into ascending aorta for airing.

- Caval anastomosis:

The superior vena cava and inferior vena cava are anastomosed while the heart is beating. Upon the pulmonary artery anastomosis, the end of the caval veins should be trimmed to avoid rudimentary tissue that may cause kinking of veins. The caval anastomosis was done in a pattern of end-to-end anastomosis by using of 4-0 polypropylene suture beginning at the posterior wall. Enough time is required for adequate reperfusion prior to the removal of cardiopulmonary bypass. the enough time for reperfusion is about 15 min for each hour of ischemic time then gradually removal of cardiopulmonary bypass. After heart transplantation, perioperative right ventricular failure develops in those with pre-existing pulmonary hypertension and has increased pulmonary vascular resistance caused by the effect of cardiopulmonary bypass. So, it is important to administrate pulmonary arteries vasodilators as inhaler nitric oxide or flolan before weaning from cardiopulmonary bypass to lowering pulmonary vascular resistant and to prevent the perioperative right ventricular failure. Some centers may use the pulmonary artery vent to prevent acute right ventricular dilatation and assist the cardiopulmonary Bypass on weaning. Also, the pulmonary dilatation may be induced by keeping pco2 between 30–35. The heart rate of implanted heart should be 100–120 beats per minute by using of pacing wire or isoproterenol to ensure adequate cardiac output from both ventricles. Also, intraoperative assessment of ventricular function and valves by using transesophageal echocardiography.

- Right atrial anastomosis:

The anastomosis of the right atrium starts at the upper border of the atrial incision by using of running suture pattern with a 3–0 polypropylene suture. Initially, the dental anastomosis should be completed by carrying of suture superiorly and inferiorly then both ends joined into the lateral atrial wall. at this point of anastomosis, the rewarming of the heart is started.

- Reperfusion:

After completing at least three of four anastomoses, the perfusion is initiated by releasing of aortic cross-clamping followed by completing of other anastomoses on the perfused heart but the surgical field will be profoundly bloody, so the blood should be cleared by using the pump sucker and then the heart is aired by using the vent followed by pacing of the heart with the help of pacing wires that put on the ventricles to initiate heart rate about 90–100 beats per minute to avoid dilatation of the ventricles, especially when the left ventricular vent is removed. Later, the heart rate should be maintained between 100–120 beats per minute to ensure adequate cardiac output and to reduce the stress on the cardiac wall by lowering the diastolic filling. During the early stage of reperfusion, transesophageal echocardiography is used for assessment of the airing adequacy because the air may accumulate in specific sites such as pulmonary veins, atrial appendages, and left ventricular apex. Continue the perfusion until normal ECG tracing and there is evidence of vigorous contraction and completed de-airing. Continuous reperfusion is aimed to reduce the ischemic time to less than 180 min. After presence of indication for cardiopulmonary weaning, the cardiopulmonary bypass should be removed slowly in a stepwise pattern starting weaning at 75%, 50%, and 25%. This gradual weaning is important for recognizing the problems that may occur during weaning as dysrhythmia or ventricular distension. Also, it is important to assess the ventricular function during weaning because ventricular dysfunction during weaning is an indication of mechanical support or increase positive inotropes. When there is a primary graft dysfunction, there is a range of manifestations starting from complete organ dysfunction to one ventricular dysfunction and then dysfunction of both ventricles, which is an indication for continuous cardiopulmonary bypass while starting interventional therapeutic measures.

After weaning from cardiopulmonary bypass, a functional deterioration may occur at specific points of time including:

- During the administration of the blood products: the pulmonary circulation may be adversely affected by platelet perfusion due to the release of vasoactive substances or volume overload or it is associated with primary graft dysfunction.

- During the administration of protamine: due to right ventricular failure or vasodilatation induced by rapid administration of protamine
- During the closure of the Chester: due to ventricular distension that leads to ventricular compression. If the sternal wires compress the ventricular surface, the chest closure is done by limited tightening of one wire, but if the chest closure induces primary organ dysfunction or hemodynamic change, a chest stenting is indicated for 24 h to overcome right ventricular function deterioration.

Checklist for weaning preparation

- Connection of positive inotropic for weaning and allow to flow in low levels for waiting of inotropic effects while the central venous line pass through dead space
- Handing off all medications that may be required
- Calibration and setting up on nitric oxide if needed
- Availability of dual chamber pacing
- Preparation of pressure transducer for left atrial and pulmonary artery pressure

Checklist for starting CPB weaning

- Resuming of ventilation
- Hemoglobin, potassium, and pH should be within acceptable ranges
- Monitoring of heart rhythm by using at least VV1 pacing but using AA1 or DDD is preferable. The rhythm should be within the acceptable range
- Assessment of de-airing by using 4/5 chamber view transesophageal echocardiography
- Flowing nitric oxide if needed
- Preparation of intraoartic balloon pump
- Siting of left atrial line is recommended to assess the left ventricular filling pressure

20　Heart injury

Causes of heart injury in donors and during donor heart retrieval:

(1) Heart donation after Brian death: during donor heart retrieval, the heart should be perfused and ventilated by using oxygenated blood until the time of retrieval. There are many insults that may cause heart injury during this stage which are including secondary injuries inherent in Brian death or iatrogenic injuries as suboptimal ventilation or fluid overload. There are some events that associated to Brian death as release of myocardial norepinephrine resulting in significant calcium overload in mitochondria, which initiates the apoptosis of myocardial cells. Also, releasing of myocardial norepinephrine may result in the release of many proinflammatory mediators which result in acute lung injury and non-cardiogenic pulmonary edema (neurogenic pulmonary edema) due to pulmonary epithelial damage and breaking of capillary–alveolar membranes [9].

(2) Donation after detection of cardiac death: according to DCD donor criteria, the suitable donors are usually patients who depend on mechanical ventilation but don't meet the criteria of brain death. They are allowed to donate only after cardiac death which is followed by the beginning of the warm ischemic time after weaning from life-sustaining therapy. This period is characterized by a critical level of hemodynamics state that is still satisfactory for organ perfusion (systolic blood pressure 50 MmHg or less). when stopping of circulation, an interval of about 5 min which called "no touch time interval" to ensure the death to allow for ensuring donation then the cold ischemic time start. during interval of warm ischemic time and non-touch Time interval, the heart may suffer from hypoperfusion and the ischemia. The donor heart condition can be optimized inside the donor by specific management (see table standard approach to donor …).

Alternatives to cold storage heart allograft preservation.

The alternatives to cold storage preservation give more advantages than cold storage preservation.

These alternatives include:

- Repetitive or continuous cold perfusion of the heart during preservation which makes preservation time longer. Some experiences on pigs showed that the heart which is preserved for 24 h gives acceptable function after transplantation
- Heart preservation in functioning, warm status by using of organ care system (OCS). This system facilitates randomized, prospective trial (known as PROCEED II trial). This system can preserve the heart beating, perfused and normothermic ex vivo. In standard groups experience, the reported ischemic time of cold storage preservation was about 195 min and 30–days survival rate was about 97% while in group of organ care system, the ischemic time was about 113 min and 30 - days survival rate was about 94% but there was no significant difference in incidence of sever rejection, cardiac adverse events and length of ICU admission in donor heart which is on organ care system can be assessed functionally, biochemically due to reduced cold storage time.so in once the heart on organ care system, can use extended criteria. An experience has done in single center reported that the using of EVHP in procedure of high-risk heart donor transplantation which defined as either recipient factors including Raised pulmonary vascular resistance, MCS or both. Or donor factors including:

  - Left ventricular ejection fraction <50%
  - Ischemic time >4 h.
  - Donor cardiac arrest.
  - Left ventricular hypertrophy.
  - Coronary artery disease.
  - Drug or alcohol abuse.

In this experience, about 30 hearts were preserved by the organ care system, of which about 26 were transplanted safely. One death was reported during the first year after transplantation. The other 25 patients reported good biventricular function. As a result, the EVHP can be used to optimize the survival rate in high-risk donor heart due to injury attenuation and allow for investigation to ensure suitability of the heart according to DCD donor criteria. During the period between weaning from life support therapy and heart harvesting, the heart experiences multiple injuries including hypoperfusion, hypoxia, and ventricular distension. A study done on pigs assessed the role of EVHP in DCD. The heart was exposed to warm ischemia for 30 minutes and then preserved in two groups. The first group of hearts was preserved for 4 h by EVHP and the second group was preserved for 4 h by standard cold storage. In the first group, 5 out of 6 hearts displayed favorable lactate profile and successfully weaned from cardiopulmonary bypass, while all hearts in the second group experienced acute severe primary graft dysfunction and couldn't be weaned from cardiopulmonary bypass. As a result, the role of EVHP in DCD heart transplantation may be related to continuous perfusion which makes the cells depend on aerobic metabolism and maintain the cellular nutrients which prevent both ischemic injury and reperfusion injury [10].

Multiple Choice Questions:

1. **The most common indication for heart transplantation is**

   A. Dilated Cardiomyopathy
   B. Coronary artery disease
   C. Recurrent cardiac arrhythmia
   D. Heart failure with pulmonary hypertension

2. **According to NYHA classification, all of the following are true except**

   A. Category I: The patient develops a symptom only During heavy activities
   B. Category II: The patient develops a symptom during ordinary activities
   C. Category III: The patient develops a symptom during maximum exercise
   D. Category IV: The patient develops a symptom at rest

3. **According to ACC/AHA classification of heart failure severity. All of the following are true except**

   A. Stage A: patients have a high risk for the development of heart failure
   B. Stage B: asymptomatic patient with structural heart disease
   C. Stage C: symptomatic patient with structural heart disease
   D. Stage D: stable patient with advanced heart failure

4. **All of the following are absolute indications of heart transplantation except**

   A. Heart failure induced hemodynamic Instability
   B. Refractory cardiogenic shock
   C. Patients with Heart failure who Completely depend on inotropic to Maintain adequate cardiac output
   D. Recurrent unstable angina unsuitable for coronary intervention

5. **All of the following are relative indications of heart transplantation except**

    A. Peak VO2 is 11–14 ml/kg/min for 55% predicted that largely Interfere with routine activities of the patient
    B. Heart failure induced hemodynamic Instability
    C. Recurrent unstable angina unsuitable for coronary intervention
    D. Recurrent fluid imbalance or renal function abnormality in patients who complained of medical therapy

6. **The positive serological test is contraindicated for heart transplantation for all of the following except**

    A. Toxoplasma gondii
    B. Hepatitis
    C. HIV
    D. Human T-cell lymphocytic virus (HTLV)

7. **All of the following are criteria for donor heart selection except**

    A. No history of heart disease or chest trauma
    B. No prolonged hypoxia or hypotension
    C. Donor age > 55 years
    D. Negative viral serology (hepatitis B and C, HIV)

8. **The average donor–recipient ratio of the size that is acceptable for heart transplantation is**

    A. 1
    B. 1.5
    C. 2
    D. 2.5

9. **The optimal ischemic time for heart transplantation is**

    A. More than 240 min
    B. Less than 240 min
    C. Less than 300 min
    D. Unclear time

10. **The most important lifestyle effect on heart transplantation is**

    A. Sedentary lifestyle
    B. High dietary fat
    C. Substance abuse
    D. Living in high amplitude

11. **The system that is used to reduce the ischemic time is called**

    A. The Trans medics Organ Care System
    B. ACC/AHA system
    C. IMPACT scoring system

D. Weiss and colleagues scoring system

12. **The accepted preservation time of the donor's heart should be**

    A. Less than 6 h
    B. Less than 240 min
    C. Just a few minutes
    D. Not limited time

13. **The most anti-fibrinolytic agents used before sternotomy during heart transplantation surgery is**

    A. Warfarin
    B. Fresh frozen plasma
    C. Heparin
    D. Tranexamic acid and aprotinin.

14. **The first step in donor's heart retrieving surgery is**

    A. Opening of inferior vena cava
    B. Ligation of superior vena cava
    C. Ventilation of the Left atrium
    D. Cross clamping of the ascending

15. **Cold ischemic time can protect the heart by all of the following mechanisms except**

    A. Prevent oxygen free radical induced injury
    B. Reduce the cell Death caused by hypothermia
    C. Prevent reperfusion injury induced by ATP store depletion.
    D. Buffering of intracellular alkalosis

16. **During Recipient cardiectomy, when the patient has a previous sternotomy, the preferable site for inferior vena cava cannulation is through which one of the following**

    A. Femoral vein
    B. Jugular vein
    C. Great saphenous vein
    D. Cephalic vein

17. **After heart implantation in the recipient's chest, the time of cross- clamping of aorta removal is**

    A. Just after left atrial anastomosis
    B. At the beginning of implantation
    C. After anastomosis of Left atrium, pulmonary artery, aorta Anastomosis then the inferior vena cava and superior vena cava
    D. At the end of implantation

18. **The heart rate of implanted heart should be**

    A. < 100 pbm
    B. 100–120 bpm
    C. >120 bpm
    D. It's not significant to set the heart rate

19. **All of the following heart structures are anastomosed by using 4–0 polypropylene suture except**

    A. Aorta
    B. Pulmonary artery
    C. Vena cava
    D. Right atrium

20. **The first step after primary graft dysfunction is**

    A. Continuous cardiopulmonary bypass
    B. Giving diuretics
    C. Giving digoxin
    D. No interventional option is needed

Answers and Explanations

1. **A.** The most common indication for heart transplantation is dilated cardiomyopathy which represents about 53%. Coronary artery disease is the second most common indication which represents about 38%. Recurrent arrhythmia is not a common indication. Heart failure in the presence of pulmonary hypertension is not an indication of heart transplantation
2. **C.** Category III: the patient develops a symptom during minimal exercise, not maximum exercise
3. **D.** Stage D: the patient has refractory heart failure
4. **D.** Recurrent unstable angina unsuitable for coronary intervention is a relative indication for heart transplantation
5. **B.** Heart failure induced hemodynamic instability is an absolute indication
6. **A.** Any donor with positive screening for Hepatitis, HIV, or HTLV is considered a contraindication for donation, while the donors who are positive for Epstein Barr virus, Cytomegalovirus, or Toxoplasma gondii are not considered as contraindication for donation but require management post transplantation
7. **C.** The donor age should be < 55 years old
8. **A.**The acceptable donor–recipients' ratio for heart transplantation is 0.8–1.2 (average is 1)
9. **B.** The optimal ischemic time for heart transplantation is less than 240 min
10. **C.** The most important lifestyle effect on heart transplantation is substance abuse (reactive drugs, alcohol, smoking)
11. **A.** The system that is used to reduce the ischemic time is called The Trans medics Organ Care System. The ACC/AHA system is a classification system for the severity of heart failure. IMPACT and Weiss and colleagues scoring system used to evaluate 3 years of mortality and the organ acceptance
12. **A.** The accepted preservation time of a donor's heart should be less than 6 h

13. **D.** Tranexamic acid and aprotinin are the most commonly used anti-fibrinolytic agents before sternotomy during heart transplantation surgery
14. **B.** The first step is ligation of the superior vena cava by using two silk ties for cessation of venous return followed by the opening of the inferior vena cava and ventilation of the Left atrium to prevent distension of the left ventricle. Subsequently followed by the cross-clamping of the ascending aorta
15. **D.** Cold ischemic time can protect the heart by buffering intracellular acidosis
16. **A.** The preferable site for inferior vena cava cannulation in a patient with a previous sternotomy is through femoral vein
17. **C.** The cross-clamping of aorta is removed after anastomosis of the Left atrium, pulmonary artery, and aorta followed by the anastomosis of inferior vena cava and superior vena cava
18. **C.** The heart rate of implanted heart should be 100–120 pbm by using Pacing wire or isoproterenol to ensure adequate cardiac output from both ventricles
19. **D.** Aorta, pulmonary artery, and vena cava are anastomosed by using 0–4 polypropylene sutures, while the right atrium is anastomosed by using 0–3 polypropylene sutures
20. **A.** The first step in the treatment of primary graft dysfunction is continuous cardiopulmonary bypass

References

1. Piperata A, et al. Marginal donors and organ shortness: concomitant surgical procedures during heart transplantation: a literature review. Journal of Cardiovascular Medicine (Hagerstown, Md.) (2021).
2. Wu Z, et al. Prompt graft cooling enhances cardioprotection during heart transplantation procedures through the regulation of mitophagy. Cells. 2021;10(11): 2912.
3. Khush KK et al. The international thoracic organ transplant registry of the international society for heart and lung transplantation: thirty-fifth adult heart transplantation report—2018; focus theme: multiorgan transplantation. J Heart Lung Transplant. 2018; 37(10):1155–1168.
4. Jha SR, et al. Reversibility of frailty after bridge-to-transplant ventricular assist device implantation or heart transplantation. Transpl Direct. 2017; 3(7).
5. Minhas A, et al. Association of hospital procedural volume with outcomes in heart transplantation. Circulation. 2021;144(1): A9998–A9998
6. Guglin M, et al. Evaluation for heart transplantation and LVAD implantation: JACC council perspectives. J Am College Cardiol. 2020;75(12): 1471–1487.
7. Roberts WC, Kietzman AT, Rao PK. Malignant ventricular tachycardia, ventricular wall ablation, and orthotopic heart transplantation. Am J Cardiol. 2021.
8. Fiore A et al. "Valvular surgery in donor hearts before orthotopic heart transplantation." Archives of Cardiovascular Diseases. 2020;113(11): 674–678.
9. Hahnel F et al. Transvenous lead extraction after heart transplantation: How to avoid abandoned lead fragments. J Cardiovascular Electrophysiol. 2020;31(4): 854–859
10. Tsamalaidze L, Elli EF. Bariatric surgery is gaining ground as treatment of obesity after heart transplantation: report of two cases. Obes Surg. 2017;27(11):3064–7.

Complications and Follow Up

Morad Al Mostafa, Qasim Mehmood, Haya Mohammed Abujledan, and Maryam Salma Babar

Abstract Heart transplant could be a life rising medical care that's related to vital complications. Adults with heart transplants had a median survival rate of 10.7 years. While early graft failure and multi-organ system disease are the leading causes of early death, late mortality is influenced by malignancy, rejection, infection, and internal organ transplant vasculopathy. When a patient has a heart transplant, chronic excretory organ disease is frequent, occurring in up to 68% of patients by year 10. Acute rejection may be a typical drawback after a heart transplant, and a heart diagnostic test can detect the rejection phase. Most rejection episodes can be reversed if caught and treated early on. Anti-rejection drugs, which prevent the body from rejecting the replacement of heart, have the unintended consequence of weakening the system and causing nephrotoxicity. Infection might be a prevalent cause of morbidity and death in heart transplant recipients.

Keywords Complications · Follow up · Graft rejection · Transplant rejection · Immunosuppression · Thrombosis · Endomyocardial biopsy · Coronary artery vasculopathy · Heart biopsy · Anti-rejection medicines

M. Al Mostafa (✉)
Jordan University of Science and Technology, Ar-Ramtha, Jordan
e-mail: morad_95@icloud.com

Q. Mehmood
King Edward Medical University, Lahore, Pakistan

H. M. Abujledan
Hashemite University, Genetic engineering, Amman, Jordan

M. S. Babar
Dubai Medical College, Dubai, UAE

1   Introduction

Cardiac transplantation is considered the gold standard treatment for patients with the most advanced stages of cardiopathy. This procedure, on the other hand, is not a permanent solution, and patients are at risk of acquiring a variety of issues throughout the post-transplant period [1].

Complications once transplant may be divided into postoperative, early, and late. Complications are linked to the denervated transplant heart's different physiology, as well as the immunological disorder drugs required to maintain graft function [1].

This chapter highlights the foremost frequent complications following heart transplant, together with rejection, viscus transplant vasculopathy, graft pathology, chronic nephrosis, infection, and malignancy. The long-term goals of heart transplantation necessitate such collaboration. Such cooperation is critical in achieving the long-term aims of cardiac transplantation.

Survival and quality of life once viscus transplantation area unit restricted by a number of adverse clinical events. These emerge commonly after viscus transplantation and show the results of the transplant procedure, alloimmune reactions to the transplanted heart, and hence the side effects of immunological disorder medications used to suppress these responses. Early adverse events embrace acute cellular rejection and infections. Later complications embrace viscus transplant vasculopathy, malignancies, and antibody-mediated rejection. Adverse outcomes linked to immunological disorders and medical treatment might occur at the same time. Changes in immunological disorder treatment regimens, as well as the deployment of diagnostic methods and medicines, may help to reduce problems and improve outcomes.

Any procedure has the potential for problems, but transplantation has its own set of risks (Fig. 9.1).

Fig. 9.1 The complications of heart transplantation

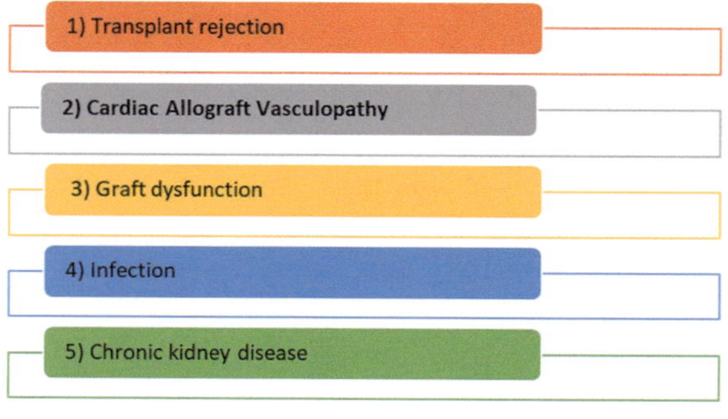

2 Transplant Rejection

Transplant rejection occurs when the recipient's system rejects the transplanted tissue, causing it to be destroyed [1]. The graft rejection response is complex, both in terms of how the graft antigens are supplied to and identified by the host leukocytes and in terms of the effector part of the response that often leads to graft harm. Rejection of a transplant occurs when the system recognizes the organ or tissue as alien, generating a reaction that may lead to the death of the transplanted organ or tissue. In transplantation, the system is extremely important. Immune processes that, under normal conditions, work to detect foreign bacteria and urge the system to eliminate them, provide a significant obstacle to flourishing transplantation.

What is heart transplant rejection?

Transplant rejection is a very regular occurrence. Even those who take all of their medications exactly as recommended are prone to it. The number of people who have been treated for rejection has decreased: According to a 2018 study from the International Society for Heart and Respiratory Organ Transplantation (ISHLT) registry, the frequency of any acute cellular rejection between discharge and one year has decreased from 30% in 2004 to 2006 to 12% in 2017 to 2018 [2]. Because the written record did not gather information on delicate rejection events (grade 1 R) or antibody-mediated rejection, this suggests that an Associate in Nursing underestimated total rejection. Furthermore, as a result of the widespread belief that mild acute cellular rejection does not require immediate therapy, the rate of treated rejection has decreased from 23% for initial transplants from 2004 to 2006 to 12.6% from 2010 to 2016. Acute cellular rejection is the most prevalent kind of cardiac transplant rejection. Rejection after a heart transplant might take a long time (chronic) [3]. Chronic rejection may take the form of coronary artery vasculopathy. The coronary arteries are affected. The inner lining of the blood vessel thickens in coronary artery vasculopathy. This might result in reduced blood flow to the heart muscle [4].

3 Etiology for Heart Transplant Rejection (HTR) Varies Based on the Onset of Rejection

- *Hyperacute rejection*

When the cross-clamp is removed during the immediate post-transplant period, hyperacute rejection can develop.

- *Acute cellular rejection (ACR).*

This is the most prevalent kind of rejection. It occurs when T cells, which are immune system cells, assault the new heart's cells. It usually occurs within the first three to six months following a transplant (Fig. 9.2).

Fig. 9.2 Rejection types

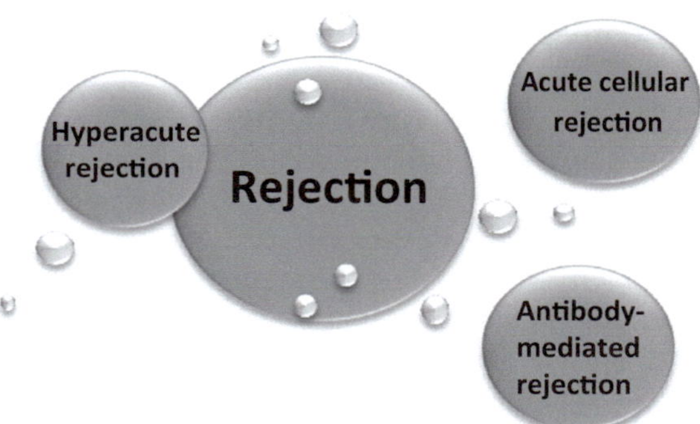

- *Antibody-mediated rejection (AMR)*

Who is at risk of having a heart transplant rejected?

The genetic mismatch between the donors and the recipients is the major risk factor for this type of rejection [5]. Younger heart recipients also are at bigger risk for each sort of rejection. Other things that specifically increase the possibilities of acute transplant rejection include:

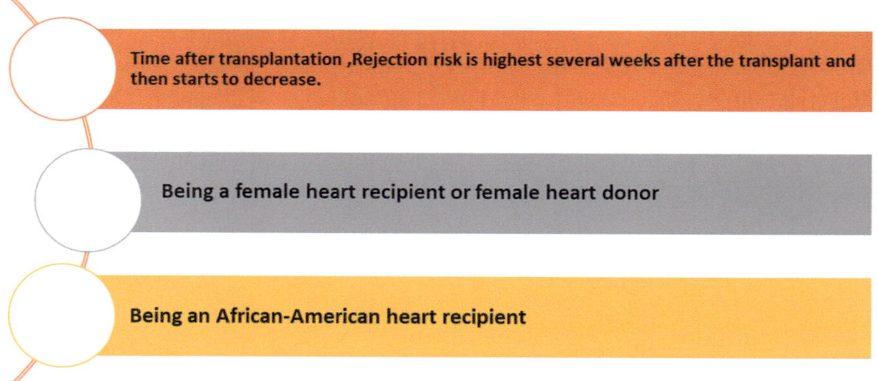

Rejection is prevalent when there are no symptoms. Because of the stringent post-transplant screening criteria, a heart attack might potentially be the major symptom.

4 Heart Transplant Rejection

Diagnosis: There are no clinical criteria that can be relied on to establish this diagnosis. Until proven otherwise, a heart transplant recipient who shows indications of cardiac failure should be considered acutely rejected. A cardiac diagnostic test is frequently used to identify acute rejection (biopsy). When you undergo a heart transplant, you will be able to have many routine biopsies. This enables people to cope with rejection. Before any symptoms appear, these biopsies frequently indicate evidence of transplant rejection. Early detection of rejection increases the chances of recovery.

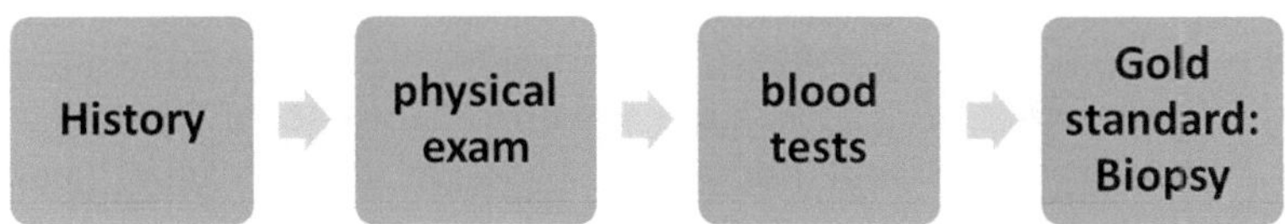

A. *History*

Symptoms of cardiac rejection are also vague and ambiguous in the early stages and include weariness and pain. Arrhythmias don't seem to be diagnostic of rejection, however, ought to increase suspicion that it's occurring.

B. *Physical Examination Findings*

Physical indicators of heart failure in any patient, as well as the development of lower-than-normal blood pressure for them, are particularly concerning.

Significant rises from a baseline heart rate have the same alarming implications as decreased blood pressure. Mental obtundation and cold, damp extremities are common indications of inadequate cardiac output in extreme instances.

In the post-transplant patient, various causes of heart failure should be investigated. Pericardial tamponade is caused by the existence of a (serosa) pericardial effusion, which is especially frequent early after surgery.

C. *What diagnostic tests ought to be performed?*

ECG (Echocardiography) is the mainstay for the diagnosis of arrhythmias and some other problems such as MI. Other diagnostic methods such as x-ray and echocardiography may help.

Echocardiogram to assess heart function

Transthoracic echocardiography is the most important diagnostic test for ruling out many issues with the pericardium or the cardiac tissue itself. If there are no other evident explanations such as ischemia or infection, a decline in systolic function of more than 10% should prompt an endocardial biopsy. There are no radiological studies that help diagnose cardiac rejection.

- Sometimes other tests are needed to diagnose chronic rejection.

"Gold Standard".

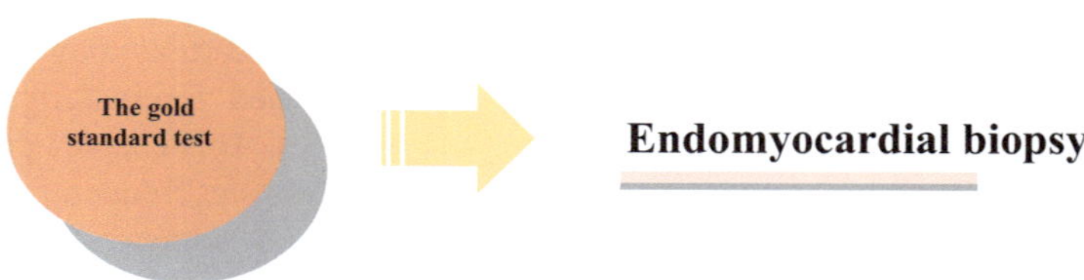

The only way to find out whether you've been refused is to get a biopsy. Approximately two weeks following transplantation, routine biopsies begin, and later as desired by the transplant cardiologist. In the hands of a trained professional, this operation is perfectly safe and has just a few minor side effects. For the histological severity of acute cardiac rejection, there is a globally recognized pathology nosological scale.

Immunohistochemistry and a serotyped test for the presence of donor-specific antibody titers should be obtained if the antibody-mediated rejection is anticipated [6].

5 Possible Alternatives

Endomyocardial biopsy has been replaced by gene expression profiling as a diagnostic tool. Gene expression profiling was shown to be non-inferior and safe in the E-IMAGE trial when compared to endomyocardial biopsy.

"Serum antibodies directed against HLA class I and II allograft antigen may accompany histologic findings in Acute Humoral/Antibody Rejection (AMR). If there is any histological evidence of antibiotic resistance. Non-HLA antibodies such as anti-endothelium, anti-vimentin, and anti-MCA/MICB are also worth in-vestigating in the absence of anti-HLA antibodies" [7].

6 Histopathology

The existence of histological evidence should be used to make a diagnosis. Noninvasive monitoring, such as troponin measurement, Doppler echocardiography, cardiac magnetic resonance imaging (MRI), imaging with radioactive lymphocytes, and antimyosin antibodies or annexin-V, is used in up to 20% of instances with negative biopsy rejection.

7   Histological Grading

(a) *ISHLT ACCR classification*

There is no proof of refusal (or) Grade 0R refers to the lack of lymphatic infiltration and no signs of cellular rejection. In essence, this is a clean biopsy that only comprises matte endocardium. Non-rejection characteristics such as the Quilty effect or biopsy site alterations may appear in one of these biopsies, but these should be reported separately and should not raise the degree of rejection. (b) a kind rejection (1R) It's characterized as interstitial and/or perivascular infiltration with a myocyte damage concentration of up to one. A modest number of perivascular lymphocytes from a highly stressed infiltrate of benign lymphocytes to more than one myocyte focus can all be seen in the infiltrate. In general, 1R-sorted biopsies do not include eosinophils or neutrophils. It's very challenging to do bilateral surgeries with a single focus on muscle cell damage. Is it possible that only one focus was discovered because the biopsy was insufficient? Is it possible that the Quilty effect is akin to muscle cell injury? When a biopsy that matches the criteria for grade 1R is especially busy or has a singular focus on myocyte damage, it is generally good to take it to the doctor.

(b) *moderate rejection (2R)*

In this type, there will be more than one site of inflammatory filtration. In the lack of widespread infiltrates, one must wonder if they are exaggerating muscle cell damage, and alternative rejection mimics should be considered. It's usually a good idea to let doctors know if there's 2R rejection in the biopsy since it necessitates immediate therapy.

(c) *extreme rejection (3R)*

In this type, which is the most serious one, there will be a widespread inflammatory response. This level of rejection is characterized by a high number of eosinophils and some neutrophils. Across the biopsy tissue, there is a significant inflammatory infiltration. This type of damage can cause edema, bleeding, and vasculitis.

Antibody-mediated rejection: Swelling of endothelial cells, macrophages filling the lumen of tiny arteries, and edema are histopathological alterations to antimicrobial resistance that may be detected on light microscopy. Immunohistochemistry or immunofluorescence staining of the split C4d product is commonly employed to assess the presence of AMR.

AM

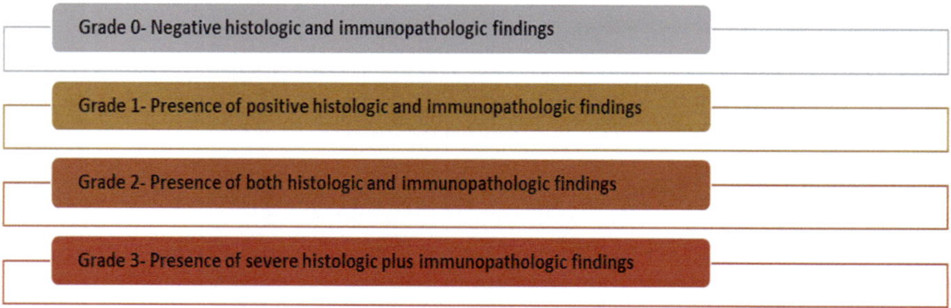

8   Prevent Rejection

To reduce the risk of rejection, antibodies are measured before and after transplantation [8].

The objective is to limit medication toxicity and infection risk while suppressing organ rejection. The type of rejection determines the treatment plan. Acute rejection persists despite the administration of powerful immunosuppressive medications immediately after heart transplantation and throughout long-term maintenance.

Post-transplant immunosuppressive medication greatly lowered the risk of rejection. Steroids, anti-proliferative treatment like cyclosporine, sirolimus/tacrolimus, and anti-metabolites like azathioprine, mycophenolate mofetil, and rapamycin are commonly used in immunosuppressive therapy. The ISHLT registry's 34th heart transplant consensus found that patients who were given tacrolimus-based immunosuppression had a lower risk of rejection than those who were given cyclosporine.

9   Acute Cellular Rejection

To prevent or control acute cellular rejection, an intravenous steroid may be used that functions by inhibiting the cells from acting or performing their actions. Another way that may be used is the anti-thymic globulin. The choice between these methods is made depending on the recipient's hemodynamic condition and the histological reality of the rejection [9].

10 Antibody-Mediated Rejection

Often, all transplant facilities choose a pulsed steroid in combination with plasmapheresis as the first therapy. Antimicrobial resistance therapy relies heavily on plasmapheresis. Plasmapheresis has long been used in conjunction with other immunosuppressive drugs; nevertheless, antimicrobial resistance can still occur if this is the only therapy. Among the most often utilized plasma separation technologies are the exchange method and double filtering technology. Both methods are non-selective, removing immunoglobulins in a nonspecific manner. Plasmapheresis with membrane adsorbent is more selective for antibody removal, but it is also costlier. Hypovolemia and infection are concerns associated with each kind of plasma cell. For individuals who require inotropic or mechanical circulatory support, cell treatment will be very beneficial. Anti-thymocyte globulin may directly decrease B cell activity, whereas cytolytic treatment may reduce B cell activation indirectly. Rituximab is a chimeric monoclonal antibody that is produced against the CD20 protein found on B cells' surfaces. Rituximab in conjunction with plasmapheresis, IVIg, or steroids has been shown to improve treatment outcomes [2]. In phase I/phase II investigations, a humanized monoclonal antibody against IL-6R (tocilizumab) was utilized to treat chronic active AMR in individuals who were resistant to high-dose IVIg.

Antimicrobial resistance prevention and treatment will rely heavily on complementary blocking. Clinical studies have looked at agents that target the C5 and C1 esterase. Eculizumab reduces complementarity by binding to the C5 protein in the complement system. It hinders the breakdown of C5 and the creation of MAC. Antibody-lowering medication should be added since eculizumab cannot reduce donor-specific antigen levels. T lymphocytes are targeted by the antibody Anti-T-Cell Globulin (ATG). This family of medicines is successful in treating ACR; as a result, it has been modified for the treatment of antimicrobial resistance, however, there is limited data on its effectiveness.

11 Long-term Management

Long-term post-treatment management of a heart transplant recipient's acute rejection episode includes careful monitoring of immunosuppressive drug levels to ensure they stay within therapeutic ranges, as well as careful monitoring of infectious complications that can occur during periods of intense immunosuppression.

Possible complications of heart transplant rejection:

The most common unintended side effects or sequelae of rejection therapy are opportunistic infections and the development of malignancy [10].

Pathogenesis

Alloantigen-independent variables and the Alloimmune System Interaction response to a response to a response to a response to a response to a response.

Chronic rejection" has been a term used to describe CAV for a long time. This phrase, however, is misleading since it ignores antigen-independent variables. Rather, the idea of 'response to damage' states that vascular lesions are the consequence of accumulated endothelial (vascular) harm caused by both malignant immune responses and nonspecific insults that are 'independent of allogenic immunity [9, 11, 12].

12 Diagnosis

A diagnosis of CAV based on the conventional symptoms of angina pectoris is doubtful because of the illegitimate innervation. If symptoms of graft impairment, such as regional wall anomalies and/or restricted diastolic dysfunction, are observed during a regular echocardiographic evaluation, it should be considered. CAV is generally in an advanced stage when they become symptomatic, and the damage to the heart muscle is irreparable. As a result, screening procedures are required to enhance early detection.

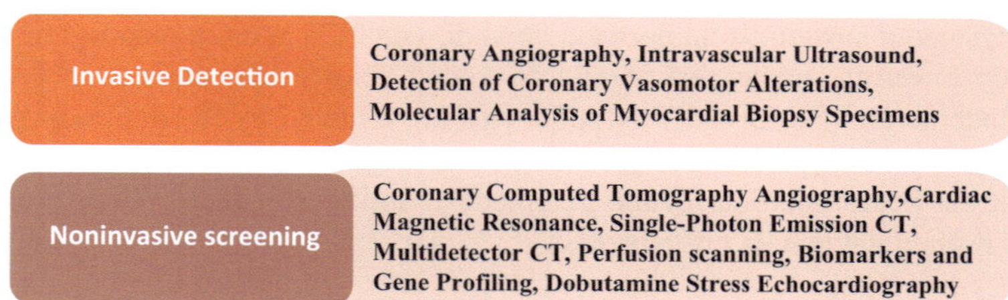

Other methods contain analysis of microvascular changes in routine endocardial biopsies and non-invasive methods such as stress echocardiography, CT coronary angiography, and measurement of blood biomarkers [13–15].

- *Angiography*

- *Intravascular ultrasound (IVUS).*

The most sensitive method for detecting CAV is intravascular ultrasonography (IVUS). IVUS enables repeated imaging of the endothelium's and media's real bore diameter, appearance, and thickness.

Internal thickness increases at the greatest pace during the first year after transplantation, with a rise in maximum internal thickness (MIT) of 0.5 mm indicating a quicker development of CAV during that time. Although IVUS can be used to assess disease risk, define prognosis, and guide treatment, this is not a widely accepted use. Conventional coronary angiography should be done yearly or biannually to check CAV advancement, according to current ISHLT recommendations [16].

Microvascular function testing has been proven to have predictive significance following heart transplantation in certain trials, but not all. Acetylcholine and substance P are used to examine endothelial-dependent vasodilation, while nitroglycerin, adenosine, and papaverine are used to assess non-endothelial-independent vasodilation.

Although a microvascular physiology measure derived from the thermal dilution of microvascular resistance was established, diabetes, ischemia duration, and a posterior confirmatory impact index of microvascular resistance alter the accuracy of microvascular tone evaluation.

Molecular analysis of myocardial biopsy samples

Endocardial biopsy samples collected during the first three months following heart transplantation indicate arterial/arterial endothelial alterations such as HLA-DR expression and tissue plasminogen activator depletion. These developments are inextricably linked to the emergence of CAV.

Noninvasive diagnostic methods

CT coronary angiography

Despite the fact that CT coronary angiography has a sensitivity of 85 to 100%, it is not currently recommended for routine CAV monitoring.

- ### *Cardiac Magnetic Resonance.*

"Cardiac magnetic resonance (CMR) is a non-invasive method that allows assessment of the epicardial coronary arteries as well as the microvasculature for CAV development" [17].

13   Management of CVA

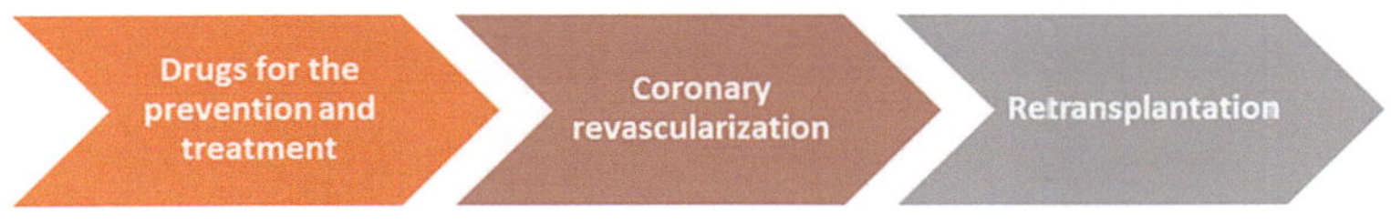

14   Early Graft Dysfunction (Primary Graft Dysfunction)

"Primary graft dysfunction (PGD) presents as severe ventricular dysfunction in the donor graft that fails to meet the hemodynamic requirements of the recipient in the immediate post-transplant period, or transplantation as severe left, right, or biventricular dysfunction occurs during the first 24 h, implant surgery for which there is no identifiable secondary cause" [18].

The incidence of early graft dysfunction ranges from 2 to 28% [19].

Risk factors of PGD:

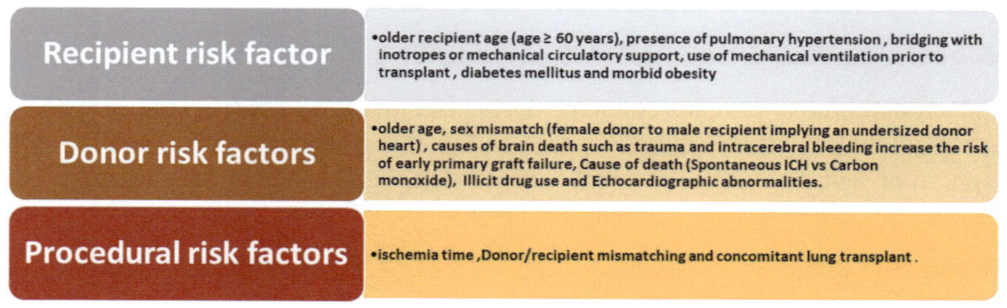

Investigations and Biomarkers

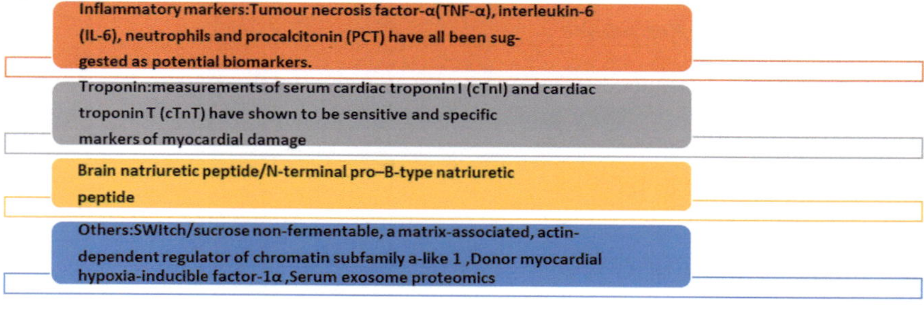

Pathophysiology of PGD

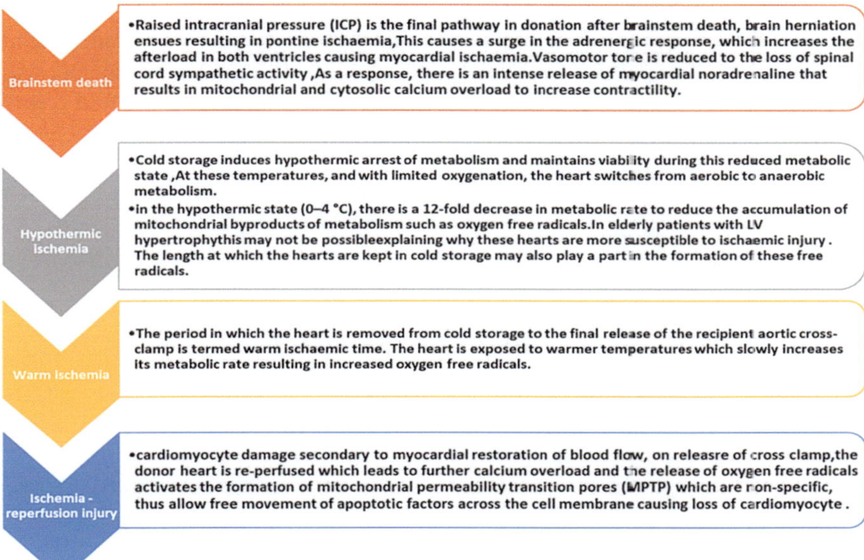

infections

After a heart transplant, infectious complications are a major source of morbidity and death, with many heart transplant patients suffering a post-transplant infection, with a cumulative rate of up to 85% after 5 years.

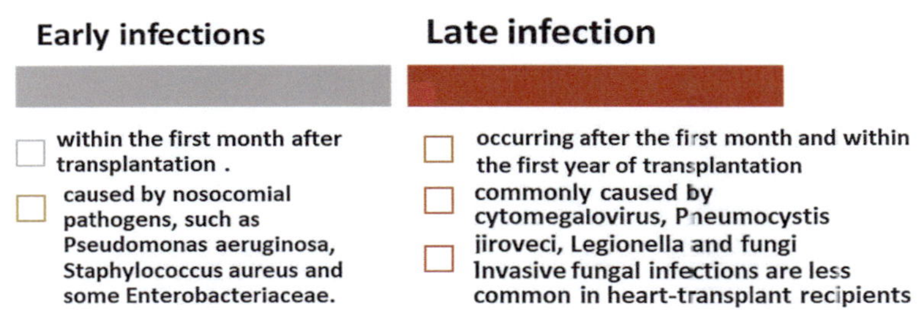

To minimize infection:

There was no significant difference in patient survival or graft function between HCV-positive and HCV-negative patients in a study evaluating heart transplant outcomes in Hepatitis C-positive recipients [5]. Furthermore, Hepatitis C virus-infected patients did not have an elevated risk of hepatic failure or accelerated coronary artery disease.

Following transplantation, ISHLT guidelines propose several antiviral layers based on the donor and recipient's CMV status, as shown in Table.

Chronic Kidney Disease

Chronic renal disease is more common in certain persons than in others. Patients with preoperative renal impairment are three times more likely to acquire infection, with a glomerular filtration rate less than 60 mL/min/1.73 m2 having a three-fold greater risk [5]. Hepatitis C virus infection, advanced age, feminine gender, and diabetes are all key risk factors.

15 Follow Up

AFTER HEART TRANSPLANT: FOLLOW-UP CARE

It requires the comprehensive involvement of the transplant surgeon and team, and the patient for mitigating post-transplant mortality and morbidity as well as increasing the chances of success and quality of the recipient's life.

After heart transplant surgery, there are certain steps the patient will take in order to recover well, live a fulfilling life, and stay healthy and out of the hospital.

Post-Op Heart Transplant Appointment Schedule

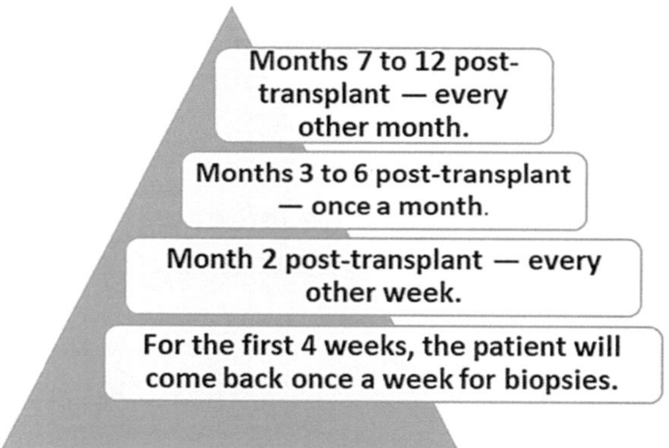

Multiple Choice Questions

1. **Cardiac transplantation is considered a treatment for**

    a. Advanced stage heart failure
    b. Myocardial infarction
    c. Pulmonary embolism
    d. Deep venous thrombosis

Answer. a

Explanation: Cardiac transplantation can be considered a gold standard treatment option for advanced stages of heart failure

2. **Complications after a heart transplant are**

a. Pre-operative complications
b. Early complications
c. Late complications
d. All of these

Answer. d

Explanation: Complications after cardiac transplantation can be divided into preoperative, early, and late complications.

3. **The most common complication after a heart transplant**

a. Rejection
b. Graft dysfunction
c. Infection
d. All of these

Answer. d

4. **Early adverse events after cardiac transplantation include**

a. Infections and acute graft rejection
b. Malignancies
c. Heart failure
d. Chronic kidney disease

Answer. a

Explanation: Early adverse events after a heart transplant includes infections and acute graft rejection.

5. **Graft rejection is**

a. A natural phenomenon
b. Immune-mediated phenomenon
c. Doesn't involve the immune system
d. None of these

Answer. b

Explanation: Graft rejection is an immune-mediated phenomenon.

6. Graft rejection can be categorized into

a. Hyperacute, chronic
b. Acute, chronic
c. Hyperacute, acute, and chronic
d. None of these

Answer. c

Explanation: Graft rejection can be categorized into hyperacute, acute, and chronic graft rejection.

7. Hyperacute graft rejection is due to

a. Electrolyte imbalances
b. Immunosuppression
c. Preformed anti-donor antibodies
d. All of these

Answer. c

8. Risk of rejection is highest in

a. First 12 years after transplant
b. First 6 months after transplant
c. Before transplant
d. None of these

Answer. b

9. Individuals at higher risk of developing rejection after heart transplant include

a. Female individuals
b. Younger individuals
c. Black individuals
d. All of these

Answer. d

10. Most common type of heart transplant rejection is

a. Hyperacute rejection

b. Acute cellular rejection
c. Subacute rejection
d. All of these

Answer. b

11. _______ is a form of chronic rejection

a. Acute kidney disease
b. Brain tumor
c. Coronary artery vasculopathy
d. All of these

Answer. c

12. Hyperacute rejection is not common now due to

a. Antibody screening before transplant
b. Blood type matching
c. Both a and b
d. None of these

Answer. c

Explanation: Hyperacute rejection is not common now due to antibody screening before transplant and blood type matching.

13. Which cells are mainly involved in acute cellular rejection?

a. B cells
b. Plasma cells
c. T cells
d. Epithelial cells

Answer. c

Explanation: In acute cellular rejection, T cells attack the cells of donor cardiac tissue.

13. Risk factors for developing antibody-mediated rejection include

a. Female gender
b. Young age
c. CMV infection
d. All of these

Answer. d

Explanation: Risk factors for developing antibody-mediated heart rejection include young age, female gender, prior, OKT3 use, prior CMV infection, artificial heart devices, etc.

14. cPRA stands for

a. Chronic per renal aneurysm
b. Chronic plasma reactive antibodies
c. Calculated panel reactive antibodies
d. None of these

Answer. c

Explanation: cPRA stands for calculated panel reactive antibodies and it quantifies the sensitization to HLA molecules prior to transplantation.

15. Risk factors for sensitization to HLA molecules prior to transplantation include

a. Previous transplant
b. Infection
c. Pregnancy
d. All of these

Answer. d

16. Risk factors for chronic rejection include

a. High cholesterol
b. Male donor
c. Older donor
d. All of these

Answer. d

Explanation: Risk factors for developing chronic rejection include high cholesterol levels, male donor, older donor, younger recipient, coronary heart disease, and insulin resistance.

17. Which of the following often have no symptoms?

a. Acute heart failure
b. Hyperacute rejection
c. Chronic heart transplant rejection
d. None of these

Answer. c

Explanation: Chronic rejection following a heart transplant often has no symptoms.

18. **Acute rejection can be diagnosed with**

a. Heart biopsy
b. Sodium levels
c. Blood sugar levels
d. None of these

Answer. a

Explanation: Acute rejection is often diagnosed with a heart biopsy

19. **In the early phase of rejection, Clinical features mostly are:**

a. Vague and nonspecific
b. Clear and specific
c. Restricted to renal findings
d. All of these

Answer. a

20. **Specific symptoms of acute heart transplant rejection include**

a. Dyspnea with exertion
b. Orthopnea
c. Edema
d. All of these

Answer. d

21. **Heart rhythm and heart function can be evaluated by ___ and ___ , respectively**

.

a. Heart transplant and rejection
b. Electrocardiogram and rejection
c. Echocardiogram and electrical imaging
d. Electrocardiogram and echocardiogram

Answer. d

Explanation: Heart rhythm can be evaluated by electrocardicgram and heart function by echocardiogram.

22. The gold standard test to diagnose or confirm a heart transplant rejection is

a. Echocardiogram
b. Electrocardiogram
c. Heart biopsy
d. None of these

Answer. c

Explanation: Endomyocardial biopsy or heart biopsy is the gold standard test to diagnose and confirm a rejection after a heart transplant.

23. The best approach for cardiac biopsy is

a. Left internal jugular approach
b. Right internal jugular approach
c. Left external jugular approach
d. Right external jugular approach

Answer. b

24. Grading criteria in ISHLT-2004 is

a. 0, 1A, 1B, 2, 3A, 3B, & 4
b. 0R, 1R, 2R, & 3R
c. 1R, 2R, 3R, & 4R
d. All of these

Answer. b

25. Rejection can be prevented by

a. Cross-matching
b. Pre-transplant antibody measurement
c. Post-transplant antibody measurement
d. All of these

Answer. d

Explanation: Rejection after cardiac transplantation can be prevented by pre- and post-transplant antibody measurement and cross-matching.

26. Most common medications for preventing rejection include

a. Analgesics
b. Anti-tussive

c. Antihistamines
d. Immunosuppressants

Answer. d

Explanation: Immunosuppressant medications help prevent rejection by suppressing the immune system.

27. **Early graft dysfunction presents as**

a. Severe edema
b. Hypersensitivity
c. Severe ventricular dysfunction
d. None of these

Answer. c

References

1. Birati EY, Rame JE. Post–heart transplant complications. Critical Care Clinics. 2014;30(3):629–637.
2. Kobashigawa J, ed. Clinical guide to heart transplantation. Springer International Publishing; 2017.
3. [Internet]. Lucris.lub.lu.se. https://lucris.lub.lu.se/ws/portalfiles/portal/22014619/Doctoral_Thesis_Ihdina_Sukma_Dewi.pdf (2022). Accessed 30 July 2022.
4. Montoya JG, et al. Infectious complications among 620 consecutive heart transplant patients at Stanford University Medical Center. Clin Infect Diseases. 2001;33(5):629–640.
5. American Transplant Congress. Executive and program planning committees and abstract review committees. Am J Transplant. 2007;7(s2):17–584.
6. Diaz B, et al. Gastrointestinal complications in heart transplant patients: MITOS study. Transpl Proc. 2007;39(7). Elsevier.
7. Gruter MO, Brand HS. Oral health complications after a heart transplant: a review. Br Dent J. 2020;228(3):177–82.
8. Atasever A, et al. Pulmonary complications in heart transplant recipients. Transplantation Proc. 2006;38(5). Elsevier.
9. Jalowiec A, Grady KL, White-Williams C. Mortality, rehospitalization, and post-transplant complications in gender-mismatched heart transplant recipients. Heart Lung. 2017;46(4):265–72.
10. Cemillan CA, et al. Neurological complications in a series of 205 orthotopic heart transplant patients. Rev Neurol. 2004;38(10):906–12.
11. Forrat R, et al. High prevalence of thromboembolic complications in heart transplant recipients: Which preventive strategy? Transplantation. 1996;61(5):757–762.
12. Lacy MQ, et al. Autologous stem cell transplant after heart transplant for light chain (Al) amyloid cardiomyopathy. J Heart Lung Transplant. 2008;27(8):823–829.
13. Zakliczynski M, et al. Surgical wound-healing complications in heart transplant recipients treated with rapamycin. Wound Repair Regener. 2007;15(3):316–321.
14. McCormick AD, et al. Generalized and specific anxiety in adolescents following heart transplant. Pediatric Transplant. 2020;24(1):e13647.

15. Van De Beek D, et al. No major neurologic complications with sirolimus use in heart transplant recipients. Mayo Clinic Proc. 2009;84(4). Elsevier.
16. Kulikowska A, et al. Infectious, malignant, and autoimmune complications in pediatric heart transplant recipients. J Pediatrics. 2008;152(5):671–677.
17. Sutcliffe DL, et al. Post-transplant outcomes in pediatric ventricular assist device patients: A PediMACS–Pediatric Heart Transplant Study linkage analysis. J Heart Lung Transplant. 2018;37(6):715–722.
18. Creating a multivariable model to predict primary graft dysfunction after heart transplantation in the United Kingdom using the 2014 International Society of Heart and Lung Transplantation consensus definition - Enlighten: Theses [Internet]. Theses.gla.ac.uk. https://theses.gla.ac.uk/79063/ (2022). Accessed 30 July 2022
19. Moro JA, et al. Impact of diabetes mellitus on heart transplant patients. Rev Esp Cardiol. 2006;59(10):1033–7.

Outcomes and Impact on Life Quality

Ilaria Tropea, Annalisa Bernabei, Giuseppe Faggian, and Francesco Onorati

Abstract Heart transplant represents the gold standard for end-stage heart failure. Through the years, the survival rate and outcomes of patients undergoing heart transplantation have progressively improved. However, short- and long-term complications still represent a fundamental challenge for the transplant physician. As years go by, the risk of acute rejection, infection, and graft dysfunction, typical of the early period after transplant, reduces to be replaced by long-term complications linked to immunosuppressive therapy and progressive chronic rejection. Chronic rejection occurs, with Cardiac Allograft Vasculopathy (CAV), in around 50% of heart transplant recipients at ten years from heart transplantation, leading to eventual graft dysfunction. Immunosuppressive therapy, through the years, is responsible for an augmented risk of malignancy, the leading cause of death after five years from heart transplant (22% of patients.). The most frequent are skin cancers, followed by post-transplant lymphoproliferative-disorders (PTLD) and other solid tumors. Progressive renal failure is another consequence of long-term immunosuppressive therapy, especially with CNIs. End-stage renal failure (defined by serum Creatinine > 2.5 mg/dl, dialysis, or renal transplant) is experienced by 50% of heart transplant recipients within 15 years from heart transplantation. Furthermore, long-term immunosuppressive therapy with corticosteroids leads to a series of metabolic derangements, including diabetes, hypertension, dyslipidemia, obesity, which are recurrent conditions in heart transplant recipients.

Keywords Heart transplantation · Long-term outcome · Cardiac allograft vasculopathy · Malignancy · Chronic renal failure · Diabetes · Metabolic disorders · Quality of life

Cardiac transplantation is the gold standard for the surgical treatment of end-stage heart failure, but after heart transplantation, a series of short- and long-term complications can occur, influencing the outcome of these patients significantly.

I. Tropea · A. Bernabei · G. Faggian · F. Onorati (✉)
Division of Cardiac Surgery, University of Verona, Verona, Italy
e-mail: Francesco.onorati@univr.it

According to ISHLT registries, median survival for adult heart recipients is 11.6 years, while in patients who undergo retransplantation, it is reduced to 8.2 years.

In the latest ISHLT report, 1-year survival increased (86.2%) in the most recent era (2012–2017) compared to the previous eras (84.2% among 2000–2005 and 2006–2011). Particularly, in North America, 1-year survival (2012–2017) was 89.1%, while in Europe and other countries was respectively 80.3% and 81.5%, and this could be a direct consequence of European recipients' characteristics (recipient older age and other risk factors). Confirming this, when analyzed distributing 1-year survival by patients age, younger patients (18–39 years) had better survival both in North America (89.9%) and Europe (85.6%) than the older ones (40–59 years and patients > 60 years).

Five years of survival (conditional on survival to one year) in the latest era (2008–2013) has improved to 87.3%, compared to previous eras (86.3% between 2002–2007 and 85.5% 1996–2001), despite the overall quality worsening of both donors and recipients. Unlike 1-year survival, 5-year conditional survival is better in Europe (88.4%) compared to North America (87.6%) and other countries (85.2%) [1].

In the first year after heart transplantation, the most frequent causes of death are related to non-CMV infections (31.8%), graft failure (17.6%), multiple organ failure (16.8%), and acute rejection (7.9%). Nevertheless, after 10–15 years from heart transplantation, the main causes of death are malignancy (21.5%), graft failure (17.3%), cardiac allograft vasculopathy (12.1%), and non-CMV infections (11.1%) (Table 1).

Statistically significative risk factors for 10-year mortality in ISHLT registries were identified in recipient characteristics like age, BMI, serum creatinine, and PRA (panel reactive antibody). Other risk factors relied on the donor and the operation itself: donor age and total ischemic time [2].

1   Chronic Allograft Rejection

Cardiac allograft vasculopathy (CAV) is the expression of chronic rejection in transplanted hearts, and it is a peculiar form of vascular disease whose pathogenesis involves both immunologic and non-immunologic factors. CAV affects heart transplant recipients exclusively and is responsible for progressive dysfunction and graft failure.

CAV is a diffuse arteritis characterized by concentric intimal thickening of coronary arteries, but in some cases, it can develop, like a native heart coronaropathy, with focal eccentric stenosis [3] (Fig. 1).

Table 1 Heart transplant recipients main causes of death

Cause of death	0–30 days (%)	31 days–1 year (%)	>1–3 years (%)	>3–5 years (%)	>5–10 years (%)	>10–15 years (%)	>15 years (%)
CAV	1.2	3.2	10.8	12.4	12.2	12.1	10.5
Acute rejection	3.9	7.9	9.8	4.7	1.9	0.9	0.5
PTLD	0	1	2.2	2.9	3.2	2.7	2.1
Malignancy	0.1	2.3	12.3	19.6	22	21.5	19.4
CMV	0	0.9	0.5	0.1	0.1	0.1	0
Infection	13.9	31.8	13.3	10.9	10.8	11.1	12.3
MOF	18.5	16.8	6.4	5.8	6.9	8.4	9.3
Graft failure	39.5	17.6	26.4	24.4	19.5	17.3	16.6
Renal failure	0.5	0.9	1.3	3.1	5.4	8	9.9

Adapted from 2019 ISHLT Registry

Abbreviations: CAV = Cardiac Allograft Vasculopathy; PTLD = Post Transplant Lymphoproliferative disorders; CMV = Cytomegalovirus; MOF – Multiple Organ Failure

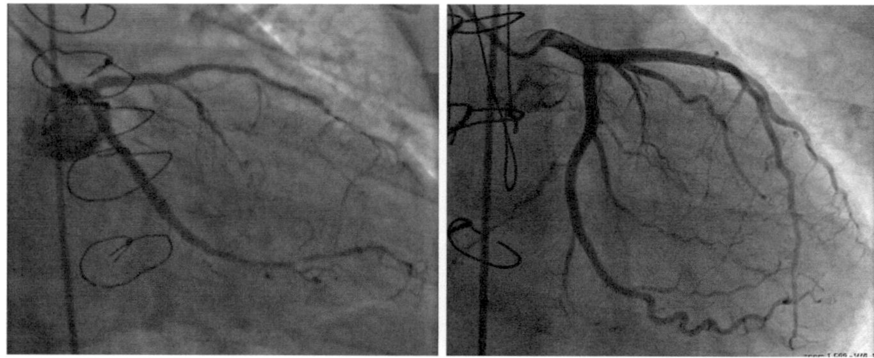

Fig. 1 Coronary angiography in heart transplant recipients

1.1 Pathogenesis

In CAV, immune and non-immune risk factors converge on endothelial injury and inflammation, leading to an excessive response to the endothelial damage, determining the accumulation of inflammatory cells, aberrant extracellular matrix, lipids deposition, and smooth muscle hyperplasia. These mechanisms result in intimal hyperplasia, fibrosis, and consequent narrowing or even occlusion of the affected vessel [4]. The histological features of CAV are expressed in both epicardial and intramural vessels, involving the intima, the media, and the adventitia, and can affect the proximal or the distal tract of the artery [5].

To identify CAV, ISHLT established a classification based on the grade of vascular involvement.

Immune Factors: After heart transplantation, the recipient immune system recognizes the donor endothelial cells as "non-self" thanks to the Human Leucocytes Antigens (HLA) system. An HLA-mismatch between the donor and the recipients predisposes to the development of CAV. The molecules belonging to the major histocompatibility complex (MHC) are located on the donor endothelial cells surface and can be detected directly by the recipient dendritic cells (Direct Allorecognition) or can be recognized, incorporated, processed, and presented to the lymphocytes by the recipient dendritic cells (Indirect Allorecognition) [6]. Both the mechanisms lead to T and B-Lymphocytes activation and proliferation, the consequent production of cytokines (IL-2, INF-γ and TGF-β) and the synthesis of donor-specific antibodies (DSA) [4]. The intima thickens, the smooth muscle cells proliferate, the extracellular matrix increases, and the fibrosis occurs [4].

Non-Immune Factors: The non-immune factors involved in the development of CAV imply a series of mechanisms and characteristics belonging both to the donor and the recipient.

Risk factors related to the donor are donor older age, male sex, previous history of smoking, and mode of donor brain death (intracranial hemorrhage is more linked to the development of CAV rather than traumatic brain death) [7].

Factors related to the recipient include traditional risk factors for coronary artery disease like hypertension, obesity, smoking, diabetes, hyperlipidemia, and ischemic cardiomyopathy [8].

Another factor contributing to the development of CAV is the ischemia/reperfusion damage during transplantation due to the production of free radicals, which can be responsible for the endothelial injury [4].

Also, patients with recurrent CMV infections have a major risk of developing CAV. A series of mechanisms have been proposed, but there is still a controversy on the effective role played by CMV. Among the mechanisms hypothesized, there is a direct endothelial dysfunction caused by the impairing of the nitric oxide synthase pathway and a consequent release of cytokines and smooth cells proliferation. Another mechanism is the cross-reaction between the viral proteins and the endothelial surface molecules, leading to T-lymphocytes activation and endothelial damage [4, 9].

1.2   Clinical Features and Diagnosis

At the moment of heart transplantation, the donor's heart is disconnected from the chains of the nervous system responsible for heart rate control, contractility, and pain sensation (angina). Heart denervation determines lack of angina in the presence of ischemia due to coronary artery disease, even though some long-term patients can refer to anginal symptoms consequent to heart reinnervation [10].

Patients affected by CAV are typically asymptomatic in the early stages of the disease but can successively develop signs and symptoms secondary to heart failure like dyspnea, edema, arrhythmias, and even sudden cardiac death [11].

Echocardiography in patients with CAV may show a preserved systolic function, a graft dysfunction, or a restrictive pattern, which is typical of CAV.

The gold standard to diagnose CAV is coronary angiography, through which CAV can be graded according to ISHLT Classification, based on the number of vessels involved, the severity of stenosis, and the eventual graft dysfunction. To prevent and assess the development of CAV, heart transplant recipients should undergo annually or biannually coronary angiography, except for those affected by chronic kidney disease, in which a less frequent evaluation may be performed [12].

A complementary method to coronary angiography to detect CAV is IVUS (intravascular ultrasound), performed inside the vessel and able to identify plaques even before they are visible on angiography.

In patients affected by chronic kidney disease, who cannot undergo coronary angiography, a series of non-invasive imaging techniques may be considered, like dobutamine stress echocardiography, myocardial scintigraphy, computerized tomography, or magnetic resonance imaging.

1.3 Therapy

Pharmacological management of CAV aims primarily to the prevention of the disease and secondly to stabilize and slow its progression. Medical therapy to prevent CAV begins at the moment of heart transplantation and is aimed at both immune and non-immune risk factors. When diagnosed, patients affected by severe CAV may undergo percutaneous revascularization procedures with drug-eluting stents, being exposed to risks linked to DAPT, with a significant likelihood of restenosis or progression of the microvascular disease. Surgical revascularization is associated with a high rate of complications; in fact, ISHLT guidelines suggest it only in selected patients and in the presence of lesions amenable to this kind of revascularization. In patients affected by advanced vasculopathy, graft dysfunction, and signs and symptoms of heart failure, retransplantation may be the only option to be considered [13].

The prevention and control of CAV through medical therapy is assured by an immunosuppressive regimen started at the moment of heart transplantation: some centers, in fact, perform an **induction therapy with ATG** (Anti-Thymocyte globulin) to reduce the activity of reactive T-lymphocytes, with the aim of delaying the administration of calcineurin inhibitors and decreasing the risk of acute kidney injury [14].

Calcineurin Inhibitors (CNIs): Cyclosporine (CsA) and Tacrolimus (TAC) constitute the main pillars of immunosuppressive therapy after heart transplantation, and their advantage is acting directly on the immune system not impairing other rapidly proliferating cells [15]. Their action is dose-dependent, and they must be titrated to obtain a therapeutic range; their main side effect is nephrotoxicity.

Although CNIs are fundamental in preventing acute rejection, they cause a series of metabolic derangements like hypertension, dyslipidemia, and diabetes, contributing consequently to the development of CAV. The concomitant use of corticosteroids can further worsen the CNIs' cardiovascular side effects. In fact, corticosteroid tapering or even suspension in selected patients may reduce metabolic disorders [15].

Antiproliferative Agents: Azathioprine (AZA) and Mycophenolate Mofetil (MMF) are used in association with CNIs and constitute the antiproliferative agents, whose action on Lymphocytes is expressed interfering with nucleotide synthesis, reducing their proliferation. Among their side effects are metabolic derangement, gastrointestinal disease, and hematologic disorders (especially leukopenia). Keogh et al. demonstrated how patients treated with MMF vs. AZA had a significant reduction in rejection and a protective effect over the development of CAV and malignancy [16].

A study by Kackzmarek et al. showed how MMF, compared with AZA, determines a better long-term survival and protection for CAV [17].

Proliferative signal inhibitors (PSI) or **Mammalian target-of-rapamycin inhibitors** (mTOR inhibitors): Sirolimus (SRL) and Everolimus (EVL) act through the inhibition of a kinase (mTOR) responsible for T-lymphocytes proliferation. Unlike CNIs, they have less nephrotoxicity and have been demonstrated to reduce the progression of CAV, having an inhibitory effect on smooth muscle cells and endothelial cells proliferation [13]. PSIs are not directly nephrotoxic, but when used with full dose CNIs, they can have a synergistic effect and potentiate the renal toxicity of CNIs [18].

PSI may be utilized through different regimens: in association with low-dose CNIs or in de-novo settings in combination with antiproliferative agents. A reduction of 61% in the diagnosis of CAV was reported in patients treated with CNIs-PSI protocol rather than CNIs-MMF/AZA [19].

A meta-analysis by Jennings et al. proved an important reduction of CAV progression and CMV infection in the PSI-CNIs regimen, but an augmentation of pharmacological side effects: wound healing-complications, hyperlipidemia, proteinuria and edema, infections, pneumonitis, and skin disorders [19].

Patients at high risk of CAV development (older donor age, established coronaropathy of the graft and retransplantation due to graft dysfunction caused by advanced CAV) may benefit from a de-novo regimen with mTOR-inhibitors; on the other hand, patients affected by uncontrolled hyperlipidemia and proteinuria > 800 mg/day should not undergo treatment with PSI [20].

2 Malignancy

Malignancy is the most frequent long-term complication and the main cause of death from 5 years after heart transplantation. Heart transplant recipients are, in fact, more prone to develop malignancy when compared with the general population.

For this increased risk, it is necessary a disease-free interval before listing a patient for heart transplantation [3].

Immunosuppressive drugs are not the only factors predisposing to malignancy since there are a series of viruses with oncogenic properties that can reactivate and proliferate, contributing to the neoplastic process. Among these viruses, a particular mention goes to Epstein-Barr virus (EBV), Human Herpes Virus 8 (HHV 8), Human Papillomavirus (HPV), and Human T cell lymphotropic virus 1(HTLV-1) [3].

ISHLT registry demonstrates how the patients deceased of malignancy (excluding post-transplant lymphoproliferative diseases—PTLD) increase as years go by, going from 2.3% by one year from heart transplantation to 22% by 10 years.

The most frequent neoplasms are represented by skin cancers (including melanoma and non-melanoma skin cancers) followed by lymphomas, prostate, and lung cancers. Though less frequent than skin cancers, lymphomas are associated with higher mortality. Survival rates at 5 years after diagnosis of skin cancer (within 3 years of transplant) are quite similar to those of patients without neoplasms, representing around 80%, while they significantly decrease to 35% in patients with a reported lymphoma.

Cardiac transplant recipients have a higher risk of developing a de novo malignancy when compared to other solid organs recipients (i.e., kidney recipients), probably because of required higher regimens of immunosuppressive therapy.

Youn et al. analyzed, from the ISHLT registry, a population of 17,587 patients undergone heart transplants between January 2000 and December 2011 and demonstrated how the incidence of de novo solid neoplasm, between 5 and 10 years from transplant, was 10.7%. In the Youn et al. study, a significative lower survival rate was confirmed in patients with a diagnosis of de novo malignancy (all types of cancer) compared with patients without a story of neoplasm. They also searched potential risk factors predisposing to malignancy: for skin cancers, a statistically significant correlation between the risk factor and the diagnosis of de novo malignancy within 5 years was found in older age recipients and a story of recent transplant. Skin cancers include squamous cell carcinomas (SCC), basal cell carcinoma (BCC), and melanoma. For non-skin solid cancers, risk factors were represented by age, height, recent transplantation, the number of hospitalizations within 1 year from transplant, recipient smoking habit, and hypertension in medical therapy. For the development of lymphoproliferative disorders, risk factors were identified in overweight, the number of hospitalizations within 1 year from transplant the use of an immunosuppressive induction therapy at the moment of transplant with anti-thymocyte globulins [21].

2.1 Skin Cancers

Represent more than 40% of all neoplasms in heart transplant recipients. The most involved areas are the head and neck district (70%), followed by the upper limbs (17%), the trunk (9%), and the lower limbs (4%) [22].

Several studies demonstrated as risk factors for skin cancer are older age at the moment of transplant, length and intensity of immunosuppressive regimen, an augmented exposure to UV, male sex, fair skin, previous HPV infection, and history of non-melanoma skin cancer. A study by Brewer et al. analyzed a population of 312 patients who underwent heart transplants from 1988 to 2006 to identify any potential risk factor for squamous cell and basal cell carcinoma. Particularly older age, male sex, previous ischemic cardiomyopathy were confirmed risk factors for SCC; on the other hand, patients treated with MMF had a major risk of BCC when compared with those in therapy with AZA. A history of HSV infection was associated with both SCC and BCC. Nevertheless, this study demonstrated how a proper screening, a consequent early diagnosis, and aggressive treatment could reduce the mortality rate associated with skin cancer [23].

The population of 6721 cardiac transplant recipients (1993–2003) examined by Alam et al., extrapolated from the Cardiac Transplant Research Database, confirmed as risk factors for skin cancer male sex, older recipient age, skin cancer history, and history of smoking within 6 months of the list [24].

2.2 Post-Transplant Lymphoproliferative Disorders

(PTLD) reunite a series of heterogenous lymphoproliferative diseases. When analyzed immunologically, they are mostly B-Lymphocytes related (87%) and less frequently T-Lymphocytes related (13%). They are typically extranodal masses localized in the gastrointestinal tract, the liver, the lungs, the skin, the central nervous system, and the transplanted graft [25] (Table 2).

An often-recurring factor in PTLDs is Epstein Barr Virus: EBV, also known as HHV-4, is a lymphocryptovirus belonging to the herpes virus family, which normally remains in a state of latency after the first infection. In the immunocompetent patient, a balance between EBV and the immune system is maintained, preventing the virus reactivation and the clinical manifestations related to the virus. In heart transplant recipients, immunosuppressive agents reduce T-Lymphocytes' action in controlling the virus replication, leading to virus reactivation and accumulation of EBV infected cells, and in rare cases, when the replication is uncontrolled, to a PTLD.

Ippoliti et al. collected a series of predisposing factors for PTLDs. Post-transplant EBV primary infection, donor-recipient CMV mismatch, and young recipient age were demonstrated risk factors for "Early lesions" development, while older recipient age and duration of immunosuppression were recurrent in "Late lesions" [26].

A study by Wasson et al. analyzed a population of 110 heart transplant recipients who had undergone heart transplants between 1989 and 2002 to evaluate the incidence of PTLDs. The incidence was 5.4%, and the interval between the operation and the diagnosis of PTLDs was 5.5 years. According to Wasson et al. study, a primary infection by EBV or CMV after transplant was more correlated to the development of PTLDs rather than the viral reactivation. Other risk factors related to PTLDs were recipient hepatitis C status, age, gender, and the grade of immunosuppression [27].

Table 2 WHO classification of PTLD

– Early lesions
Florid follicular hyperplasia or non-infectious mononucleosis-like lymphoid hyperplasia
Plasmacytic hyperplasia
Infectious mononucleosis-like lesion
– Polymorphic PTLD
Same ICD-O codes as those for the respective lymphoid or plasmacytic neoplasm
– Monomorphic PTLD
B cell neoplasms (Diffuse large B cell Lymphoma, Burkitt lymphoma, Plasmacell myeloma, Plasmoacytoma-like lesion)
T cell neoplasms (Peripheral T cell lymphoma, NOS, Hepatosplenic T cell lymphoma)
– Classical Hodgkin lymphoma Type PTLD
Adapted from WHO Classification

2.3   Other Solid Tumors

Solid tumors in heart transplant recipients are less frequent than skin cancers and PTLDs, and their incidence is not significantly higher when compared to the general population.

A study by Keller et al. analyzed a population of 851 patients who had undergone heart transplants from 1997 to 2004 at Columbia Presbyterian Hospital. Exclusion criteria were history of cancer before transplant and PTLD after transplant. All the patients were periodically screened with blood chemistry and instrumental tests (chest X-ray, mammograms, and colonoscopy). De novo solid tumors developed in 8.5% of the population, the most frequent of which was prostate cancer (31%), followed by lung cancer (11%), and breast cancer (8%). The study also demonstrated a similar incidence of solid tumors in heart transplant recipients and the general population; only cancers involving a viral infection in the oncogenic process were more frequent in the heart transplant recipient. Older age at the moment of the transplant was recognized as a risk factor for the development of solid tumors [28].

A post-transplant malignancy was diagnosed in 2673 patients (11.5%). Skin cancers were the most frequent (50%), followed by lung (10.9%) and prostate (10%) cancers and PTLD (8.5%).

2.4   Cancer Prevention

Heart transplant recipients are more prone to develop malignancy rather than the general population because of the higher regimens of immunosuppressive therapy; for this reason, cancer screening and prevention play a fundamental role in the early diagnosis and therapy of malignancy [12].

3   Chronic Kidney Disease (CKD)

Chronic Kidney Disease (CKD) is a common complication after heart transplantation, and it represents a relevant determinant of mortality and long-term quality of life.

It is the consequence of a series of factors and mechanisms, including pre-transplant renal disease, acute damage during extracorporeal Circulation at the time of intervention, nephrotoxicity linked to CNIs, and progressive renal function derangement consequent to hypertension and diabetes [29].

ISHLT registries show how renal failure constitutes a cause of death in 3.1% of patients at 5 years, increasing to 5.4% at 10 years and 9.9% after 15 years from heart transplantation. Freedom from severe renal dysfunction, defined by serum Creatinine > 2.5 mg/dl, dialysis, or renal transplant, is around 75% at 5 years, reducing drastically to 50% at 15 years after transplant. According to ISHLT registries, statistically significant risk factors for the development of severe renal dysfunction within 5 years from heart transplant were recipient serum creatinine and bilirubin at the moment of heart transplantation [2]. Furthermore, the augmented risk of death in patients affected by chronic kidney disease is not restricted only to the presence of end-stage renal failure, but it also involves patients with mild or moderate renal failure if compared to those without renal impairment. Patients with end-stage renal failure on dialysis can benefit from a kidney transplant.

3.1 Pathogenesis

After a heart transplant, renal function impairs following a biphasic trend: an initial rapid worsening of renal function occurs in the first year after the operation, followed by a slow deterioration through the years.

Patients with a pre-existing renal failure, who undergo extracorporeal Circulation (ECC) during heart transplant, may develop an acute renal injury in the immediate post-operative period related to initial hemodynamic instability. A series of pre-transplant characteristics have been recognized as predisposing factors for the development of post-operative renal failure: age at the moment of heart transplantation, pre-existing cardiovascular risk factors (hypertension, dyslipidemia, diabetes, ischemic cardiomyopathy), female sex, and preoperative left ventricular assist device (LVAD). In these patients, hemodynamic instability, post-operative bleeding and mediastinal re-exploration, primary graft dysfunction and acute rejection, sepsis, and the use of nephrotoxic antimicrobial agents can further worsen a pre-existing impaired renal function. On the other hand, a fundamental role in the progressive decline of renal function through the years is played by CNIs (Cyclosporin and Tacrolimus), whose nephrotoxicity has been known for years. CNIs act on the renal glomerulus determining afferent arteriolar vasoconstriction, which induces glomerular ischemia, augmentation of oxidative stress, and cellular apoptosis. These mechanisms lead to nodular arteriolar hyalinosis and glomerular sclerosis through the years. Furthermore, CNIs are responsible for direct tubular toxicity, which causes tubular atrophy and interstitial fibrosis, deteriorating further renal function.

3.2 Measures of Prevention

Patients with an end-stage heart and renal failure (on dialysis or not) may be listed for both heart and renal transplant, undergoing a combined or a sequential heart-kidney transplant.

To prevent acute kidney injury in the immediate post-operative period, it is fundamental to maintain adequate hemodynamics, avoid hypotension and anemia, and introduce inotropic agents if necessary to improve kidney perfusion.

After hospital discharge, a series of precautions must be taken through the years to slow the progressive renal decline typical of most heart transplant recipients: a strict blood pressure control, through the use of oral antihypertensive agents, to prevent hypertensive nephropathy and a blood glucose control from reducing the risk of diabetic nephropathy are required [29].

Immunosuppressive agents like CNIs should be lowered as possible to reduce their nephrotoxicity, and conversion from AZA to MMF may be considered when possible. Otherwise, to slow the progressive decline of renal function, blood pressure (ACEi and ARBs are recommended in these patients, and CCBs are the alternative when ACEi and ARBs cannot be used) and blood glucose must be strictly controlled according to international guidelines [12].

3.3 *Outcomes*

Confirming the role of renal function in the overall outcome of heart transplant recipients, ISHLT registries assert that 1-year survival rate in patients with pre-existing renal dysfunction (eGFR < 30 ml/min/1.73 m^2) does not reach 80%, while it overcomes 90% in patients with an eGFR > 60 ml/min/1.73 m^2. At 5 years from heart transplant survival in patients with eGFR < 30 ml/min/1.73 m^2 is around 83%, while it slightly increases to 87% in patients with eGFR > 60 ml/min/1.73 m^2 [1].

Regardless of the presence of pre-existing renal insufficiency, a series of studies analyzed heart transplant recipients' renal function through the years, confirming a progressive decline in most of the cases.

A multicenter study conducted by Janus et al., through the CARIN Study (Cardiac transplantation and Renal Insufficient), reported chronic kidney disease in 59.6% of the population within 36 months from heart transplantation, particularly patients who lost 15–19% of their initial eGFR [30]. In a study conducted by Roest et al. 614 patients, undergone heart transplant between 1984 and 2016 were investigated to evaluate the trend of renal function through the years: 19.7% of the patients developed end-stage renal disease (ESRD), the median time between hospital discharge after heart transplantation and the diagnosis of ESRD was 7.7 years. Among 614 patients, 19 received kidney transplants, of which 15 underwent pre-transplant dialysis.

Grupper et al. conducted a retrospective study on 268 heart transplant recipients to evaluate the outcome following heart and kidney transplant after a diagnosis of ESRD vs. heart transplant recipients without ESRD. During a period of 76 months, 19% of the patients developed ESRD, and 39 of them (77%) underwent kidney transplants. Prolonged therapy with CNIs has been confirmed a risk factor for ESRD. Overall median survival was 16.3 years after heart transplantation. When compared, red survival of patients with ESRD treated with kidney transplants was better than those with ESRD who were maintained on dialysis (17.5 vs. 7.3 years). Furthermore, the median survival of patients who had undergone kidney transplants was similar to patients without ESRD (17.5 vs. 17.1 years) [31].

4 Metabolic Disorders After Heart Transplant

Metabolic disorders (overweight, hyperglycemia or diabetes, hypertension, and dyslipidemia) are frequent conditions in patients listed for heart transplantation, especially in those developing end-stage heart failure consequents to ischemic cardiomyopathy.

4.1 Diabetes

Patients undergoing heart transplants may be affected by pre-existing Diabetes Mellitus (DM) or can develop diabetes in the following period, the so-called new-onset diabetes after transplant (NODAT), because of the metabolic derangements caused by immunosuppressive agents and the post-operative stress linked to surgery. The latest ISHLT Registry states that 28.2% of patients who have undergone heart transplants already had a diagnosis of diabetes [1].

Diabetes plays a fundamental role in heart transplant recipients' clinical course. In fact, several studies affirm that patients with normal pre-transplant glycemia are less prone to develop acute rejection, infections, and NODAT, having a better outcome consequently compared to patients with pre-existing diabetes [32].

Furthermore, a target glycemia between 80–100 mg/dl has been demonstrated to decrease mortality and morbidity in the immediate post-operative period (in the Intensive Care Unit) when hyperglycemia is controlled through insulin therapy [33].

ISHLT registry states that 12 years-survival of heart transplant recipients without diabetes is 55.9% vs. patients with pre-existing diabetes was 43.1% [1].

NODAT can be diagnosed using the usual criteria for DM, and risk factors related to its development are the same as DM, including overweight, older age, and history of hyperglycemia. In addition to these predisposing factors, post-operative stress and immunosuppressive agents' action can further contribute to hyperglycemia.

In fact, they determine insulin resistance and increase hepatic gluconeogenesis, causing hyperglycemia. In the early post-operative period, high doses of corticosteroids are required, and hyperglycemia is very frequent, but as time goes by, corticosteroids may be tapered, reducing their hyperglycemic action.

Although antiproliferative agents have no hyperglycemic effects, CNIs' mechanism of action can interfere with insulin secretion and sensitivity, contributing to altering blood glucose control.

After heart transplantation, when high doses of immunosuppressive agents are used, patients are treated following a basal/bolus insulin schema to have proper control of glycemia (in Intensive Care Unit). After discharge, patients with a pre-existing history of diabetes can restore their previous hypoglycemic therapy, while patients with a diagnosis of NODAT can continue a basal/bolus insulin schema and then switch to oral hypoglycemic drugs. Some patients without previous diabetes may return to normal glucose levels, only leading to a healthy lifestyle and diet [32].

ISHLT guidelines recommend periodic screening for diabetes after heart transplantation by measuring blood glucose levels and $HgbA_{1C}$ planning the frequency of controls according to risk factors, and immunosuppressive therapy. In patients with long-term diabetes, annual screening for hyperglycemia complications should be performed: ophthalmologic issues, vascular complications, neuropathy, etc. [12].

Kim et al. analyzed 391 patients who underwent heart transplants from 1992 to 2013, dividing the population into no diabetes (n = 257), pre-existing diabetes (n = 46), and new-onset diabetes after transplant (n = 88). A total of 25.5% of the non-diabetic patients developed diabetes after transplant. This study determined how patients with new-onset diabetes, compared with the non-diabetes group, had an increased risk for overall death and chronic kidney disease. Furthermore, the new-onset diabetes group had a worse survival rate than the non-diabetes group but similar to pre-existing diabetes one [34].

4.2 Corticosteroids Side Effects

Corticosteroids were among the first drugs utilized as immunosuppressive agents and still represent one of the best treatments to prevent rejection, but their use is responsible for a series of metabolic disorders as side effects. They are administrated as induction, maintenance, and antirejection therapy in heart transplant recipients, requiring high doses of corticosteroids in the early period of transplant, going through progressive tapering until definitive suspension in some cases. Patients treated with long-term corticosteroids therapy develop most of the typical adverse effects. In fact, they interfere with the normal function of the hypothalamus-Hypophysis-adrenal axis, altering the normal metabolism of both glucocorticoids and mineralocorticoids and determining chronic adrenal suppression. They cannot be suddenly suspended but require progressive tapering to avoid adrenal insufficiency.

Typical metabolic derangements consequent to corticosteroids therapy are hypertension, diabetes, hyperlipemia, salt and water retention, osteoporosis, and weight gain (with typical trunk obesity). Furthermore, they act on the psychological sphere, determining emotional lability or eventual depression and psychosis.

A series of effects concerning esthetics are peculiar to patients undergoing therapy with corticosteroids like typical "moon face", acne, hirsutism, cataracts, skin fragility, easy bruising, and slow wound healing. Fat disposition is characteristic: there is proximal myopathy and truncal obesity [35]. Corticosteroids also have effects on the gastrointestinal tract, including peptic ulcers, gastritis, esophagitis, and pancreatitis.

A correct lifestyle, including weight loss, diet, physical activity, is fundamental in heart transplant recipients suffering from hypertension, diabetes, and dyslipidemia.

When hypertension needs specific drug therapy, the drug choice is typically empiric and depends on blood pressure response: Calcium Channel blockers (CCBs) are the most used, followed by ACEI/ARB.

According to ISHLT guidelines, bone mass density (BMD) in patients affected by corticosteroid-induced bone disease should be evaluated periodically through a dual-energy X-ray absorptiometry (DEXA). Patients with low BMD should be treated with bisphosphonates, the drugs of choice, while all heart transplant recipients should undergo a chronic treatment with Calcium and Vitamin D. After the first year of transplant, if corticosteroids are discontinued and BMD is in the range of normality, bisphosphonates may be interrupted maintaining a proper follow-up for osteoporosis [12].

5 Quality of Life After Heart Transplant

Outcomes after heart transplantation can be measured by evaluating long-term survival and complications rate, but a fundamental role is being acquired by the quality of life (QoL) and functional recovery [36].

According to the WHO definition, QoL is the individual's perception of their position in life in the context of the culture and value systems in which they live and in relation to their goals, expectations, standards, and concerns [37].

The term "Quality of life" was introduced to define the satisfaction of people's needs, referring not only to the presence or absence of a disease but also to the physical, psychological and social aspects of patients. In this perspective, patients' outcome does not involve only the clinical result but also the patients' feelings towards their health status [38].

A sample of 884 patients, transplanted between 1990 and 1999 in four different medical centers, was enrolled by Grady et al. to evaluate QoL 5–10 years after transplant. The most common co-morbidities reported were hypertension (87%), dyslipidemia (78%), chronic kidney disease (37%), malignancy (27%), and diabetes (27%), while cardiac allograft vasculopathy was evidenced in 42% of the population. According to this report, at 5–10 years from heart transplantation, patients were satisfied with their overall QoL, and predictors of more satisfaction were less depression, less fatigue, being married and not having family-related stressful events, not working, and particularly not having complications related to heart transplant like CAV, malignancy, rejection episodes [39].

A series of the study show how QoL after heart transplantation is not only influenced by clinical features and events related to the graft dysfunction, therapy, and its complications, but a particular focus should be kept on the psychological aspects following heart transplants. They are recognized as risk factors for depression NYHA classes II to IV, corticosteroids-based therapy, and a recently reported episode of acute rejection. Predisposing factors for anxiety were instead female sex and singlehood [40].

The disorders of the sexual sphere can influence QoL, and particularly in end-stage heart failure, they are very frequent because of both organic and psychological causes. A study by Basile et al. demonstrated how a sexual impairment was still present in patients who had undergone heart transplants, and even those with a former active sexual life were not completely satisfied. For this reason, heart transplant recipients can benefit from psychotherapeutic support to restore normal sexual life [41].

ISHLT guidelines provide a series of recommendations concerning sexual life and disorders in heart transplant recipients. For men with erectile dysfunction, the use of phosphodiesterase inhibitors can be considered, and when they are ineffective or contraindicated, patients may be referred to a specialist to undergo intra-cavernous injection of prostaglandin E1. For women desiring pregnancy, a multi-disciplinary team involving maternal and fetal physicians, cardiologists, anesthesiologists, psychologists is fundamental. The pregnancy must be planned to take into consideration the status of the mother and the function of the graft: the risk of acute rejection, infection, and the toxicity of immunosuppressive therapy must be carefully evaluated. Pregnancy should be discouraged in the presence of severe CAV and graft dysfunction, and in any case, it is not recommended within 1 year after transplant.

Multiple Choice Questions.

1. **1-main treatment for advanced heart failure is**
   (A) left ventricular assist device
   (B) bi-ventricular assist device
   (C) heart transplant
   (D) Diuretics

   Ans/c
2. **What are the factors that affect heart transplant?**
   (A) malignancy
   (B) graft failure
   (C) donor selection
   (D) all

   Ans/D
3. **First dual transplantation done in 1983 is**
   (A) heart and liver
   (B) heart and kidney
   (C) heart and lung
   (D) heart and bone

   Ans/A
4. **Survival rate for kidney and heart transplantation in 1 year is**
   (A) %76
   (B) %67
   (C) %50
   (D) %90

   Ans/A
5. **Survival rate for heart and liver transplant in 5 years is**
   (A) %72.8
   (B) %83.4
   (C) %50

(D) %30

Ans/A

6. **Main cause of death among heart transplant patient in first 30 days is**
    (A) acute rejection
    (B) infection
    (C) graft failure
    (D) all

Ans/D

7. **Main cause of death among heart transplant patient after 12 months is**
    (A) Vasculopathy
    (B) rejection
    (C) graft failure
    (D) none of them

Ans/A

8. **COVID-19 and heart failure**
    (A) heart transplant not affected by COVID-19
    (B) COVID decrease survival rate of heart transplant
    (C) COVID-19 increase survival rate of heart transplant
    (D) none of them

Ans/B

9. **COVID-19 is associated with fatality rate of**
    (A) %25
    (B) %40
    (C) %60
    (D) %10

Ans/A

10. **The most vulnerable people for doing heart transplant is**
    (A) advance heart failure
    (B) cardiomyopathy
    (C) valvular heart disease
    (D) none of them

Ans/A

11. **11- Heart transplantation is**
    (A) major surgery
    (B) minor surgery
    (C) neither minor or major

Ans/A

12. **In the past, was regarded as gold standard therapy for heart failure:**
    (A) Medications
    (B) LVAD
    (C) Heart transplantation

    (D) Stem cell therapy

Ans/C

13. **Number of candidates in the waiting list for transportation is**
    (A) increasing
    (B) decreasing
    (C) stable

Ans/A

14. **Nowadays, is no longer termed as a bridge to transplant:**
    (A) Medications
    (B) Stem cell therapy
    (C) LVAD

Ans/C

15. **New LVAD technology devices are**
    (A) Need transcutaneous drive line
    (B) have more complications compared to before
    (C) wireless with less complications

Ans/C

16. **The recent technological changes in LVAD made it more:**
    (A) difficult to use
    (B) more presented with complications
    (C) easy to use

Ans/C

17. **Mortality rate of COVID-19 in patients with chronic co-morbidities is**
    (A) slightly increased
    (B) Decreased
    (C) not changed
    (D) Doubled

Ans/D

18. **Mortality rate of COVID-19 in patients with transplantation is increased due to**
    (A) Immunosuppression
    (B) Co-morbidities
    (C) Both
    (D) none

Ans/C

19. **Morbidity and mortality risk of COVID-19 infection compared to COVID-19 vaccine is**
    (A) Low
    (B) have same morbidity and mortality rate
    (C) high

Ans/C

20. **Post-transplant patients receive their vaccinations:**
    (A) before the transplant by 2 weeks
    (B) Second dose at least one month after transplant if first dose was taken before the transplant
    (C) immunosuppressive agent reduction is mandatory for the vaccine's improved efficacy
    (D) all above

    Ans/D

21. **Regarding survival after cardiac transplantation?**
    (A) Older aged recipients >60 has similar survival outcome as younger recipients.
    (B) Female donor to male recipient carries bad survival outcome.
    (C) Pretransplant Mechanical support does not affect the outcome
    (D) The most critical period for survival is 3-years post-transplant.

    Ans: B

22. **Optimized Immunosuppression regimens for heart transplant management are**
    (A) Induction therapy
    (B) Maintenance therapy
    (C) Treatment of rejection
    (D) All

    Ans: D

23. **Regarding survival after hear transplantation commonest cause of death is**
    (A) Allograft dysfunction
    (B) Rejection
    (C) Allograft vasculopathy
    (D) Renal failure

    Ans: D

24. **Main leading cause of death early after heart transplantation is**
    (A) Cardiac allograft vasculopathy
    (B) Primary graft dysfunction
    (C) Renal failure
    (D) Malignancy

    Ans: B

25. **One of the major long-term complications following cardiac transplantation is**
    (A) Cardiac allograft vasculopathy
    (B) Primary allograft dysfunction
    (C) Hypertension
    (D) All

    Ans. A

26. **Following malignancies are frequent in transplanted patients but rare in non-transplanted general population.**
    (A) Kapposi sarcoma
    (B) Colorectal cancer
    (C) Lung cancer
    (D) Sequomous carcinoma
    Ans. C
27. **Morbidities from immunosuppression toxicity include**
    (A) Renal insufficiency
    (B) Hypertension
    (C) Diabetes.
    (D) All

    Ans. D
28. **Lifestyle after transplantation is**
    (A) greatly affected
    (B) slightly affected
    (C) not affected at all

    Ans. A
29. **Immediately after transplant surgery, the patient needs**
    (A) admission to CPICU
    (B) Vital observation
    (C) IV-line insertion and pain medication
    (D) All above

    Ans. D
30. **Post-transplantation, the patient**
    (A) should be screened closely
    (B) Left without follow-up
    (C) instructed personally for home recovery
    (D) A & C

    Ans. D

References

1. Khush KK, Hsich E, Potena L, Cherikh WS, Chambers DC, Harhay MO, Hayes D Jr, Perch M, Sadavarte A, Toll A, Singh TP. The international thoracic organ transplant registry of the international society for heart and lung transplantation: thirty-eighth adult heart transplantation report — 2021; focus on recipient characteristics. J Heart Lung Transplant. 2021.
2. Khush KK, Cherikh WS, Chambers DC, Harhay MO, Hayes D Jr, Hsich E, Meiser B, Potena L, Robinson A, Rossano JW, Sadavarte A, et al. The international thoracic organ transplant registry of the international society for heart and lung transplantation: thirty- sixth adult heart transplantation report — 2019; focus theme: donor and recipient size match. J Heart Lung Transplant. 2019;3:1.

3. Chang D, Kobashigawa J, Luu M. Outpatient management and long-term complications in heart transplantation. In: Kobashigawa J, editor. Clinical guide to heart transplantation. s.l.: Springer; 2017. p. 171–84.

4. Lee F, Nair V, Chih S. Cardiac allograft vasculopathy: insights on pathogenesis and therapy. Clin Transplant. 2020;1–13.

5. Rahmani M, Cruz RP, Granville DJ, McManus BM. Allograft vasculopathy versus atherosclerosis. Circul Res. 2006;801–15.

6. Schmauss D, Weis M. Cardiac allograft vasculopathy recent developments. Circulation. 2008;2131–41.

7. Ram E, Lavee J, Freimark F, Maor E, Kassif Y, Sternik L, Kogan A, Peled Y. Improved long-term outcomes after heart transplantation utilizing donors with a traumatic mode of brain death. J Cardiothorac Surg. 2019.

8. Labarrere CA, Jaeger BR, Kassab GS. Cardiac allograft vasculopathy: microvascular arteriolar capillaries ("capioles") and survival. Front Biosci. 2017;110–28.

9. Spartalis M, Spartalis E, Tzatzaki E, Tsilimigras DI, Moris D, Kontogiannis C, Iliopoulos DC, Voudris V, Siasos G. Cardiac allograft vasculopathy after heart transplantation: current prevention and treatment strategies. Eur Rev Med Pharmacol Sci. 2019;303–11.

10. Hoffman FM. Outcomes and complications after heart transplantation: a review. J Cardiovasc Nurs. 2005;31–42.

11. McCartney SL, Patel C, Del Rio JM. Long term outcomes and management of the heart transplant recipient. Best Pract Res Clin Anaesthesiol. 2017.

12. Costanzo MR, Dipchand A, Starling R, Anderson A, Chan M, Desai S, Fedson S, Fisher P, Gonzales-Stawinski G, Martinelli L, McGiffin D, et al. The international society of heart and lung transplantation guidelines for the care of heart transplant recipients. J Heart Lung Transplant. 2010;14–56.

13. Spitaleri G, Torres MF, Sabatino M, Potena L. The pharmaceutical management of cardiac allograft vasculopathy after heart transplantation. Expert Opin Pharmacother. 2020;1367–76.

14. Zhang R, Haverich A, Strüber M, Simon A, Bara C. Delayed onset of cardiac allograft vasculopathy by induction therapy using anti-thymocyte globulin. J Heart Lung Transplant. 2008;603–9.

15. Keogh A. Calcineurin inhibitors in heart transplantation. J Heart Lung Transplant. 2004;202–6.

16. Keogh A. Long-term benefits of mycophenolate mofetil after heart transplantation. Transplantation. 2005;45–6.

17. Kaczmarek I, Ertl B, Schmauss D, Sadoni S, Knez A, Daebritz S, Meiser B, Reichart B. Preventing cardiac allograft vasculopathy: long-term beneficial effects of mycophenolate mofetil. J Heart Lung Transplant. 2006;550–6.

18. Bellumkonda L, Patel J. Recent advances in the role of mammalian target of rapamycin inhibitors on cardiac allograft vasculopathy. Clin Transplant. 2020.

19. Jennings DL, Lange N, Shullo M, Latif F, Restaino S, Topkara VK, Takeda K, Takayama H, Naka Y, Farr M, Colombo P, Baker WL. Outcomes associated with mammalian target of rapamycin (mTOR) inhibitors in heart transplant recipients: a meta-analysis. Int J Cardiol. 2017.

20. Zuckermann A, Manito N, Epailly E, Fiane A, Bara C, Delgado JF, Lehmkuhl H, Ross H, Eisen H, Chapman J, Valantine H. Multidisciplinary insights on clinical guidance for the use of proliferation signal inhibitors in heart transplantation. J Heart Lung Transplant. 2008;141–9.

21. Youn J, Stehlik J, Wilk AR, Cherikh W, Kim I, Park G, Lund LH, Eisen HJ, Kim D, Lee SK, Choi S, Han S, Ryu K, Kang S, Kobashigawa JA. Temporal trends of De Novo malignancy development after heart transplantation. J Am Coll Cardiol. 2018.

22. Lateef N, Basit K, Abbasi N, Murtaza S, Ansari AB, Shah M. Malignancies after heart transplant. Exp Clin Transplant. 2016.

23. Brewer JD, Colegio OR, Phillips PK, Roenigk RK, Jacobs MA, Van de Beek D, Dierkhising RA, Christopher WK, McGregor GA, Kremers CCO. Incidence of and risk factors for skin cancer after heart transplant. Arch Dermatol Res. 2014.

24. Alam M, Brown RN, Silber DH, Mullen GM, Feldman DS, Oren RM, Yancy CW, Cardiac Transplant Research Database Group. Increased incidence and mortality associated with skin cancers After Cardiac Transplant. Am J Transplant.2011;1488–97.
25. Kobashigawa JA, Kittleson M. Long term care of the heart transplant recipient. Curr Opin Organ Transplant. 2014;515–24.
26. Ippoliti G, Rinaldi M, Pellegrini C, Vigano M. Incidence of cancer after immunosuppressive treatment for heart transplantation. Crit Rev Oncol Hematol. 2005.
27. Wasson S, Zafar MN, Best J, Reddy HK. Post-transplantation lymphoproliferative disorder in heart and kidney transplant patients: a single-center experience. J Cardiovasc Pharmacol Ther. 2006;77–83.
28. Kellerman L, Neugut A, Burke B, Mancini D. Comparison of the incidence of De Novo solid malignancies after heart transplantation to that in the general population. Am J Cardiol. 2009;562–6.
29. Gonzalez-Vilchez F, de Prada JAV. Chronic renal insufficiency in heart transplant recipients: risk factors and management options. Drugs. 2014.
30. Janus N, Launay-Vacher V, Sebbag L, Despins P, Epailly E, Pavie A, Obadia J, Pattier S, Varnous S, Pezzella V, Trillaud L, Deray G, Guillemain R. Renal insufficiency, mortality, and drug management in heart transplant. Results of the CARIN study. Transpl Int. 2014;931–8.
31. Grupper A, et al. Kidney transplantation as a therapeutic option for end stage renal disease developing after heart transplantation. J Heart Lung Transplant. 2017;297–304.
32. Wallia A, Illuri V, Molitch ME. Diabetes care after transplant. Med Clin North Am. 2016;535–50.
33. van den Berghe G, Wouters P, Weekers F, Verwaest C, Bruyninckx F, Schetz M, Vlasselaers D, Ferdinande P, Lauwers P, Bouillon R. Intensive insulin therapy in critically ill patients. N Engl J Med. 2001;1359–67.
34. Kim HJ, Jung S, Kim JJ, Yun TJ, Kim JB, Choo SJ, Chung CH, Lee JW. New-onset diabetes mellitus after heart transplantation - incidence, risk factors and impact on clinical outcome. Circ J. 2017.
35. Lindenfeld J, Miller GG, Shakar SF, Zolty R, Lowes BD, Wolfel EE, Mestroni L, PageII RL, Kobashigawa J. Drug therapy in the heart transplant recipient. Circulation. 2004;3858–65.
36. Karam VH, Gasquet I, Delvart V, et al. Quality of life in adult survivors beyond 10 years after liver, kidney, and heart transplantation. Transplantation. 2003;1699–704.
37. WHO.int. https://www.who.int/tools/whoqol.
38. Burra P, De Bona M. Quality of life following organ transplantation. Transpl Int. 2007;397–409.
39. Grady K, Naftel DC, Kobashigawa J, Chait J, Young JB, Pelegrin D, Czerr J, Heroux A, Higgins R, Rybarczyk B, McLeod M, White C, Kirklin J. Patterns and Predictors of quality of life at 5–10 years after heart transplantation. J Heart Lung Transplant. 2007;535–43.
40. Loh AZH, Tan JSY, Tam JKC, Zhang MW, Ho RC. Post-operative psychological disorders among heart transplant recipients: a meta-analysis and meta-regression. Psycosomatic Med. 2020;689–98.
41. Basile A, Maccherini M, Diciolla F, Balistreri A, Bouklas D, Lisi G, Toscano T, Mondillo S, Biagioli B, Simeone F, Papalia U. Sexual disorders after heart transplantation. Transplant Proc. 2001.

Heterotopic Heart Transplantation

Mohammed Mohammed Hussein

Abstract Heterotopic heart transplantation is major cardiac procedure that includes implanting the donor heart in recipient thorax in connection with recipient heart which means keeping the native heart in place functioning along with graft in the body circulation. This procedure was first pioneered by. Dr. Barnard and Dr. Losman in 1975. It is an alternative to the orthotopic type of heart transplantation in several conditions specially in the pre-cyclosporine era of heart transplant as a solution for the acute rejection failure. The procedure rate declined due to introduction of immunosuppressive therapy protocol to heart transplantation field, and it is limited to a few certain indications like the condition of severe pulmonary vascular resistance in which orthotopic type is not considered an option. The procedure includes multiple complications, and the statistical studies show variable information regarding its success rate in comparison to the orthotopic type. The operation requires special steps that are performed in the operative theater, and it is discussed in detail in the chapter.

Keywords OHT · Orthotropic Heart Transplantation · HHT · Heterotopic Heart Transplantation · IVC · Inferior Vena Cava · SVC · Superior Vena Cava · RA · Right Atrium · LA · Left Atrium · LV · Left Ventricle · RV · Right Ventricle · PV · Pulmonary Vein · PA · Pulmonary Artery · PVR · Pulmonary vascular resistance

1 Introduction

For many decades till now, orthotropic heart transplantation is regarded as the standard surgical therapeutic protocol for the cases of heart failure in its end stage severity, in which the first orthotropic heart transplant was performed by Dr. Christiaan Barnard in Cape Town, South Africa on December 3, 1967, which considered as one of the most innovative surgical procedures and advances in the twentieth century [1]. Despite that, the OHT faces many difficulties in that era, especially the

M. M. Hussein (✉)
College of Medicine, University of Baghdad, Baghdad, Iraq
e-mail: Mohammed.Mohammed1700d@comed.uobaghdad.edu.iq

  199
H. T. Hashim et al. (eds.), *Heart Transplantation*,
https://doi.org/10.1007/978-3-031-17311-0_11

complications regarding the immune response, graft failure and rejection with many technical and anatomical obstacles in some cases that OHT was not a possible option for them. Another innovative procedure emerges within years after that in spite facing those difficulties and offering alternative treatment in those cases, which is known as Heterotopic Heart Transplantation. HHT in surgical terms means transplanting the donor heart in the recipient body with the reservation of the native recipient heart, without removing it from the recipient thoracic cavity and connecting both of them into the blood circulation [2]. This unique technique was first performed on humans also by Dr. Barnard and Dr. Losman in 1975 for many indications that demand this type of procedures will be discussed later in this chapter.

2 Historical Perspectives

In fact, the attempts that are concerned with cardiac transplantation in general, started with idea of implanting the donor's heart in the circulation without removing the native heart, those attempts are carried on initially on animal models. Such studies through time provide valuable information regarding the aspects of anatomy, physiology, pathology, immunology, and technically of the field of cardiac transplantation.

With respect to these trials, it is possible to classify them into three stages according to the functional, physiological, and anatomical rules of the grafted heart. The first stage of experiments started implanting the donor heart in the recipient body in animal model as an accessory organ without applying the pumping function of the donor heart into the recipient circulation. The Second stage was concerned with putting workload on the donor heart and putting its functionality into the recipient circulation as auxiliary pump. The third stage includes the attempts to implanting the donor heart inside the thoracic cavity with direct connection with recipient heart and working parallelly together to assist the recipient circulation firstly in animal model then human model and using the donor heart as living allograft ventricular assisted device as what is known in the present day.

The first experiment was performed by Dr. Alexis Carrel and Dr. Charles Claude Guthrie in 1905 as a part of many surgical experiments regarding cardiac, vascular surgery, and transplantation of tissues and whole organs in which regards his work, the 1912 Nobel Prize in Medicine and Physiology was assigned to Carrel and the following studies were extensively based on their work. The transplantation performed by implanting the donor heart in the neck of recipient in dog model, the heart was relatively small to the recipient. The attempts followed many different techniques until reaching the most suitable one, which is including the attachment of native carotid artery with the donor right atrium and attachment of donor pulmonary artery with the native jugular vein. In respect to the left side of the heart, the donor aorta was connected with the native jugular vein and one of the donor pulmonary vein with the native carotid artery, in addition, the ligation of openings of the graft superior vena cava and the remanent pulmonary veins [3].

After the end of the procedure which lasted about 75 min, the donor coronary system was circulated with blood after 20 min of reinitiating the circulation. The ventricular contractions started effectively after one hour of the procedure with a heart rate of 88 beats per minute which is considered slightly low regarding the normal heartbeat in the model which was 100 beats per minute [3, 4]. Regarding implanting the donor heart in the neck of the recipient, the techniques regarding attachments and anastomoses had been modified and developed, Mann and his colleagues started new technique in which the graft aorta connected to the host common carotid artery, which in fact providing the donor coronary circulation with oxygenated blood, while the drainage of the deoxygenated blood that is coming from donor coronary sinus, right atrium and ventricle along with the pulmonary artery, is drained into the jugular vein of the recipient body [5]. The heart rate after performing the procedure and establishing the coronary perfusion was 100 to 130 beats per minute with no changes unexpectedly even when the model is in state of exertion. The authors perform many experiments without stating their number, with average of four days regarding the duration of survival of the donor graft and a maximum of eight days in one of the experiments. The hearts were removed after the cessation of pulsation or multiple attacks of fibrillation, and they were examined postoperatively. Grossly, the exam revealed clotting in the left atrium and dilation in the right atrium and ventricle, and the heart tissue infiltrated with lymphocytes and other immunocytes histologically. Mann technique was useful to an extent in some following studies like Downie experiments in 1953 which was implied to study the nature of tachycardia in dog models [6]. The technique had gone through a lot of modifications during the consequential experiments, some of them had some improvements like the studies of Chiba in 1961 and 1962, respectively [7, 8].

Therefore, the interests of making the donor heart using its pumping function in the recipient circulation not only as an accessory organ, but also had been raised with multiple trials. In the attempts of making the donor heart able to supply its coronary system without direct perfusion of oxygenated blood from the recipient vessels, in which contains implement of workload on the donor heart, Marcus had developed a technique of anastomosis that applied anastomosing the recipient proximal common carotid artery to the donor left atrium (which is called Marcus II technique) after slightly different and modified version of Mann technique as first attempt (which is called Marcus technique I) which has implied a workload and pump functioning on the right ventricle of the donor heart [9]. Abdominal transplantation of the donor heart in animal models was bringing more attention in the sixties of the twentieth century, the technique was also involving connection of the donor ascending aorta with the recipient abdominal aorta, giving the perfusion to the donor coronary system [10, 11].

In 1965, Stansel and Terino performed a new technique regarding the heterotopic heart transplant in the abdomen using single anastomosis with many modifications in the procedure with survival rates up to 36 days in the models, they also add immunosuppressive drugs in the experiments which aided the opportunity to reach this survival rate [12].

Transplanting a working model of the graft as an assisting additional pump to the circulation necessitates the intrathoracic transplantation of the donor heart in animal model which begun with Demikhov experiments as heterotopic heart transplant with the graft connected to a native lung lobe in 1950, heart-both lungs transplantation in multiple trials in the fifties of previous century which ended by intrathoracic heart transplantation only without the lungs in 1962 [13, 13].

In 1964, Reemtsma defined a technique in which the graft is transplanted into the recipient thorax as a model of a working pump with support to the native circulation [15].

After one year in India, Sen studies outlined an additional method in which the graft involved only in the systemic circulation of the host [16]. Other techniques were also invented regarding the intrathoracic auxiliary pump model in the following time.

Regarding the introduction of Heterotopic heart transplantation as surgical procedure in human-operated cardiac surgery, it occurred lately due to the increasing interests and experiments in regard to the orthotopic type in the sixties which are crowned by the first man to man heart transplant in 1967. Due to the complications that faced OHT, especially in that time when immunosuppression did not enter the field of solid organ transplantation, the demands of developing of new technique that overcome these difficulties were increasing. These demands are fulfilled by Bernard and Losman work by outlining the operation of heterotopic heart transplantation which is firstly performed on two patients by Barnard and Losman in 1975 in which they added additional surgical methods carrying more benefits but with some restrictions in comparisons with OHT [17]. The operation when first performed has no intraoperative mortality or postoperative complications. Furthermore, HHT became used in cases with severe cardiac failure where OHT is not a suitable option.

3 Indications of HHT

In fact, orthotopic heart transplant was invented before the era of application of immunosuppressive therapy in solid organ transplantation protocols especially cyclosporin, in spite of that, OHT was complicated by the acute immune rejection of the donor graft, which was a major disabling issue regarding the success of the procedure and survival rate of the patients [18]. In contrast, HHT is offering a solution that keeps the native heart functioning, aids in the circulation, and decreases the severity of the clinical status in case of the rejection of the donor heart; this was the main indication for HHT in that time [17]. If hyperacute rejection takes place, the native's heart has crucial rule in the body circulation viability [18]. The native's heart will then offer some sustainability of the circulation during recovery in case of reversible acute rejection or sustains life to the time when another graft can be transplanted. After the emerging of application of the immunosuppressive drug cyclosporine in transplantation protocols, the frequency of abrupt graft failure owing to acute rejection reduced, consequently abolishing one of the main indications of HHT [19].

Other cases were facing more complicated problem, the excessive pulmonary vascular resistance that may end in ventricular failure of the donor graft, in which the condition is fatal and OHT resembles inapplicable or contraindicated especially patients that have high index of pulmonary vascular resistance, which are considered suitable candidates for HHT [20]. This problem was overcome by either heterotopic heart transplantation or heart–lung transplantation. But due to the limited and small numbers of lung grafts and the poor outcomes of OHT in those cases, HHT became the procedure of choice in these situations [21]. This indication of HHT was limited to the patients who have PVR index greater than 6 Wood units despite medical management by pre-operative catheterization in order to use pharmacological agents to decrease the PVR index and reduce it below 6 Wood units, because the if the PVR is reduced below the mentioned level before, the OHT become a better approach with more favorable outcome [22]. Also, Performing HHT for those who have high PVR index, was limited to the adult age group due to the small size of the thoracic cavity in pediatric age group which may not tolerate the procedure [23], but some studies suggest that it can be applied safely in those cases [24].

Orthotopic heart transplant has poor results in cases that have donor-recipient mismatch regarding the height and weight. Some studies suggest that HHT can be a good alternative to the level of 20 per cent donor-recipient mismatch, but that is still controversial that some studies suggest that it has increased rates regarding morbidity and mortality compared to OHT. This indication must be considered and applied with caution [25, 26].

4 Complications of HHT

As early as the patient leaves the operative theater, the complications may arise. The earliest complication to be recognized is Atelectasis. Atelectasis and collapsing of the middle and inferior lobes of the right lung due to the mechanical compressive pressure that is applied by the donor heart, are known complications postoperatively in case of HHT [27]. Atelectasis could be lethal in this situation because it makes the lung susceptible to infection and deterioration of respiratory function and subsequently, ventilatory impairment. The pathology here is hard to be detected on a simple chest radiograph due to the opacification applied by the graft, computed tomography is indicated to assess the lungs radiologically for atelectasis and also to search for other pathologies that may arise regarding fluid collections and consolidations [27]. Atelectasis can be prevented intraoperatively by clearing and suctioning the respiratory secretions in the bronchi via bronchoscopy which can be regarded as aggressive approach [27].

As the HHT is regarded as major open cardiothoracic surgery, endocarditis is very possible complication. The rate of infection arises especially with patients suffering from immunosuppression or those who have prosthetic valve which is considered as an absolute contraindication for HHT [27].

Patients with HHT can develop recipient heart failure or deterioration of native heart function. Due to multiple risk factors including progression or severity of the underlying pathology in native, prolonged ischemia and the asynchronicity and dysregulated inotropic and chronotropic activity to both graft and native heart, the recipient heart more liable to ejection failure caused by the abnormal backward flow of the blood due to valvular incompetency in the mitral and aortic valves, respectively, which are almost continuous. This can be recognized by making an echocardiographic study. Some studies suggest that the complication can be prevented by using permanent pacing by linking both hearts to a pacemaker which can be resulted in enhanced hemodynamic and rhythmical stability that prevents premature failure of the recipient's heart [28, 29].

After HHT procedure, the patients could suffer from ventricular arrhythmia, many reported cases inform that tachyarrhythmias occurred in both native and donor's heart [30].

Due to hemodynamic causes, dilation of recipient heart and ventricular arrhythmia, thromboembolic events have increased the rate in HHT cases as high as 20% in some studies. The embolic events include mainly cerebral vascular events, peripheral embolism, and pulmonary embolism. This can be prevented by anticoagulation therapy with warfarin to decrease the morbidity rate on the long-term perspectives to decrease the morbidity rate [30, 31].

Patients with ischemic heart disease can suffer from recurrence of episodes of ischemic cardiomyopathy and angina. This complication could occur postoperatively, during the follow-up period or being a possible complication regarding long-term perspectives. Ischemic cardiomyopathy can be prevented in the recipient's heart by performing myocardial revascularization or coronary bypass grafting alongside with HHT procedure [32].

As the consequence, cases with HHT suffer decreased cardiorespiratory endurance and exercise capacity in comparison to OHT which can be explained by the competitive chronotropic activity in regards of both hearts or as result of the persistent ischemic attacks that are mentioned above. This complication can be prevented also by implanting pacemakers [33].

Also, rejection of the donor's heart was a complication after HHT procedure due to the immune response of the host, but that is abolished after the introduction of the immunosuppressive agents [34].

5 Postoperative Care in HHT

The aims in follow-up of HHT patients are assessing the clinical status, observing the functionality of both heterotopic and native hearts, monitoring the risks for complications in the purpose of preventing it, evaluating the quality of life and the outcomes of the procedures. Post-operative care starts from the first hour in the ICU by assessing the respiratory function and serial radiological assessment of the chest in case of possible complication of atelectasis, electrocardiographic (ECG) recordings for the electrical activity monitoring of the hearts. But ECG monitoring can be ineffective or misleading because of the indistinguishability and interference of electrical waves parts of both hearts on ECG recording [35]. This can be solved, and the monitoring is done more accurately via pacing temporary pacing wire in the right ventricle of each heart respectively and separately. Like OHT, HHT is also requiring monitoring central venous pressure, right atrial pressure, pulmonary wedge pressure, arterial blood pressure (via invasive method), and arterial oxygen saturation with respect to serial assessments of drains records and fluids and blood input. In addition, postoperative care includes measurement of cardiac output parameters, performing esophageal echocardiography, and urinary output measurement by continuous assessment. Furthermore, the patient status requires reevaluation continuously for signs of postoperative infection, endocarditis, thromboembolism in addition to other postoperative care measures [36].

Chest drains can be removed if there is no risk of further bleeding, pneumothorax, or fluid collection such as pleural effusion. Intravenous and arterial catheters and cannulations should be taken off as soon as the circumstances allow to decrease the hazard of infection especially in population of heart transplant patients with serial specimens' collection, swabs, and culturing of drains and body fluids to monitor the possibility of the postoperative infection [36].

Regarding the evaluation of graft status and function, endomyocardial biopsy, right heart catheterization, and coronary angiography are required. These procedures are invasive and contain difficulties in patients with HHT, but a study suggests that these procedures can be done harmlessly and successfully without reporting any mortality or any other subsequent significant morbidity [37]. As OHT patients, patients with HHT need postoperative immunosuppressive protocols, chest physiotherapy, pharmacological and interventional measures regarding dysrhythmias, postoperative pain, bleeding, infections, fluid retentions, thromboembolism, and measures to prevent psychological isolation in ICU.

6   Statistical Comparison Regarding HHT and OHT

During early years of performing HHT in practice, there were 44 HHTs done in 40 patients from 1974 to 1981 which are collected to be known as HHT Cape Town series in parallel to OHT Series in Cape Town (1967 to 1973) [38].

Regarding the clinical status of the patient preoperatively, all patients were diagnosed with terminal and severe cardiac failure, 21 of them (53%) were diagnosed with ischemic heart disease, 16 cases of cardiomyopathy (42%), and other causes aortic regurgitation and Rheumatic heart diseases. Four cases required retransplantation due to the graft rejection with no operative deaths.

Regarding survival rate, in terms of patients' numbers and survival length, it increased in comparison to the Cape Town series of OHT. Regarding 6 months survival rate, it was 63.2%. Also, it was 54.5% for one year, 41.5 for two years, 38% for 5 years survival rate [38, 38]. However, a study done with series of HHT surgeries between 1993 and 1999 indicated that HHT in undersized graft match has lower survival rate significantly in comparison to OHT and similar survival rate regarding size-matched cases [40].

Regarding the mortality, the rate was 70% with the most common cause being infection in a percentage of 42% of total deaths. The most frequent organisms were clostridium perfringens, Enterobacter, Escherichia coli, and multiple other microorganisms. Infection was followed by graft rejection with 11 cases (28%) divided into 3 cases of acute rejection and 8 cases of chronic rejection. Other causes were cerebrovascular accident, pancreatitis, pulmonary embolism, and iatrogenic causes [38, 38].

Regarding series of 10 HHT and 27 OHT were performed in Texas Heart Institution, the ages in HHT surgeries were variable between 36 and 65 years, these cases were indicated for transplantation due to ischemic cardiomyopathy in 8 cases and dilated cardiomyopathy in 2 cases. Postoperatively, 6 cases suffered from infections, 1 patient from immune rejection, and single case of internal bleeding in the gastrointestinal tract. No postoperative deaths in HHT group in contrast to the OHT group which had 5 deaths divided into 2 postoperative and 3 after patients' discharge [41].

A study in the United States in 2014 included a total 32,361 OHT and 111 HHT cases, separately, were registered. In total, 1-, 5-, and 10-year survival were significantly improved in OHT (87.7%, 74.4%, 54.4%) than HHT cases (83.8%, 59%, 35.1%) [42, 43].

7 The Surgical Technique of HHT

During performing the operation, several steps are required, starting with the removal of the donor heart from the body in similar manner to the OHT techniques but with slight differences, followed by the preparation of both the graft and the recipient thorax and ended by connecting the graft and recipient heart by several anastomosis [44, 45]. This operation also requires many further procedures that will be discussed also in the chapter.

7.1 Harvesting the Donor Heart

The step is accomplished in similar manner to the classic donor cardiectomy in OHT but with few modifications, these modifications include azygos vein ligation and division to obtain longer superior vena cava and dissecting extensively of the ascending aorta and the pulmonary arteries.

7.2 Donor Heart Preparation

This step is accomplished in a solution of cold saline. The IVC and right PVs are over-sewn. After that, create single large opening into the LA with 4 cm diameter by an excision of the tissue between the left pulmonary veins.

After that, 6 cm length incision is done in SVC's posterior aspect and widely through the RA to make satisfactory size for the RA opening.

7.3 Preparation of the Recipient Thorax

The key initial method is a complete median sternotomy but there were attempts to perform it through right-sided thoracotomy. It is crucial to have a safety distance of 2 cm away from the phrenic nerve. Secure hemostasis near the flap edges at that point. Another reflection is done similarly and upward to the previous one, widely advancing the pleuro-pericardial flap towards the superior vena cava, with extreme cautions to not make a damage to the phrenic nerve. A pleuro-pericardial space in the right side is made when the flap falls back to the lung.

7.4 Recipient Cannulation and Cardioplegia

Snares are used and subsequently, the cross-clamping of the native's aorta. After that, a cardioplegic solution is added and adding more is an option depending on the situation requirements throughout the operation. The operation can similarly be accomplished by fibrillation of the native heart, permitting incessant perfusion through coronary circulation.

7.5 The Atrial Anastomosis

To connect both hearts, the initial step is making anastomosis between the donor and native left atria by doing left atriotomy with an incision in the recipient left atrium near the groove of Waterson. After that, evaluation of the edge of right pericardium is crucial. If there is any condition that indicates constriction of left atrial pathway between the native to donor heart, more the right pericardial relaxation is done. Nevertheless, at separation from cardiopulmonary bypass, no gradient must exist through this anastomosis.

7.6   The Aortic Anastomosis

Aorto-aortic anastomosis in an end-to-side manner. Perform aortotomy by doing longitudinal incision with smaller length to some extent than of the graft aorta's end. When the anastomosis between the aortae is done, removing of the cross-clamps takes a place by putting the patient steep Trendelenburg position.

After this step, many procedures are indicated including de-airing, also defibrillation, ventilation, and performing transesophageal echocardiography.

7.7   Anastomosing the Graft Main PA with Recipient RA

An end-to-side anastomosis is performed between graft main PA to native RA free wall with identical incisions in regard to size and diameter on both sides of the anastomosis. Doing this step in that manner gives the possibility of performing right ventricular biopsy of the graft and offers decompression on coronary sinus in regard to the graft.

7.8   The Superior Vena Cava Anastomosis

This anastomosis is done in end-to-end manner. The purpose here is to establish a conduit to make cardiac biopsy possible. A crucial point in this step is making the anastomosis large until it can accommodate the size of the graft SVC and the obtainable SVC of the host.

7.9   Post-Anastomosis Procedures

Furthermore, a series of procedures take place, defibrillation is sometimes needed with direct application of paddles on both hearts, performing the de-airing in the position of steep head down, removing cross-clamp on the aorta, cardiac resuscitation of both hearts during rewarming takes a place before of cardiopulmonary bypass discontinuation, elevation and aspiration of both hearts apices then closure of the aspirated openings and finally, performing transesophageal echocardiogram to ensure the de-airing and assessing if there is retained air.

Multiple Choice Questions:

(1) **A 55 years old patient suffering from severe congestive heart failure with increased pulmonary vascular resistance, the severity from pulmonary vascular resistance that makes him a good candidate for HHT should be**

   a. Higher than 2 wood units
   b. Higher than 4 wood units
   c. higher than 6 wood units
   d. Higher than 8 wood units

(2) **61 years old female diagnosed with stage IV heart failure with increased pulmonary vascular resistance, the PVR score is 6 wood units, what is the best step could be offered to this patient?**

   a. The patient is indicated for Heterotopic heart transplant
   b. OHT should be preferred over HHT
   c. Decreasing the PVR through pharmacological agents
   d. None of the above

(3) **48 years old male patient with heart failure due to severe pulmonary hypertension, the PVR score is 4 wood units, his condition showed improvement after pharmacological trials, he is indicated for a cardiac transplant:**

   a. The patient is a good candidate for OHT
   b. HHT is the procedure of choice
   c. The PVR score should be decreased more to perform OHT
   d. None of the above

(4) **72 years old patient presented with severe dyspnea and cyanosis on day 0 after heterotopic heart transplantation surgery, ECG was normal, echocardiographic indicate no new pathologies in the native heart and no visible lesions in the graft and a chest radiograph was taken but the graft opacify the view on the right lung and the left side was clear with no lesions, the first differential diagnosis to think about in this case:**

   a. Postoperative atelectasis
   b. Pulmonary embolism
   c. Failure of the graft
   d. Pneumonia

(5) **Following the case above, the cause may be due to**

   a. Mechanical compression on the right lung by the graft
   b. Disruption in the pulmonary circulation
   c. Increased pulmonary vascular resistance
   d. None of the above

(6) **After 1 year of a heterotopic heart transplantation surgery, 76 years old patient complains of frequent palpations, decreased endurance for exercises, and dyspnea on exertion. On physical examination, there is continuous murmur on auscultation.**

   a. This condition regarded as normal in case of patients undergo HHT
   b. This condition is result of the asynchronicity between the native heart and the graft
   c. The patient may suffer from valvular incompetency as complication of HHT
   d. B & C

(7) **In the previous case, the condition could be prevented by**

   a. permanent pacing by linking both heart to a pacemaker
   b. Performing valvular replacement at the time of HHT surgery
   c. giving immunosuppressive drugs
   d. it is inevitable, and cannot be prevented

(8) **A 66 years old patient is suffering from severe ischemic heart disease and is not fit for OHT, indicated for heterotopic heart transplant surgery. Regarding this case:**

   a. Modifying the anti-ischemic therapy protocol of the patient
   b. myocardial revascularization or coronary bypass grafting should be performed alongside HHT
   c. Strictly postoperative observation with conservative intervention if the anginal episodes intervene
   d. No other intervention is needed, HHT is enough for his condition

(9) **A 56 years old patient with heterotopic heart transplant admitted to the hospital for evaluation of the graft viability and function, all of the following procedures are needed except**

   a. endomyocardial biopsy
   b. right heart catheterization
   c. Loop recorder implantation
   d. coronary angiography

(10) **the records showed that patients that undergo heterotopic heart transplantation surgery are at high risk for thromboembolic events as high as 20% in some studies, this is maybe explained due to**

   a. asynchronicity between the native heart and the graft
   b. Increased coagulopathy in the subjects of these studies
   c. dilation of recipient's heart and ventricular arrhythmia
   d. Immuno-reaction as acute rejection of the graft

(11) Regarding the first days of performing heterotopic heart transplantation, the major cause of mortality is

    a. Donor-recipient mismatch
    b. Infection
    c. Acute rejection
    d. Post-operative cardiovascular event

(12) Regarding the recent data review of the outcomes of the survival rate in heterotopic heart transplantation, which statement is true:

    a. HHT has much better outcome than OHT
    b. Both HHT and OHT have indistinguishable results with respect to the outcome
    c. OHT by far has better survival rate
    d. Cannot be stated due to lack of data

(13) Regarding the historical overview of Heterotopic heart transplantation, the first trials were about

    a. Implanting the graft as functioning unit in the circulation
    b. Connecting the donor heart as non-functioning unit
    c. The donor heart was partially connected to the recipient's circulation
    d. None of the above

(14) In First trials of HHT, the surgical site that used to implant the donor heart in HHT procedure was

    a. Thorax
    b. Abdomen
    c. Cervical site
    d. None of the above

(15) The main necessitate to make HHT procedure functional in the circulation of the recipient body require

    a. Intrathoracic implanting of the graft
    b. It depends on the type of the anastomosis not the site
    c. Abdominal implantation of the graft offers the same functionality as in intrathoracic implantation.
    d. None of the above

(16) The main indication for inventing heterotopic heart transplantation procedure in its first days was:

    a. Mismatch-related complications
    b. Acute immune rejection in case of OHT
    c. Failure of OHT in ischemic cardiomyopathies
    d. None of the above

(17) **The rate of performing heterotopic heart transplantation was declining due to**

    a. Using of cyclosporine and immunosuppressive therapy in OHT
    b. Increased Failure rate of the procedure
    c. Increased incidence of the postoperative complications
    d. The complexity of procedure and its requirements

(18) **If both OHT and HHT are contraindicated in case with increased pulmonary vascular resistance, the alternative option is**transplantation

    a. Heart-Lung transplantation
    b. Conservative approach with pharmacotherapy
    c. Both a & B
    d. None of the above

(19) **The main problem that faces the procedure of Heterotopic heart transplantation in pediatric age group:**

    a. The intolerability of body for the changes in the circulation
    b. Increased rate of postoperative complications
    c. The small size of thoracic cavity
    d. High rate of immunologic rejections

(20) **To prevent the postoperative atelectasis in HHT, the surgeon should**

    a. Intraoperative suctioning of the secretions via bronchoscopy
    b. Close Monitoring postoperatively of the respiratory function
    c. Can be predicted intraoperatively
    d. Cannot be prevented in case of HHT

(21) **One of the absolute contraindications of heterotopic heart transplantation is**

    a. When the recipient heart has a prosthetic valve
    b. PVR less than 4 wood units
    c. History of severe comorbidities
    d. A case with previous HHT

(22) **Regarding heterotopic heart transplantation, all of the following are false except:**

    a. No need for immunotherapy in case of HHT
    b. The patient should be on immunosuppressive protocol
    c. Endomyocardial biopsy has no benefit in assessing status of the graft
    d. Acute Rejection mostly does not occur for the graft in HHT

(23) **Regarding the assessment of the graft in case of HHT, which investigation could be used:**

    a. Right heart catheterization
    b. Endomyocardial biopsy
    c. Cardiac magnetic resonance imaging
    d. Both a and c

(24) **In the beginning of trials of HHT in animal models, Marcus II technique involved:**

    a. The donor aorta connected to the recipient common carotid artery,
    b. Connecting the recipient proximal common carotid artery to the donor left atrium
    c. Including the attachment of native carotid artery with the donor right atrium
    d. None of the above

(25) **The main problem that faces OHT and favors HHT over OHT in case of increased pulmonary vascular resistance is**

    a. Ventricular failure of the donor graft
    b. Patients with Increased PVR are more to develop acute postoperative complications
    c. A procedural failure due to technical considerations
    d. None of the above

(26) **Regarding atrial anastomosis in the procedure of HHT, if there is constriction of the native to donor heart left atrial pathway, which statement is true:**

    a. more relaxation of the right pericardium is performed
    b. Considered as normal with no further procedure to do in regard to this step
    c. Further pericardial relaxation has no benefit in this case
    d. None of the above

(27) **Regarding the anastomosis of Superior vena cavae of recipient and donor heart, metallic clips are kept in place, the indication of this step is**

    a. This step gives more stability for the anastomosis
    b. Guidance for the endocardial biopsy later on
    c. A Leading point intraoperatively in the next steps
    d. None of the above

(28) **After establishing the anastomosis between aortae of both recipient and donor heart, it is crucial to**

    a. Performing Intra-operative transesophageal echocardiography
    b. De-airing and disposing of all the air on the site
    c. Cardiac defibrillation
    d. a and c

e. All of the above

(29) Having prosthetic valve in the recipient's heart is absolute contraindication in regard to HHT, this contraindication is due to

a. Increased risk of endocarditis
b. Possible effect on the circulation postoperatively
c. Increased risk of tachyarrhythmias
d. These patients are more liable to develop thromboembolic events

(30) It is crucial to prevent or treat atelectasis postoperatively as soon as diagnosed in case of HHT, regarding this situation which statement is false:

a. It is crucial because of the infection, sepsis, and ventilatory dysfunction
b. Chest radiograph is enough to diagnose it
c. It could be prevented by intraoperative bronchoscopic suctioning
d. Need further evaluation by computed tomography imaging

Answers:

1. C
2. B
3. A
4. A
5. A
6. D
7. A
8. B
9. C
10. C
11. B
12. B
13. B
14. C
15. A
16. B
17. A
18. A
19. C
20. A
21. A
22. B
23. D
24. B
25. A
26. A
27. B

28. E
29. A
30. B

References

1. Kempa ME. Christiaan Neethling Barnard–pionier transplantacji serca u człowieka. (W 30 rocznice pierwszego w świecie przeszczepu serca) [Christiaan Neethling Barnard–pioneer in human heart transplantation (on the 30th anniversary of the first heart transplantation]. Polski merkuriusz lekarski : organ Polskiego Towarzystwa Lekarskiego. 1997;3(15):152–4.
2. Barnard CN, Wolpowitz A. Heterotopic versus orthotopic heart transplantation. Transpl Proc. 1979;11(1):309–12.
3. Carel A. The transplantation of vein and organs. Am Med (Philadelphia). 1905;10:1101.
4. Carrel A. The surgery of blood vessels, etc. Johns Hopkins Hosp Bull. 1907;18(190):18–28.
5. Mann FC, Priestley JT, Markowitz J, Yater WM. Transplantation of the intact mammalian heart. Arch Surg. 1933;26(2):219–24.
6. Downie HG. Homotransplantation of the dog heart. AMA Arch Surg. 1953;66(5):624–36.
7. Bing RJ, Chiba C, Chrysohou A, Wolf PL, Gudbjarnason S. Transplantation of the heart. Circulation. 1962;25(2):273–6.
8. Chiba C, Wolf PL, Gudbjarnason S, Chrysohou A, Ramos H, Pearson B, Bing RJ. Studies on the transplanted heart: Its metabolism and histology. J Exp Med. 1962;115(4):853–66.
9. Wong S. Homologous heart grafts; transplantation of the heart in dogs. In: Surgical forum; 1951. p. 212–7.
10. Marcus E, Wong SN, Luisada AA, Liu WC. Homologous heart grafts: I. Technique of interim parabiotic perfusion II. Transplantation of the heart in dogs. AMA Arch Surg. 1953;66(2):179–91.
11. Cooper D. Experimental development of cardiac transplantation. BMJ. 1968;4(5624):174.
12. Stansel HC, Terino EO. A single-anastomosis heterotopic cardiac homotransplant. Arch Surg. 1965;90(3):444–8.
13. Demikhov VP. A new and simpler variant of heart-lung preparation of a warm-blooded animal. Bull Eksp Biol Med. 1950;7:21–7.
14. Adams W. Experimental transplantation of vital organs. By VP Demikhov. Authorized translation from the Russian by Basil Haigh, MA, MB, B. Chir. Cloth. Pp. 285, with 74 illustrations. Consultants Bureau, 227 W. 17th St., New York City, 1962. Anesthesiology. 1963; 24(3).
15. Reemtsma K. The heart as a test organ in transplantation studies. Ann N Y Acad Sci. 1965;120(2):778–85.
16. Cooper DKC. Clinical orthotopic and heterotopic heart transplantation: aspects of the University of Cape Town experience. Master's thesis, Faculty of Health Sciences;1985.
17. Losman JG, Barnard CN. Heterotopic heart transplantation: a valid alternative to orthotopic transplantation: results, advantages, and disadvantages. J Surg Res. 1982;32(4):297–312.
18. Cooper DKC, Novitzky D, Becerra E, Reichart B. Are there indications for heterotopic heart transplantation in 1986? Thorac Cardiovasc Surg. 1986;34(05):300–4.
19. Baumgartner W, Achuff S. Heart and heart-lung transplantation. Philadelphia, PA: WB Saunders; 1990. p. 284–92.
20. Addonizio LJ, Gersony WM, Robbins RC, Drusin RE, Smith CR, Reison DS, Reemtsma KEITH, Rose EA. Elevated pulmonary vascular resistance and cardiac transplantation. Circulation. 1987;76(5 Pt 2):V52–5.
21. Wang SS, Chu SH, Ko WJ, Chen YS, Chou NK. Heterotopic heart transplantation for severe pulmonary hypertension. Transplant Proc. 1998;30:3408–9.

22. Cochrane AD, Adams DH, Radley-Smith R, Khaghani A, Yacoub MH. Heterotopic heart transplantation for elevated pulmonary vascular resistance in pediatric patients. J Heart Lung Transplant. 1995;14(2):296–301.
23. Reichart B. Size matching in heart transplantation. J Heart Lung Transplant. 1992;11(4 Pt 2):S199-202.
24. Desruennes M, Muneretto C, Gandjbakhch IRADJ, Kawaguchi A, Pavie A, Bors V, Piazza C, Rabago G Jr, Leger P, Vaissier E. Heterotopic heart transplantation: current status in 1988. J Heart Transplant. 1989;8(6):479–85.
25. Parry A, Large S. Donor-recipient size match in heart transplantation. J Thorac Cardiovasc Surg. 1994;108(6):1150–1.
26. Sethi GK, Lanauze P, Rosado LJ, Huston C, McCarthy MS, Butman S, Copeland JG. Clinical significance of weight difference between donor and recipient in heart transplantation. J Thorac Cardiovasc Surg. 1993;106(3):444–8.
27. Kadner A, Chen RH, Adams DH. Heterotopic heart transplantation: experimental development and clinical experience. Eur J Cardiothorac Surg. 2000;17(4):474–81.
28. Hildebrandt A, Reichenspurner H, Gordon GD, Horak AR, Odell JA, Reichart B. Heterotopic heart transplantation: mid-term hemodynamic and echocardiographic analysis–the concern of arteriovenous-valve incompetence. J Heart Transplant. 1990;9(6):675–81.
29. Akasaka T, Lythall D, Cheng A, Yoshida K, Yoshikawa J, Mitchell A, Yacoub MH. Continuous aortic regurgitation in severely dysfunctional native hearts after heterotopic cardiac transplantation. Am J Cardiol. 1989;63(20):1483–8.
30. Neerukonda SK, Schoonmaker FW, Nampalli VK, Narrod JA. Ventricular dysrhythmia and heterotopic heart transplantation. J Heart Lung Transplant. 1992;11(4 Pt 1):793–6.
31. Kotliar C, Smart FW, Sekela ME, Pacifico A, Pratt CM, Noon GP, DeBakey ME, Young JB. Heterotopic heart transplantation and native heart ventricular arrhythmias. Ann Thorac Surg. 1991;51(6):987–91.
32. Ridley PD, Khaghani A, Musumeci F, Favaloro R, Akl ES, Banner NR, Mitchell AG, Yacoub MH. Heterotopic heart transplantation and recipient heart operation in ischemic heart disease. Ann Thorac Surg. 1992;54(2):333–7.
33. Cowell RP, Morris-Thurgood J, Coghlan JG, Ilsley CD, Mitchell AG, Khaghani A, Paul VE, Yacoub M. Effects of paced counterpulsation on exercise capacity and hemodynamics after heterotopic heart transplantation. Am J Cardiol. 1995;75(5):415–7.
34. Perrault LP, Bidouard JP, Janiak P, Villeneuve N, Bruneval P, Vilaine JP, Vanhoutte PM. Time course of coronary endothelial dysfunction in acute untreated rejection after heterotopic heart transplantation. J Heart Lung Transplant. 1997;16(6):643–57.
35. Housmans PR, Rietman GW, Wellens F, Verbeke J, Nollet G. Ventricular dysrhythmia in the native heart after heterotopic heart transplantation: diagnosis with selective electrocardiography. J Am Soc Anesthesiol. 1996;85(4):936–9.
36. Karp RB. Heart transplantation: the present status of orthotopic and heterotopic heart transplantation. JAMA. 1985;254(6):834–834.
37. Lowry RW, Bitar JN, Carter Grinstead W, Young JB, Noon GP, Vardan S, Cocanougher B, Kleiman NS. Heterotopic heart transplantation: catheterization, endomyocardial biopsy, and coronary angiography of the donor heart. Cathet Cardiovasc Diagn. 1994;32(1):18–26.
38. Losman JG. Review of the Cape Town experience with heterotopic cardiac transplantation. Cardiovasc Dis. 1977;4(3):243.
39. Barnard CN. The present status of heart transplantation. S Afr Med J. 1975;49(7):213–4.
40. Bleasdale RA, Banner NR, Anyanwu AC, Mitchell AG, Khaghani A, Yacoub MH. Determinants of outcome after heterotopic heart transplantation. J Heart Lung Transplant. 2002;21(8):867–73.
41. Konertz W, Sheikhzadeh A, Weyand M, Friedl A, Bernhard A. Heterotopic heart transplantation: current indications for the procedure, with results in 10 patients. Tex Heart Inst J. 1988;15(3):159.
42. Jahanyar J, Koerner MM, Ghodsizad A, Loebe M, Noon GP. Heterotopic heart transplantation: the United States experience. Heart Surg Forum. 2014;17(3):E232–40.

43. Cockrell HC, O'Brien R, Carter KT, Shaw TB, Baran DA, Kutcher ME, Copeland JG, Copeland H. Better together: a reappraisal of heterotopic heart transplantation. Transplant Int. 2021.
44. Novitzky D, Cooper DKC, Barnard CN. The surgical technique of heterotopic heart transplantation. Ann Thorac Surg. 1983;36(4):476–82.
45. Copeland J, Copeland H. Heterotopic Heart Transplantation: Technical Considerations. Oper Tech Thorac Cardiovasc Surg. 2016;21(3):269–80.

Artificial Heart, Cellular, Regenerative, and Xenotransplantation

Ali Talib Hashim, Ibrahim Dheyaa Al-Hasani, and Rebecca Caruana

Abstract The Artificial heart is a system which regulates cardiovascular circulation and oxygenation in the body. Any system which replaces the heart is in fact an artificial heart system. There are over 100,000 normal genes in the nucleus of a skeletal myoblast that affect the cell's normality and features. In vitro, skeletal myoblasts preserve their myogenic ability. During the healing process, they aid in muscle regeneration.

Keywords Artificial heart · Cellular · Regenerative · Xenotransplantation · Barriers

1 Introduction

Any system which replaces the heart is in fact an artificial heart system. In 1982, Jarvik-VII was the first successfully implanted artificial heart. The procedure was performed by Willem Johan Kolff and Robert Jarvik. And their team [1].

Modern Medicine's main scientific studies and research rotate around finding an alternate heart substitute. Reducing the need for heart transplants would be the obvious advantage of a functional artificial heart, since the organ demand often exceeds the supply significantly. The heart represents subtleties that with synthetic materials and power supplies challenge clear mimicry. The effects of these problems include extreme foreign-body rejection and mobility-limiting external successions. The life span of early human recipients was reduced by these complications to hours or days [1].

A. T. Hashim (✉)
Golestan University of Medical Sciences, Gorgan, Iran
e-mail: talibhashim42@gmail.com

I. D. Al-Hasani
College of Medicine, University of Baghdad, Baghdad, Iraq

R. Caruana
Medicine and Surgery Department, University of Malta, Msida, Malta
e-mail: rebec-ca.caruana.15@um.edu.mt

H. T. Hashim et al. (eds.), *Heart Transplantation*,
https://doi.org/10.1007/978-3-031-17311-0_12

In 1937, the Soviet scientist Vladimir Demikhov rendered the first artificial heart.

Around that same time the University of Utah also created a similar patent artificial heart device yet Winchell's heart was cited initially [2].

At the meeting, Liotta acknowledged dog implantation as three forms of orthotopic (within the pericardial sac) TAHs, respectively, each one was making use of a different external energy source.

2 Initial Clinical Indication for the Use of a Permanent Artificial Heart

Paul Winchell independently developed and patented a ventricle with a similar shape and after donated it to the Utah program. During that period, Robert Jarvik who was still a student combined multiple modifications at the University of Utah. His studies and research involved creating an ovoid form to be able a suitable size for the human chest. William DeVries rooted the artificial heart on December 2, 1982 into the retired dentist Barney Bailey Clark who died on March 23, 1983, living 112 days with the implant. The second recipient was Bill Schroeder and he lived for a total of 620 days [2].

As a bridge to transplantation, it has been implanted in over 1,350 individuals. In the mid-1980s, it was dishwasher-sized pneumatic power sources which powered the artificial hearts. Furthermore, two catheters had to deliver pneumatic pulses to the implanted heart. This significantly increased the risk of infections. To accelerate the creation of new technological generations, the National Heart, Lung, and Blood Institute created a competitional aspect for implantable electrically powered artificial hearts. It was Cleveland Clinic in Cleveland, Ohio; Pennsylvania State University's College of Medicine in Pennsylvania; and Danvers, Massachusetts' AbioMed, Inc. who earned funding. The Cleveland program was withdrawn subsequently after the first five years, even though it was quite successful at the time [3, 4].

3 Heart–Lung Machine

This process is necessary to sustain life in both high-demand organs, i.e., the brain, heart, lungs, kidneys and liver and even in those of lower demand. Those areas of the body which have a lower entails the pumping of 5 L or more per minute. This process is important for open-heart surgery procedures.

In 1953, the American surgeon John H. Gibbon, Jr. announced the first effective use for the heart-lung machine [3].

Since then, with smaller and more powerful oxygenators, heart-lung devices have been significantly improved, enabling them to be used by adults and even in children and newborns.

4 Mechanical Hearts

When implanting a full artificial heart requires both ventricles of the lower chambers must be removed.

Only after all other medical management has failed are artificial hearts implanted. They can be used after cardiac arrest for heart resuscitation, after heart surgery for recovery from cardiogenic shock. The aim is to provide a secure, efficient system which permits the donor to move around easily, therefore promoting and enriching the quality of life of that patient. Most VAD donors in fact benefit from prolonged life and return to their normal routine, work, and regular physical activities [3].

Synthetic materials were created during the 1970s, which greatly improved the growth of permanent artificial hearts. In 1982, American surgeon William C who was first user lived 112 days and his death occurred because of multiple implant-caused physical complications. There was no change or much worse in subsequent patients, so the use of the Jarvik-7 was discontinued [3].

Carmat heart sensors were also used to monitor blood flow and heartbeat [1–3, 5].

5 Carmat Bioprosthetic Heart

The prototype was composed of "biomaterials" or a "pseudo-skin" of biosynthetic, chemically treated animal tissues, microporous materials, using embedded electronic sensors [2].

Two chambers are each separated by a membrane in Carmat's design, which carries hydraulic fluid on one side. In and out of the chambers, a motorized pump pushes hydraulic fluid, causing that membrane to move. This results in blood to pass on the other side of each membrane. To make the system more biocompatible, the blood-facing the membrane side is composed of the sac tissue of a cow's heart [3].

The Carmat system often uses valves which are composed of a cow's heart tissue and which has sensors within the device which sense any elevated pressure. It is capable of altering flow rate unlike the older models which are only capable of maintaining a continuous flow rate.

Unlike previous designs, the Carmat device was mainly directed for the use of end stage heart failure [1–3].

6 Soft Artificial Heart

Cohrs and his colleague's main aim were that of creating an artificial heart roughly a similar size of the patients' heart to imitate his/her heart's form and function as close as possible. In a hybrid model, the model does move and function like the real heart yet it only beats for around 30,000 beats. This corresponds to only 30 to 50 beats per minute [5].

7 Hybrid Assistive Devices

Ventricular assist devices (VAD) may be indicated for patients who have some residual heart function yet requires assistance to function, maintain, and preserve life. It was Domingo Liotta who invented the first Left Ventricular Assist Device (LVAD) system in 1962 at the Baylor College of Medicine.

The Kantrowitz CardioVad, which was designed by Adrian Kantrowitz, is another example of VAD which supports the patient's native heart by taking up more than 50% of the heart's function.

Another important benefit of a VAD is that if the artificial pump had to stop functioning, the patient will be capable to maintain the function of the natural heart which can act as temporary back-up support. This can provide ample time to provide a plan for the patient's care [5].

In August 2006, a 15-year-old teenage girl at Stollery Children's Hospital was implanted with an artificial heart. It was planned to serve as a temporary fixture before it was possible to find a donor heart [3, 5].

8 Cellular Heart Implantation

There are over 100,000 normal genes in the nucleus of a skeletal myoblast that affect the cell's normality and features. In vitro, skeletal myoblasts preserve their myogenic ability. During the healing process, they aid in muscle regeneration. The cause of myogenic development, on the other hand, is unknown. Mononucleated skeletal myoblasts merge naturally to produce multinucleated myotubes during myogenesis and muscle regeneration, and so share a common gene pool. However, unlike previous cell fusions, the nuclear membranes are not broken. The nuclei of the fusing cells on no occasion do fuse together, therefore their nuclear components are never mixed together. Myotubes evolve into myofibrils and then into myofibers after establishing neuronal and vascular connections. If these myotubes do not form any of these connections, they will degenerate. The myoblast population isolated from skeletal muscle biopsies is not identical. The skeletal myoblasts which were transplanted are capable to endure and live within the host's myocardium, according to the majority of researchers. In a pig model of chronic cardiac ischemia, the grafted transgenic skeletal myoblasts continued to live for further than 10 weeks within the host's cardiac muscle after transplantation. One of the potential drawbacks of employing skeletal myoblasts is that their electromechanical properties differ from those of cardiomyocytes. The cardiomyocytes are joined together in the myocardium's architectural set-up by intercalated disks, which are cell junctions. Gap junction proteins are expressed sooner in skeletal myoblasts. During the differentiating process, however, its expression is suppressed. As a result, it's unlikely that grafted adult skeletal muscle will form electromechanical connections with the host myocardium. As a result, skeletal myoblasts that express high levels of Connexin-43 may be superior candidates for cardiac transplantation. The exact mechanism through which myoblast transplantation improves heart function has yet to be determined [6].

The results showed that heart function had improved overall. Ten ischemic heart failure patients who were reported to have infarcted, non-viable and a myocardium which was non-revascularized were injected with autologous skeletal myoblasts within the myocardium region during the CABG procedure. Ventricular tachyarrhythmias occurred in three cases. Explanted hearts underwent histological analysis, which revealed the development of viable grafts in damaged myocardial tissue [6].

9 Problems in Skeletal Myoblast Transplantation

Primary cell death, low survival cell rate, and restricted translocation from the injection site are all limiting aspects in myoblast transplantation for tissue healing. According to one study, up to 80% of transplanted cells perish in the first 24–48 h after transplantation in vivo. Myoblasts modified to express anti-inflammatory interleukin-I had higher posttransplant survival, according to Qu et al. 67. The findings on skeletal myoblasts show that the population of developing myogenic cells is heterogeneous. The cells that cycle quickly in vitro, on the other hand, are the ones that die after transplanting. Important characteristics to look for are the sources of the skeletal myoblasts and the ability of these myoblasts to express desmin. Pre-Irradiation of the recipient muscle is a concept that does not exactly mimic the actual clinical condition. In immunocompromised animal models, better results were obtained, with no problem of rejection and the donor cells surviving for longer periods of time. The administration of immunosuppressants in cases of allogeneic cell transplantation has therapeutic implications due to immunosuppression's negative effects. The allogeneic myoblasts are retained in the host tissue for a longer period of time after receiving a transitory immunosuppressive treatment. The success of cell transplantation is impossible without proper immunosuppression before and after the procedure. Different immunosuppressants had different efficacies in suppressing immunological responses against donor cells, according to studies. When compared to other medications, cyclosporine has been proven to produce effective immunosuppression. The variation within the major histocompatibility complex (MHC) molecules has a crucial influence on immunological rejection of cellular transplants. It's also impossible to rule out the possibility of small antigen molecules influencing the cell surface. Furthermore, the deposition of C3 complement has been linked to the transplanted cells' early death. Transplantation of myoblasts causes cellular and humoral responses, leading to graft rejection, according to data from human research and immunocompetent animal models like mice. The disparity in survival between cultured and injected skeletal myoblasts and those implanted directly suggests that some feature of the tissue culture conditions is harmful to the cells. The most common method of delivery is to introduce skeletal myoblasts directly into the normal and damaged heart by direct intramural injection. More research is needed to increase and outline arterial myoblast administration efficacy. Improved heart function after transplantation may be depending on donor cell dosage [7].

A linear relationship between the functional outcome of the cell transplantation process and the sum of cells which were grafted exists. The degree in improvement of cardiac function depends mainly on the number of injected myoblasts. Yet further research is required to establish the exact and ideal number of cells which needs to be injected and the time period within these cells need to be injected post-infarction. Time injectable period is fundamental since if the cellular transplantation is delayed cellular remodeling would be established and therefore the process would be irreversible. On the other hand, early, cellular transplantation may lead to rapid cellular death because it promoted inflammatory actions at the site of injury [7].

For the effectiveness of skeletal myoblast therapy, a better understanding of all of these characteristics, as well as a better understanding of the immunobiology of cell transplantation, is required.

10 The Second Generation: Blood and Bone Marrow-Derived Cells

After 5–9 days of an episode of an acute ST-elevation MI, a percutaneous transluminal coronary angioplasty (PTCA) was performed in 10 patients. These patients were infused with autologous mononuclear bone marrow cells. When after 3 months these patients were followed-up and compared with 10 other patients who did not have an implant and hence were the control in the study the transplanted patients were found to have exhibited smaller infarcts and also a lower left ventricular end-systolic volume. This was linked to an improved infarct contractility and also perfusion of the myocardium [6, 7].

11 Xenotransplantation Heart Transplant

Baboons who had their hearts replaced with genetically engineered pig hearts lived for up to 195 days after the procedure. Bruno Reichart and colleagues developed an adapted protocol for the transplantation of cross-species (xenotransplantation) that is a significant improvement over previous efforts—the longest survival time of a pig-to-baboon heart replacement was only 57 days. Patients with terminal cardiac failure have no other alternative except to undergo a heart transplant. The results of human heart transplantation are positive, and life is not only extended but also improved in quality. Yet a significant organ scarcity worldwide, and the quantity of organs available for heart transplantation does not meet the increased demand. "Xenogeneic heart transplants are doable and surprisingly easy to treat in the long run, especially when using cutting-edge, non-nephrotoxic immunosuppression," he says [8].

Multiple Choice Questions:

1. **What are the barriers that can lead to the failure of the heart transplant from pig to human?**

(A) Immune barriers.

(B) Infectious disease barrier.

(C) Physiological barriers.

(D) Immune barrier, physiological barrier and infectious disease barriers.

Answer: Immune barrier, physiological barrier and infectious disease barriers.

2. **Which one of the following is false regarding the barriers for pig to human heart transplantation**

(A) Delayed xenograft rejection (DXR) occurs within hours after transplantation.

(B) Despite intensive immunosuppression, thrombodysregulation is sufficient to elicit DXR in immunologically tolerized GalTKO organ recipients and GalTKO.hCPRP organ recipients.

(C) Immunological barriers are caused by antibodies against carbohydrates.

(D) DRX includes organ xenograft malfunction and recipient damage.

Answer: Delayed xenograft rejection (DXR) occurs within hours after transplantation. because DXR normally occurs within days to weeks after transplantation.

3. **The process of replacement of nonfunctional heart of human with healthy and genetically engineered pig heart called:**

(A) replacement therapy.

(B) transplantation.

(C) repair and replacement.

(D) all of the above.

Answer: transplantation.

4. **The transfer of pigs' heart to humans is called:**

(A) Allograft.

(B) Autograft.

(C) Syngeneic graft.

(D) Xenograft.

Answer: Xenograft.

5. **The immunological barrier can be solved by**

(A) Genetic engineering strategies have been employed to prevent hyperacute rejection and DXR.

(B) Expressing one of three human complement pathways regulating proteins on the surface of pig cells and organs reduces complement-mediated cell damage and prolongs pig cell and organ survival.

(C) By Immunosuppressive medications.

(D) All of the above.

Answer: all of the above.

6. **Which one of the following is not a solution for immunological barrier:**

(A) Triple knockouts (TKOs).

(B) Antiviral medication.

(C) single gene knockout (KO).

(D) all of the above.

Answer: Antiviral medication.

7. **Heart-Lung machine can be used:**

(A) only in adults.

(B) only in children.

(C) only in infants.

(D) adults, children, infants.

Answer: adults, children, infants.

8. **About Heart-Lung machine, all the following are true except:**

(A) The oxygenator replaces the function of the lung during heart surgery.

(B) Heart catheterization is one of the indications to use a Heart–Lung machine.

(C) Heart-lung machine is used for fixing or removing the valve, repairing defects within the heart, or revascularizing blocked arteries.

(D) The Heart–Lung machine has an ability to pump Up to 5 L (1.3 gallons) or more of blood per minute.

Answer: Heart catheterization is one of the indications to use a Heart–Lung machine.

9. **Which one of the following is considered to be contraindicated for ventricular assistance device use:**

(A) severe renal, pulmonary, liver, or neurological disease.

(B) after cardiac arrest.

(C) chronic heart failure patients.

(D) after heart surgery for recovery from cardiogenic shock.

Answer: severe renal, pulmonary, liver, or neurological disease.

10. **Heart–lung machine:**

(A) is a mechanical machine that pumps blood during heart surgery.

(B) An oxygenator is not necessary during surgery.

(C) blood cannot reach a highly demanded area like the brain.

(D) not useful during open-heart surgery.

Answer: is a mechanical machine that pumps blood during heart surgery.

11. **Which of the following was made from silicone:**

(A) Hybrid assistive devices.

(B) Soft Artificial heart.

(C) Carmat bioprosthetic heart.

(D) Mechanical Hearts.

Answer: Soft Artificial heart.

12. **In cellular heart transplantation the two available graft cells are**

(A) skeletal myoblast cells and bone marrow-derived cells.

(B) heart myoblast cells and bone marrow-derived cells.

(C) smooth myoblast cells and bone marrow-derived cells.

(D) heart myoblast cells and skeletal myoblast cells.

Answer: (A) skeletal myoblast cells and bone marrow-derived cells.

13. **Various delivery routes and modes have been used. The most common method of delivery is.**

(A) introduce skeletal myoblasts directly into the normal and damaged heart by direct intramural injection.

(B) Direct intramural injection of skeletal myoblasts into the normal and injured heart is used to introduce them indirectly.

(C) intramural injection of cardiac myoblasts into the normal and injured heart.

(D) intracoronary injection of skeletal myoblasts.

Answer: (A) introduce skeletal myoblasts directly into the normal and damaged heart by direct intramural injection.

– according to the recent researches, the most common method of delivery is to introduce skeletal myoblasts directly into the normal and damaged heart by direct intramural injection.

14. **Different immunosuppressants had different efficacies in suppressing immunological responses against donor of skeletal myoblast cells, according to studies. When compared to other medications, has one of the following has been proven to produce effective immunosuppression:**

(A) prednisone.

(B) cyclophosphamide.

(C) mycophenolate.

(D) abatacept.

Answer: (B) cyclophosphamide.

– Different immunosuppressants had different efficacies in suppressing immunological responses against donor cells, according to studies. When compared to other medications, cyclosporine has been proven to produce effective immunosuppression.

References

1. Latrémouille C, et al. A bioprosthetic total artificial heart for end-stage heart failure: results from a pilot study. J Heart Lung Transplant. 2018;37(1):33–7.
2. Gautier SV, et al. Artificial heart in Russia: past, present, and future. Artif Organs. 2021;45(2):111–4.
3. Netuka I, et al. First clinical experience with the pressure sensor-based autoregulation of blood flow in an artificial heart. ASAIO J. 2021;67(10):1100.
4. Pal, S. Design of the total artificial heart. In: Design of artificial human joints & organs. Boston, MA: Springer;2014. https://doi.org/10.1007/978-1-4614-6255-2_16
5. Briasoulis A, et al. Trends in utilization, mortality, major complications, and cost after total artificial heart implantation in the United States (2009–2015). Hellenic J Cardiol. 2020;61(6):407–12.
6. Isomi M, Sadahiro T, Ieda M. Progress and challenge of cardiac regeneration to treat heart failure. J Cardiol. 2019;73(2):97–101.

7. Cathery W, et al. Concise review: the regenerative journey of pericytes toward clinical translation. Stem Cells. 2018;36(9):1295–310.
8. Fernández-Ruiz I. Breakthrough in heart xenotransplantation. Nat Rev Cardiol. 2019;16:69. https://doi.org/10.1038/s41569-018-0151-4.
9. Cooper DKC, et al. Perspectives on the optimal genetically-engineered pig in 2018 for initial clinical trials of kidney or heart xenotransplantation. Transplantation. 2018;102(12):1974.
10. Fernández-Ruiz I. Breakthrough in heart xenotransplantation. Nat Rev Cardiol. 2019;16(2):69–69.
11. Pierson III, Richard N, et al. Pig-to-human heart transplantation: who goes first? Am J Transplant. 2020;20(10):2669–74.
12. Pierson III, Richard N, et al. Progress toward cardiac xenotransplantation. Circulation. 2020;142(14):1389–98.

Multi-organ Transplantation

Fahtiha Nasreen, Tasnia Noor Salim, Avishek Kunda, Ibad Ur Rehman, Maryam Aman, and Rebecca Caruana

Abstract Organ transplantation is one of the many wonders of the world of medicine; multi-organ transplantation even more so. Among various methods of prolonging life, organ transplantation is the only one backed by hefty results. In the last few decades, it has been gauged to be one of the most prolific ways to guarantee a prolonged life, especially in patients suffering from end-stage diseases. Almost all major organs of the body are being transplanted these days successfully. Organs in different combinations are transplanted by a team of specialists in specialized OTs, these include surgeons, nurses, anesthesia specialists, and many more participants. Depending on the type of organs involved, success rate of these transplants varies. Even in successful transplants, the majority of the patients do still have to cope with complications of surgery. The most important concern in organ transplantation is the selection and availability of donors. Apart from the basics of blood type matching, donor needs to fulfill a set of requirements for the process to go ahead. One of the major concerns in the transplant procedures is allotment and distribution of organs without disparity. The solution to this concern is an open public distribution system in which the transplantation process is done on merit. Multiple recommendations and suggestions are in process of implementation, which when achieved will make these transplants a lot more successful and common occurrence.

F. Nasreen (✉)
Armed Forces Medical College, Dhaka, Bangladesh
e-mail: Fnas24@gmail.com

T. N. Salim · A. Kunda
Bangladesh Medical College, Dhaka, Bangladesh

I. Ur Rehman
Shifa Tameer E Millat University, Shifa College of Medicine, Islamabad, Pakistan
e-mail: Fnas24@gmail.com

M. Aman
Shifa College of Medicine, Shifa Tameer E Milat University, Islamabad, Pakistan

R. Caruana
Medicine and Surgery Department, University of Malta, Msida, Malta
e-mail: rebecca.caruana.15@um.edu.mt

Keywords Multi-organ transplant · Donors · Process of implementation · Rotationplasty · Isograft

1 Introduction

Multi-organ transplants can be defined as the transfer of two or more organs from donors to recipients. These transfers are utilized to treat a few falling flat or ailing organs by supplanting them with sound ones, typically from a similar giver. People might be considered for this operation when every single other treatment and medicine has been ineffective in improving the condition of the patient.

Multi-organ transplant is beneficial to certain recipients since it avoids having multiple surgeries. Tragically, advancements in extending the organ pool have not been similarly fruitful, prompting ever-lengthening holding up records and holding up occasions. In the setting of organ shortage, multi-organ transplantation is a field that presents open doors for reexamining key moral ideas around assignment change [1, 2].

The normal reason for various organ disappointments can be a multisystem illness called amyloidosis. This condition can prompt the development of irregular proteins in organs, for example, the kidneys, heart, or liver. Specialists utilize creative strategies in multi-organ relocate a medical procedure and different kinds of relocate a medical procedure, with astounding outcomes. In various clinic studies, specialists found that individuals who required and got heart–kidney transfers had fantastic long-haul results. The practice of multi-organ transplant has become a quite popular procedure, but it is striking heterogeneity in the choice of patient's choice in different countries which uncovers the issues of value and utility. Reforms ought to remember a decrease in impetuses to perform multi-organ transplants, invent new ways of examination, and more readily build up very few clinical criteria for such transplants. Qualification and a straightforward public cycle for deciding distribution needs for this should be conducted as well. Changes to organ allotment policies and practices should address moral standards just as the particular clinical conditions for various sorts of multi-organ transplants [1].

2 Background of Organ Transplantation

For patients who have end-stage illness, transplantation regularly gives them simple opportunity to endurance. Indeed, even before the primary transfer was performed, unmistakably OT must be effective in using a multidisciplinary team approach [2].

3   The History of Organ Transplantation

The history of OT procedures dates back to old Greek, Rome, Chinese, and Indian history. Alexis Carrel performed vascular anastomoses and he was also successful in kidney transfers in canines successfully starting vessel recreation and cold graft preservation. Sedation and Perioperative Care for Solid Organ Transplantation also forms part of the BMC Anesthesiology. In fact, this aspect of surgery was set up in an attempt to give anesthesiologists the opportunity and basic consideration pros to introduce their work in the field of organ transplantation [1, 2].

Expanded consciousness of organ gift has expanded the accessibility of perished benefactors, and it has supported the open doors for treating patients with numerous organ brokenness. All the while supplanting two organs gives favorable circumstances for single medical procedure, lower immunosuppression portion, and preferable endurance over when one organ alone is relocated.

4   Organ Transplantation Records

In 1954, the kidneys were the first human organs to be relocated successfully. In the end of the1960s, the liver, heart, and pancreas transfers were also successfully transferred, while the lungs and intestinal organs relocated techniques were started later during the period of the 1980s.

Types of Organ Transplant:

1.   Single Organ Transplantation
2.   Multi-organ Transplantation.

Organs that are Transplanted:

1.   **Heart Transplant**

A heart relocation is a therapy choice for irreversible, dangerous heart infections that can't be overseen by other clinical or careful strategies. These pathological conditions range from:

- Cardiomyopathy;
- Severe coronary artery disease;
- Congenital heart defects;
- Heart valves defects which may cause severe congestive heart failure.

A solid heart from a contributor who has endured mind demise is utilized to supplant the patient's harmed or infected heart.

2. Lung Transplant

Indications of Lung Transplantation:

- Chronic obstructive pulmonary disease (COPD)
- Cystic fibrosis
- Interstitial lung diseases

    - Alpha 1-antitrypsin deficiency

- Pulmonary hypertension

As a result of severe clinical measures for reasonableness of lung contributors, very few lung transfers are performed. Besides, the selection of candidates for a lung transplant is also very difficult. Such a recipient is chosen on the criteria of chances of more survival after the surgery.

Manpower required for lung transplant prior, during and after surgery:

- Transplant surgeons
- Nurses
- Pulmonologists
- Pharmacists
- Dietitians
- Social workers
- Physical and occupational therapists
- Psychologists
- Rehabilitation specialists.

3. Liver Transplant

Live is one of the most transplanted organs and it can be transplanted from donors who are brain-dead or from healthy individuals by taking some parts of the liver. It needs a good genetic mismatch.

4. Pancreas Transplant

This sort of relocation is regularly done on type 1 diabetic patients as their pancreas is not functioning appropriately. Transplantation of the pancreas not only improves the patient's quality of life but also reduces the risk of patients who are type 1 diabetics and have severe episodes of hypoglycemia.

5. Cornea Transplant

Corneal gift reestablishes vision to those patients who because of corneal illness have lost their vision. A harmed or shady cornea can be supplanted precisely with a sound, typical cornea during a corneal transplantation.

6. Trachea Transplant

Trachea transplantation can help patients who experience the ill effects of solidifying and contraction that hinder their respiration.

7. **Kidney Transplant**

It is a very important option for end-stage renal failure with multiple sessions of dialysis.

8. **Skin Transplant**

Skin also can be transplanted either from the same patient but different region or from other individuals.

9. **Vascular Tissues Transplant**

Relocating vascular tissues which are responsible for blood circulation can help alleviate indications of sleepiness and lightheadedness in patients with serious cardiovascular disorders. Vascular tissues can be given as long as 24 h after death.

Different organ transplantation can be effective if benefactor and beneficiary dwell in a similar organ dissemination unit; notwithstanding, such a large number of chances for various organ transplantation have been missed because of an absence of correspondence between organ dispersion units and activities that were not in the soul of OPTN strategy 3.9.3, which suggests willful sharing of the subsequent organ.

5 Modes of Transplant

- Autografts are tissues or organs which are transplanted from one part of the body to another part. Therefore, in this case, the donor is also the recipient. Autografts may be excess tissue, recoverable tissue, and tissue which is required somewhere else, for example, as can be seen in vein extraction procedure in CABG procedure. In some cases, an autograft procedure is done to excise tissue and that same tissue is then treated before it is introduced back to the patient. This can be seen when incorporating undifferentiated cell autograft and putting away blood ahead of time for a medical procedure.

  Because of the hereditary distinction between the organ and the beneficiary, the beneficiary's insusceptible framework will distinguish the organ as unfamiliar and endeavor to annihilate it, resulting in transfer dismissal. The danger of relocating dismissal can be assessed by estimating the Panel receptive immunizer level.
- Xenograft & Xenotransplantation—A transfer of organs or tissue starting with one animal variety and then onto the next. The model may be a porcine heart valve relocation or piscine-primate (fish to monkeys) relocation of islet (for example, pancreatic or separate) tissue. The last exploration study was expected to introduce this method for human utilization if effective [3].
- Contingent upon the individual on the holding up rundown, this has now and again been rehashed for up to six sets, with the last contributor giving to the individual at the first spot on the list. This technique permits all organ beneficiaries to get a transfer regardless of whether their living benefactor isn't a match to them. This further advantages individuals beneath any of these beneficiaries on holding up

records, as they draw nearer to the first spot on the list for an expired contributor organ.

- ABO incompatible transplants—Children under the age of 12–24 months have non-developed immune systems.

6 Multi-organ Transplants

Heart–Lung Transplantation:

At the point when all other treatment choices have fizzled in individuals with both heart and lung disappointment, a joined heart–lung relocation is required.

Unquestionably, different components have added to the improvement in results yet none has had a more significant effect than the immunosuppressive specialist cyclosporine, which came into inescapable use in the mid-1980s. However, the sensational expansion in long-term endurance inferable from cyclosporine has adequately exposed its most huge disadvantage: permanent nephrotoxicity. To be sure, renal inadequacy has surfaced as a main source of horribleness and mortality among heart and lung relocate beneficiaries, as an expected 2–18% of nonrenal relocate beneficiaries experience clinically critical nephrotoxicity. A big part of these patients progresses to plain renal disappointment within 10 years of transplantation these patients are now increasingly being indicated for renal transplantation. [3].

Need of Heart–Lung Transplant:

Conditions that regularly need a heart–lung relocation include.

- Pulmonary hypertension.
- Intrinsic coronary illness (birth deformities of the heart that influence the lungs).

The utilization of both DCD (Donation After Cardiac Death) cardiovascular and pneumonic unions was begun in the US in 1993. Despite the fact that DCD (Donation After Cardiac Death) hearts and lungs have been effectively relocated. [4].

Finding Donor's Heart:

To diminish the opportunity of dismissal, you should be combined with a heart that matches as close as conceivable to your tissue type. Body size is additionally significant, as the heart must have the option to fit easily inside the beneficiary's rib confine. Individuals hanging tight for a contributor heart are allotted a status code that shows how direly they need a transfer.

Typically, the heart can't get by outside of the body longer than 6 h. Thus, contributor hearts are frequently given to individuals anticipating transfer who live in nearness to the medical clinic where the organs are recuperated. As a component of a clinical preliminary, a strategy called benefactor after circulatory demise, or DCD, utilizes another compact organ care framework that keeps the heart suitable longer, improving admittance to giver hearts.

Evaluation for Heart Transplantation:

Prior to being considered for a heart relocation, you should go through a complete assessment to decide whether you are an up-and-comer and to preclude elective treatment choices. The assessment will incorporate an actual test just as blood and heart testing, drug screening, tissue composing, ultrasounds, and chest X-beam.

Heart-Kidney Transplant:

Joined heart and kidney transplantation (HKTx) is performed in patients with extreme cardiovascular breakdown and progressed renal inadequacy. Heart and kidney transplantation should be considered in patients with advanced renal and cardiac failure [4].

Fate of Heart Kidney transplant:

After heart transplantation, kidney failure may occur. Kidney failure also is associated with the increased mortality rate post-operatively.

Clinical Implications:

Heart and kidney transplantation are protected and practical, with incredible results in more seasoned and more youthful patients, with or without dialysis, and in sharpened patients.

Heart Liver Transplant:

Clinical studies have concluded that patients who received heart–liver transplants had equal results to those patients who received a heart transplant alone. In these cases, priorities are set based on the "Sickest first" principle where the person who is the sickest among the recipients receives the transplant first.

7 Indication for Heart–Liver Transplantation

Patients with essential coronary illness who experience auxiliary cardiovascular cirrhosis brought about by persistent hepatic venous outpouring check: This gathering incorporates patients with innate heart absconds that necessary Fontan strategy who at last reformist hepatic fibrosis from their circulatory physiology. These patients are at expanded danger for improvement of hepatocellular carcinoma (HCC) and require cautious assessment and reconnaissance.

- Patients with a finding of genetic transthyretin amyloidosis prompting cardiomyopathy: Liver transfer is simultaneously performed to eliminate the essential wellspring of foundational transthyretin protein.

  Patients with essential signs for liver transfer with simultaneous coronary illness.

8 Patient Selection

Tolerant choice is significant, and focuses seeking after CHLT ought to have a point-by-point institutional convention. It is important that heart relocate competitors are screened for hazard factors for liver fibrosis dependent on history, actual assessment, lab esteems, and imaging examinations. Patients in danger are painstakingly surveyed by the hepatology/liver transfer group. Liver biopsies might be performed to survey the level of fibrosis if cirrhosis is viewed as conceivably dependent on clinical discoveries. Transjugular biopsy is favored due to worries for seeping from clogged livers, particularly with continuous utilization of anticoagulation in this patient populace. Furthermore, hepatic venous weight estimations can be acquired to give an extra appraisal of hepatic hold [5].

Lung–Kidney Transplant:

The first case of a successful double lung–kidney transplant was reported in 1998. The procedure was performed on a patient who suffered from pulmonary lymphangioleiomyomatosis and kidney angiolipomas after having a unilateral nephrectomy. The patient was reported to have an adequate creatinine clearance; therefore, a possible postoperative renal failure could be avoided [5].

Helpless results after thoracic transplantation with simultaneous renal brokenness are all around portrayed: without transplantation or with thoracic-just transplantation, patients face unsatisfactorily high mortality. Results after joined lung-kidney transplantation (LKT) remain to a great extent not studied. The United Network for Organ Sharing/Organ Procurement and Transplantation Network information base was questioned to distinguish all kung–kidney transplantations, lung transplantations, and kidney transplantations (KTs) acted in the US from 1995 to 2013. Endurance was determined utilizing the Kaplan–Meier strategy and looked at utilizing log-rank tests or Cox relapse models. 31 LKTs were performed. The mean beneficiary age reported was of 45.4 ± 13.5 years, i.e., 48.3 percent were male.

Life Expectancy After Lung–Kidney Transplantation:

Although some patients have lived 10 years or more after a lung transplant, only about half or the patients who underwent the transplant procedure are in fact still alive after 5 years. Combined lung and kidney transplant is a surgically possible intervention at present. Yet post-operative management of the patient may be quite difficult particularly because a balance must be drawn of strict fluid restriction for the prevention of pulmonary edema and adequate fluid intake to maintain renal function. Furthermore, immunosuppressive treatment, especially anti-calcineurin frugs for lung transplantation, must be improved to decrease nephrotoxicity.

Liver–Lung Transplant:

Most of the patients with cardiac failure, who also have liver disease, have some sort of lung diseases involved with them as well. There is currently no organ allocation policy for these patients and, therefore, this requires addressing. Combined lung–liver transplant (CLLT) is an alternative for patients who have end-stage lung and liver disease. Yet long-term post-operative outcomes of CLLT patients are still unknown.

Since 1994, 67 CLLTs with 50 CLLLTs have been achieved since May 4, 2005. 2005 to date is in fact referred to as the LAS era. The most common indication for CLLT is Cystic Fibrosis.

It is necessary for a proper listing of outcomes regarding such transplant to determine whether double allocation of organs to a single recipient is justifiable.

Cause of Death in such patients:

The causes of death were mainly related to:

1. Failure of the primary graft
2. Bronchiolitis obliterans syndrome
3. Large cell adenocarcinoma of the lung
4. Cholestatic liver disease
5. Pneumonia nocardia
6. Systemic nocardia

Liver–Kidney Transplant:

CLKT is the method of decision for patients with both liver and kidney failure. Use of calcineurin inhibitors, sepsis, and hemodynamic insults might be the cause of renal failure in the patients with liver transplantation. CLKT is the most ideal alternative for patients who need transplantation of the two organs, particularly when living benefactor is inaccessible. With various preferences, it gives preferred outcomes over when done consecutively. Severe abstract standards should be followed as there is long rundown for one or the other organ.

Selection of Donor & Operative Management:

To oblige for applicants needing multi-organ transfers, Organ Procurement and Transplantation Network (OPTN)/UNOS strategy directs that when the essential organ is a heart, lung, or liver, patients who get a proposal for one of these three essential organs typically get the second, nonprimary organ from that benefactor, paying little heed to their wait-list need for that subsequent organ, if the contributor is situated with a similar organ acquirement association (OPO) where the beneficiary up-and-comer is enrolled (21).The capacity to pull an auxiliary organ from another OPO is subject to neighborhood strategy and practice. The CHLT applicants get standard heart need without an extra need for the consolidated heart-liver status. CHLT join assignment is quite often dependent on the heart need with the liver after the heart. Hypothetically, if the patient has essential liver sickness with a high Model for End-Stage Liver Disease (MELD) or MELD special case focus, OPO strategy can introduce the situation of distribution driven by MELD with the heart pulled by the liver. There is progressing conversation with respect to whether this distribution is suitable or reasonable, and there are contentions that these patients should be given higher need due to expanded demise on the standby list 8. There have been worries that joined designation can contrarily influence those on the standby list; however, no current information upholds this case. The capacity to pull an auxiliary organ from another OPO is subject to neighborhood strategy and practice. The CHLT applicants get standard heart need without extra need for the consolidated heart-liver status. CHLT join assignment is quite often dependent on the heart need with the liver after the heart. Hypothetically, if the patient has essential liver sickness with a high MELD or MELD special case focus, OPO strategy can introduce the situation of distribution driven by MELD with the heart pulled by the liver. There is progressing conversation with respect to whether this distribution is suitable or reasonable, and there are contentions that these patients should be given higher need due to expanded demise on the standby list. There have been worries that joined designation can contrary influence those on the standby list; however, no current information upholds this case. The capacity to pull an auxiliary organ from another OPO is subject to neighborhood strategy and practice. The CHLT applicants get standard heart need without extra need for the consolidated heart–liver status. CHLT join assignment is quite often dependent on the heart need with the liver after the heart. Hypothetically, if the patient has essential liver sickness with a high MEL or MELD special case focus, OPO strategy can introduce the situation of distribution driven by MELD with the heart pulled by the liver.

There is progressing conversation with respect to whether this distribution is suitable or reasonable, and there are contentions that these patients should be given higher need due to expanded demise on the standby list. There have been worries that joined designation can contrarily influence those on the standby list; however, no current information upholds this case. The capacity to pull an auxiliary organ from another OPO is subject to neighborhood strategy and practice. The CHLT applicants get standard heart need without extra need for the consolidated heart–liver status. CHLT join assignment is quite often dependent on the heart need with the liver after the heart. Hypothetically, if the patient has essential liver sickness with a high MELD or MELD special case focus, OPO strategy can introduce the situation of distribution driven by MELD with the heart pulled by the liver. There is progressing conversation with respect to whether this distribution is suitable or reasonable, and there are contentions that these patients should be given higher need due to expanded demise on the standby list. There have been worries that joined designation can contrarily influence those on the standby list; however, no current information upholds this case [6].

Giver/Recipient coordinating measures, for example, age, size, and separation are chosen by the two groups and steady for the two organs. As a result of the more drawn-out ischemic time required for the liver, a unit of good quality is required, and in this way harder to get. At the point when a fitting giver is distinguished, both cardiovascular and liver groups make temporary acknowledgments subsequent to evaluating the organs. Last acknowledgment is made after conversation among groups, and acquisition timing is composed. Two recuperation groups are dispatched for heart and liver obtainments. Standard human leukocyte antigen (HLA) composing is finished at the hour of heart relocation assessment. On the off chance that fundamental, a virtual cross-match for beneficiary/benefactor similarity is performed when a potential giver is being thought about. [7].

Post-Operative Immunosuppression: (Mostly in case of Heart–Liver Transplant)

Liver allografts have for quite some time been seen to be more "lenient" to HLA bungle and alloimmune wounds. Also, liver allografts exhibit some level of resistant insurance in joined organ transplants. CHLT beneficiaries typically don't get acceptance treatment. They get high-dose steroid at cardiovascular allograft reperfusion followed by tightening. Also, upkeep treatment with calcineurin inhibitor and mycophenolate mofetil is started post-operatively. Convention endomyocardial biopsies are performed to keep an eye on for cell and antibody-mediated dismissal. Routine post-transplant blood testing at predefined stretches is performed to screen for the advancement of donor-specific antibodies. In our patients, we have noticed fundamentally less patients in the CHLT partner encountering cell dismissal of the cardiovascular allograft contrasted and heart relocate alone (unpublished information), proposing immune-protective properties of the corresponding liver allograft [8].

9 Advantages of Multi-organ Transplants for the Candidates

The short- and long-term results of multi-organ transplants have been similar to that of single organ transplant in some cases. The chances of organ rejection and dysfunction in cases of multi-organ transplants are also seen less compared to single organ transplants in research [6].

However, due to ethical reasons, we must take into consideration the situation of all the candidates who are on list to receive an organ rather than only those who need multi-organ transplant [4, 5, 9].

10 Steps to Standardize Multi-organ Transplant at the Transplant Centers

It is seen that after a single organ surgery, if the patient dies, the performance of the transplant center is affected as the mortality rate after a transplant is increasing, but in the case of multi-organ transplant, if the patient dies, it doesn't affect the overall performance of the transplant centers [7].

Besides, there is another problem that is faced while the question of standardizing the transplant centers is concerned [7].

11 Recommendations for Multi-organ Transplant Standardization

It is very important to understand that eligibility criteria are very much needed for multi-organ transplant to be more successful and also to establish equity and utility.

However, if this field is neglected, people will feel less motivated in working towards such multi-organ transplant and this sector will be abandoned. This will reduce the chances of success in life-saving operation procedures that are possible.

Steps should also be taken to prevent the centers to avoid such complicated but live-saving cases due to fear of failure or outcomes of such procedures. More research is actually needed about patients and benefits they are receiving before and after the multi-organ and also solitary organ transplant to understand the efficiency and the risk–benefit ratio in both the cases. This work could appear as imminent execution of strict versus tolerant measures for multi-organ transplants at various focuses. The potential for randomized preliminaries or quasi-experimental plans ought to likewise be deliberately considered by partners, including the Health Resources and Services Administration.

12 Alternatives of Transplant

Specialists likewise are considering the chance of living-organ transplant starting with one animal variety and then onto the next (xenotransplantation). Xenotransplantation research incorporates hereditary designing of pigs so their organs are viable for transplantation to people. Furthermore, specialists are taking a gander at treating infections through moving qualities into tissues (quality treatment). For instance, quality treatment may treat dismissal of a heart transplantation [10].

The instance of multi-organ transplant shows how strategies that favor debilitated patients can subvert value and utility in settings of shortage. It has increased the chance of survival of patients who had very less chances to live without such procedures. The transfer network has the occasion to align practice with morals through changes that limit the transplants as indicated by straightforward models and by diminishing motivations for multi-organ transplants in situations where single transplant can solve the problem [6, 7].

Multiple Choice Questions:

1. **When and where was the first human-to-human transfer performed?**

    A. 1903 in the United Kingdom.
    B. 1913 in the United Nations.
    C. 1923 in the Soviet Union.
    D. 1933 in the Soviet Union.

2. **Dr. Carrel was famous for carrying out?**

   A. kidney transfers in canines.
   B. liver transfers in canines.
   C. brain transfers in canines.
   D. vascular transfers in canines.

3. **When were the lung and intestinal organ relocation techniques started?**

   A. 1920s.
   B. 1940s.
   C. 1960s.
   D. 1980s.

4. **The most suitable patients for pancreas transplant are:**

   A. Type I diabetics with malfunctioning pancreas.
   B. Type II diabetics with malfunctioning pancreas.
   C. Patients with cardiomyopathy
   D. Patients with Cystic fibrosis

5. **Which country gave record corneal tissue from neighborhood and unfamiliar contributors for relocation in 2016?**

   A. Singapore.
   B. United Kingdom.
   C. United States.
   D. Pakistan.

6. **Solidifying and narrowing of windpipe is an indication of:**

   A. Lung transplant.
   B. Liver transplant.
   C. Trachea transplant.
   D. larynx transplant.

7. **Which of the following diseases have the ability to survive for many years through dialysis without any kind of transplants?**

   A. Chronic renal diseases.
   B. Myocardial infarction.
   C. Cirrhosis of liver.
   D. Cystic fibrosis

8. **Most human tissue and organ transfers are**

   A. Allografts.
   B. Autograft.
   C. Xenograft.
   D. Xenotransplantation.

9. **Which technique permits all organ beneficiaries to get a transfer regardless of whether their living benefactor isn't a match to them?**

   A. Great Samaritan" kidney transplant.
   B. Liver transplant.
   C. Lung transplant.
   D. Lens transplant.

10. **Which One is the Need of Heart Lung Transplant?**

    A. Pulmonary hypertension.
    B. Myocardial infarction.
    C. Cirrhosis of liver.
    D. Cystic fibrosis

11. **Which organ is donated most frequently after DCD (Donation After Cardiac Death) along with heart?**

    A. Cornea.
    B. Larynx.
    C. Lungs.
    D. Trachea.

12. **For how many hours the heart can get by outside of the body**

    A. No longer than 10 h.
    B. No longer than 12 h.
    C. No longer than 6 h.
    D. No longer than 8 h.

13. **Which option is most suitable for patients with advanced heart and kidney failure?**

    A. Heart and kidney transplantation (HKTx).
    B. Coronary arteries and kidney transplantation (HKTx).
    C. Heart and abdominal aorta transplantation (HKTx).
    D. Heart and suprarenal gland transplantation (HKTx).

14. **Which of these is a common factor associated with increased mortality after heart transplantation?**

    A. Gut complications.
    B. Liver failure.
    C. Lug failure.
    D. Renal failure.

15. **Which one of the following is the most common complication which follows Liver–Lung Transplant?**

    A. Primary graft failure.
    B. Liver failure.

C. Lung failure.
D. Hypovolemic shock.

16. **Which of the following involves the removal of the diseased portion of the small intestine to replace it with a healthy and viable small intestine from a donor?**

A. Isolated Intestinal Transplantation.
B. Multi-visceral Transplantation.
C. Modified Multi-visceral Transplantation.
D. Domino transplants.

17. **Which of the following is correct sequence of Multi-visceral transplantation?**

A. Readiness Sedation incision Assessment removal implantation closure.
B. Sedation Readiness incision Assessment removal implantation closure.
C. Assessment removal implantation Readiness Sedation incision closure.
D. Assessment implantation removal Readiness Sedation incision closure.

18. **Which of the Following is the Main Task of the National Organ Transplant Act (NOTA)?**

A. Keeps record of cornea gifts.
B. Keeps up the organ library.
C. Reflects mortality risk on the waiting list.
D. Sorts 1 diabetic whose pancreas doesn't work appropriately.

19. **Which of the following is main task of the United Network for Organ Sharing (UNOS)?**

A. Keeps up the organ library.
B. Sorts 1 diabetic whose pancreas doesn't work appropriately.
C. Reflects mortality risk on the waiting list.
D. Matches available organs with recipients.

20. **Standard human leukocyte antigen (HLA) composing is finished:**

A. After fours hour of heart relocate assessment.
B. After three hours of heart relocation assessment.
C. After two hours of heart relocation assessment.
D. at the hour of heart relocation assessment.

21. **When will a virtual cross-match for beneficiary/benefactor similarity is performed?**

A. When a potential giver is being thought about.
B. To draw out ischemic time required for the liver.
C. To evaluate the organ.
D. To implant the organ.

22. **Which test is performed to screen for the advancement of donor-specific antibodies?**

    A. Routine post-transplant blood testing.
    B. Histopathology.
    C. CT scan.
    D. MRI scan.

24. **Which of the following is action of immunosuppressants on transplanted organs?**

    A. Decrease killer cells.
    B. Increase T cells.
    C. Prevent infection.
    D. Weaken the immune system to prevent rejection.

25. **Which of the following will likely have to be taken for the rest of their lives so that their bodies don't reject their donor organs?**

    A. Immunosuppressant.
    B. Antivirals.
    C. Antibiotics.
    D. Antihypertensives.

26. **The Human Organ Transplant Act (HOTA) considers the kidneys, heart, liver and corneas to be eliminated in case of death from individuals who are?**

    A. 21 years old.
    B. 31 years old.
    C. 11 years old.
    D. 41 years old.

27. **What part of the eye can be given through donation?**

    A. Cornea.
    B. Sclera.
    C. Optic nerve.
    D. Ciliary body.

28. **Which of the following tissue was utilized for the first time by the Italian spe-cialist Gasparo Tagliacozzi in the sixteenth century?**

    A. Skin transplant for plastic remaking.
    B. Aorta for vascular grafts.
    C. Bone for joint replacement.
    D. Cartilage for regeneration of trachea.

29. **Which of the following is a must regarding Manpower required for lung transplant prior, during & after Surgery without which transplant is not possible?**

    A. Transplant surgeons.
    B. Pharmacists.
    C. Dietitians.
    D. Social workers.
    E. Rehabilitation specialists.

Answers:

1. D
2. A
3. D
4. A
5. A
6. C
7. A
8. A
9. A
10. A
11. C
12. C
13. A
14. D
15. A
16. A
17. A
18. B
19. D
20. D
21. A
22. A
23. D
24. D
25. A
26. A
27. A
28. A
29. A

References

1. Goldfarb SB, et al. The international thoracic organ transplant registry of the International Society for Heart and Lung Transplantation: twenty-first pediatric lung and heart–lung transplantation report—2018; Focus theme: multiorgan transplantation. J Hear Lung Transplant. 2018;37(10):1196–1206.
2. Khush KK, et al. The International Thoracic Organ Transplant Registry of the International Society for Heart and Lung Transplantation: thirty-fifth adult heart transplantation report—2018; focus theme: multiorgan transplantation. J Hear Lung Transplant. 2018;37(10):1155–1168.
3. Wong K, Tecson K, Cedars A. Outcomes of multi-organ transplant in adult patients with congenital heart disease. J Am Heart Assoc. 2019;8(22):e014088.
4. Rossano JW, et al. The international thoracic organ transplant registry of the International Society for Heart and Lung Transplantation: twenty-first pediatric heart transplantation report—2018; Focus theme: Multiorgan transplantation. J Hear Lung Transplant. 2018;37(10):1184–1195.
5. Rossano JW, et al. The international thoracic organ transplant registry of the International Society for Heart and Lung Transplantation: twenty-first pediatric heart transplantation report—2018; Focus theme: Multiorgan transplantation. J Hear Lung Transplant 2018;37(10):1184–1195.
6. Morris-Stiff G, et al. Transmission of donor melanoma to multiple organ transplant recipients. Am J Transplant. 2004;4(3):444–6.
7. Sibal A, et al. Experience of 100 solid organ transplants over a five-yr period from the first successful pediatric multi-organ transplant program in India. Pediatr Transplant. 2014;18(7):740–745.
8. Patcai JT. Inpatient rehabilitation outcomes in solid organ transplantation: results of a unique partnership between the rehabilitation hospital and the multi-organ transplant unit in an acute hospital. Open J Ther Rehabil. 2013;1(02):52.
9. Giani T, et al. Cross-infection of solid organ transplant recipients by a multidrug-resistant Klebsiella pneumoniae isolate producing the OXA-48 carbapenemase, likely derived from a multiorgan donor. J Clin Microbiol. 2014;52(7):2702–2705.
10. Chambers DC, et al. The International Thoracic Organ Transplant Registry of the International Society for Heart and Lung Transplantation: thirty-fifth adult lung and heart-lung transplant report—2018; focus theme: multiorgan transplantation. J Hear Lung Transplant. 2018;37(10):1169–1183.

Ethical Issues of Heart Transplantation

Tonazzina Hossain Sauda, Myesha Maliha Binte Mamun,
Asadur Rahman Nabin, Monzer Ousseily, and Sarah Meribout

Abstract As the world advances in the fields of medicine and healthcare, what also increases is the emergence of newer ethical issues with increase in ambiguity of the code. One such ethical dilemma the world of medicine faces today is the idea of Heart transplantation, and was concluded that a donor is considered legal when determined to be brain dead. The process of comprehending all the risks and benefits of a medical procedure is known as informed consent that is the main moral principle guiding the donation of organs. Moreover, religion is often the guide to establishing ethical principles for individuals and most religions will allow this act when it is selflessly performed without the expectation of any reward.

Keywords Multiorgan transplant · Informed consent · Presumed Consent · Organ donor · Organ recipient · Ethical issues · Heart donor · Potential donors · Consent policies · Dead donor rule

1 Introduction

The Hippocratic Oath, is one of the oldest binding documents in history, which is held sacred by physicians while treating the ill. It is also known as the code of medical ethics. However, as the world advances in the fields of medicine and healthcare, what also increases is the emergence of newer ethical issues with an increase in ambiguity of the code. An ethical conflict during the professional practice of healthcare or medicine arises when it compromises the conduct and reputation of the professional

T. H. Sauda (✉)
University of Illinois, Urbana Champaign, Champaign, IL, USA
e-mail: saudath008@gmail.com

M. M. B. Mamun · A. R. Nabin
Bangladesh Medical College, Dhaka, Bangladesh

M. Ousseily
Faculty of Medical Sciences, Lebanese University, Hadat, Beirut, Lebanon

S. Meribout
Faculty of Medicine, University of Constantine III, El Khroub, Algeria

© The Author(s), under exclusive license to Springer Nature Switzerland AG 2022
H. T. Hashim et al. (eds.), *Heart Transplantation*,
https://doi.org/10.1007/978-3-031-17311-0_14

or it compromises with the interests and wellbeing of the consumer. We recognize an ethical problem when there is a confusion in determining whether a decision is right or wrong, because several elements and interests need to be taken into consideration, and it becomes necessary to deliberate each moral conflict in order to reach the most 'righteous' course of action and the best path to be followed, which again needs to be continuously reevaluated. What we have to understand is that there is no mathematical formula for solving an ethical problem. Rather it requires creativity and collective thinking in order to brainstorm new solution alternatives, and this needs to be a constant process. One such ethical dilemma the world of medicine faces today is one surrounding the idea of Heart transplantation [1].

In this chapter, we will address the ongoing conversation of the ethics of heart transplantation such as its history, the dead donor rule, the ethical conflict between informed consent and presumed consent, ethical justification of financial incentives to donors and what religion has to say regarding transplantation and its ethics.

History:

Organ transplantation is regarded as one of the "miracles" seen in medical advancements. The idea of substituting a vital organ that is dead or dying (e.g., heart or kidney) may have seemed an impossibility to the human mind once upon a time. However, this concept was realized when two doctors of Peter Bent Brigham Hospital, Drs. Joseph Murray and John Merrill succeeded in transplanting a kidney from one monozygotic twin to another on December 23, 1954 [2].

It was dubbed "one of the peaks of modern scientific achievement" by The New York Times. Denise Darvall, the 25-year-old donor, was hit by a drunk driver the day before. She had become unconscious following severe trauma to the head. At the Groote Schuur Hospital a case of multiple skull fractures was diagnosed, which the attending doctor declared to be "beyond treatment". After hearing what the doctor had to say, Denise's father consented to the surgeons to remove his daughter's heart and transplant it into a stranger. He did this because he believed that's what Denise would have done if she could have had a say in the matter. "If you can't save my daughter, you must try and save this man," he said. Then in the 1950s, another advancement of medical science happened. This was Mechanical Ventilation, a new invention that allowed to sustain human life, by helping a dying man breathe. This led to more questions. The ethical dilemma was that ventilator-dependent donors were themselves alive and collecting vital organs from them would lead to their death. One commentator said, "As the need for donors grows larger, the definition of death must be carefully redefined. When are you dead enough to be deprived of your heart?". The solution was to come up with a new definition of death [1–3].

The definition of brain death is the permanent loss of all brain functions, including the brainstems. Coma, the absence of brainstem reflexes, and apnea are the three hallmarks of brain death. It was agreed that a patient who was determined to be brain dead was also regarded as legally and clinically dead. This new definition helped disregard the idea that doctors were 'killing' to obtain an organ for transplantation.

Brain dead patients became legal donors. The concept of brain death allowed the transplant community to enforce a new rule that is today known as the "dead donor rule" (DDR) [3].

2   What is the "Dead Donor Rule"?

The removal of a single kidney or a liver lobe would be examples of exceptions to this rule, as neither would be expected to end the life of the donor. The dead donor rule has been a topic of significance in the organ procurement literature for at least the past twenty-five years.

Is the Dead Donor Rule ethical?

Supporters of the dead donor rule are with a view that the rule is indeed ethical. However, there is a matter that comes into discussion here, and that is the right a person has to his or her own body. This is known as the principle of autonomy. The autonomy principle refers to a person's right to control their own body. The right to refuse an undesirable invasion of one's own body is a crucial part of human dignity. While still living, anyone can opt out of an organ donation [1, 2].

This takes us to the idea of consent. After organ transplantation evolved, talks regarding its ethics did as well. At first, we see that there were debates about whether it is ethical to remove a beating heart from a person altogether where a beating heart could be regarded as a sign of life. Now the world seems more accepting of organ transplants but human rights issues such as consent comes into play. Is it fair to remove organs from a body without the prior consent of the individual?

The next section highlights the existing types of consent and how they are used by countries worldwide to create policies regarding organ removal and transplantation [3].

3   The Types of Consent

What is Informed/Expressed consent?

Doctors are expected to give details to their patients about a particular procedure and explain everything related to it from the first and make it very simple to the patients and after that ask them to give their consent, and sign on the papers [4].

Why is it important?

- Informed consent is an ethical and legal requirement
- Informed consent provides all required information to a competent individual so that they can make a conscious decision
- It reflects the practical application of autonomy

- It is proof that the individual's opinion is respected
- It is the legal document that shows the individual has voluntarily contributed to an important decision.

While the importance of informed consent is well understood and applied in case of live donors, for organ donations of kidney or a lobe of liver or other tissues, the issue is much more complex when we speak of cardiac transplantation that can only be done from deceased donors.

Why is that?

It is because the principles of Informed consent only apply to a donor while they are still alive; we may ponder about death, but how often do we ponder about organ donation after death to make a conscious decision about it?

4 The Principles of Informed Consent

- To make the decision, you must be competent.
- You must be able to understand the pertinent information.
- You must give consent willfully, without intimidation or coercion.

Considering the above factors, a cardiac transplantation requiring an Informed / Express-Consent would mean that the donor has expressed his desire to be a donor while the donor still had the ability to willfully express his opinion- either by officially registering as a Donor in a recognized donor system (for e.g., has a donor card), or by mentioning it in his will, or by expressing his wish to family members/friends at a time before his death. Usage of Expressed Consent puts a limit to organ donors and a limited number of people take the time to register as donor. Families also find it difficult to say yes to donating organs of their deceased loved ones. The donor's family is not permitted to intervene with the decision to donate under the foregoing description of presumed consent. However, this is a more stringent form of presumed consent [4].

Expressed/Informed VS Implied/Presumed Consent in case of heart donors. Since the first successful transplant surgery decades ago, there has been a severe and ongoing scarcity of organs available for transplant. Nations all across the world employ various tactics to address this issue, with differing degrees of success.

The Unites States' system is based on the principle of expressed consent. This signifies that until a person has stated otherwise, he or she will not be an organ donor. Potential donor autonomy is respected, but the expressed consent paradigm is not thought to be as effective in expanding supply to match demand [5].

Some countries, on the other hand, embrace the notion of presumed (instead of expressed) consent for organ procurement, assuming that people want to give their organs when they die unless they declare a preference otherwise. In the next section, we will take a look into the existing Consent Policies in the world [5].

However, donation rates are far less than that which is required. In 2015, Spain ranked first in the world for organ transplantation, with 40 donors and more than 100 transplant surgeries per million people. How was this achieved? Spain passed its presumed-consent in the year 1979. A potential donor must be declared "brain dead" by three doctors under the presumed-consent law. The effectiveness of Spain's organ procurement program can be attributed to this structure, which is combined with positive recognition and encouragement for organ donors. Belgium passed and implemented a similar presumed-consent law in 1986. According to this rule, anyone who objects to their organs being harvested after death must document his or her opposition with the Belgian Central Health Authority. However, they are free to change their decision at any point in life [4–6].

In Belgium, healthcare professionals are not required by law to obtain the donor family's agreement to remove the organs, or even to notify them if such a choice is made. Nevertheless, if a family member expresses an open opposition to organ recovery, the physician is unable to proceed with the surgery [6].

The Caillavet Law, which was approved in December 1976, allows a third party to speak on behalf of a deceased donor by voicing any concerns the donor may have had, even if the donor did not register them. "There shall be a legal presumption of donation if a person has refrained from exercising his right to object to the removal from his body of anatomical organs or parts during his lifetime," according to a Columbian law. Organs can be recovered in Norway after the treating physician has spoken with the patient's relatives, and only the patient's direct relatives have the legal right to object [5].

When residents of Singapore reach 18, they are issued a letter from the government stating that if they do not express an objection, they are believed to consent to donate organs. Muslims are excused from this policy, and are considered objectors regardless, unless they state otherwise. On the other side of the spectrum, nations such as the United States, Denmark, the United Kingdom, Canada, and Brazil follow a system of expressed or informed consent for organ donation [7].

The question is, if it is proven that nations with presumed consent have better rates of transplant success, why are there so many different policies regarding consent existent worldwide? To put it simply, the conflicting policies exist because of the prevalent ethical dilemma of whether to choose the donor's right to autonomy or the receiver's right to live [1–3].

In the next section, we will analyze the moral justifications of presumed and expressed consent for cardiac transplantation.

5   The Ethical Arguments in Favor of Presumed Consent

1. Efficiency:

Increasing the supply of organs. To think simply, increasing supply of available organs and saving the life of another individual through transplantation should be the primary target set even if it compromises goals and values of other individuals, within limits. This is in line with the concept of choosing the "Greater Good".

2. Asking for Consent can be Brutal:

Consent from the family is very important, although, some families refused even if the patient himself or herself agreed to donate before death. So, it is justified to ease the family of this difficulty by presuming consent from the deceased donor [8].

3. Individual Conscience is Deserving Respect:

Presumed consent does give the option to an object of organ donation to state his anti-donation preference at any time before his or her demise. So, the argument in favor is that it is respecting human principles and individual choice.

4. Individuals owe it to Society to Make the Effort to Register their Disapproval:

It is viewed that individuals who do not support organ donation should take the trouble of notifying the authorities of their preferences since they are depriving another member of the public the right to an organ if they need it. Taking this into consideration, it is argued that objectors to organ donation are the ones who should bear the responsibility of conveying their opposition.

6   The Ethical Arguments Against Presumed Consent

1. False Positives:

Under a policy of "presumed consent, "there is a possibility of false positives. Certain individuals who are against organ donation because of personal preference/morals/beliefs may have not registered their preference with public authorities for many reasons. One such factor may be ignorance. Individuals may not be aware of the fact there is an option to register a refusal for organ donation prior to the event of their death. If information about donations such as opting for refusals are being sent to individuals through mediums such as postcards/letters/ media announcements one can never be sure if all citizens are receiving the information.

2. Problems in Registration and Transferring the Status of Dissent:

There are likely to be faults in the process of registering and communicating opposition status. Because persons may incur sudden brain death outside of their state of residence.

3. Autonomy:

Their decision may be influenced by the fact that they have to express their opinion publicly. Some argue that it should not be a moral obligation for a citizen to express that they have an objection.

4. Consent is not a dichotomous variable only applicable to the individual:

Individuals should be able to transfer decision-making authority to their family members. Presumed consent would allow organs to be harvested from a donor who had willfully authorized his family to decide such a thing for him.

What is then the solution or the ultimate answer? Is it ethically justified to presume consent or not?

Presume-Consent national Policies cannot be changed overnight, despite existing conflicts. A reasonable solution, therefore is to familiarize the public about transplantation procedures, and to motivate and encourage them through planned advocacy so that they may become more positive about the idea of organ donation. On the other hand, countries wishing to stick to Express-Consent Policies should focus more on making the process of registration simpler and should spread awareness regarding organ donation in order to increase their number of potential donors.

A wide range of public discussions are held to improve the laws governing organ recovery as well as for redefining the goals and objectives of procurement organizations. A summary of some significant ways to combat the existing moral turpitude include:

- Extensive education and collaboration among involved stakeholders
- In House Coordinators (IH(C): Recruiting Statutory in-patient coordinators in hospitals and the usage integrated healthcare systems can significantly improve consent and donation rates. Health care coordinators can act as a liaison between patients and physicians and can offer support, guidance and information to patients. This may help to give the encouragement patients need to consider organ donation. A health care coordinator can be hired and expected to screen for potential donors, coordinate timely referrals, educate hospital personnel, help with family consent, provide family support and help the authorities with potential donor management. An IHC (In house coordinator) program should be regarded as a considerable option that could help match the high organ demand with sufficient supply [6].
- The use of Social Media: On May 1, 2012, popular Social Network Facebook, added a new addition to its Profile where members could specify themselves as "Organ Donor". If a profile was edited according to the new update, it would be provided with a link to the state registry where they could submit an official designation. "Facebook friends" would receive a notification when a fellow friend became registered as a donor. On the first day of the Facebook organ donor initiative, 13,054 new online registrations were performed which was 21.1-fold compared to the baseline average of 616 registrations. It can thus be inferred that Social media can be used to form a donor registry and encourage communication between friends and families and act as positive motivation for organ donation. There should be further research conducted to determine if Social Media can be a durable method to improve organ donation rates.

However, the solutions listed above are very long term and results cannot be found overnight. Perhaps this is why efforts to increase the number of organ donors have become increasingly focused. One technique advocated to boost the availability of organs for transplant by compensating donors with a financial incentive for donating. This has been adopted in numerous systems around the world, but there is still disagreement because an ethical dilemma exists here as well [6].

7 Arguments Supporting Financial Incentives

1. Demand:

The simple and straightforward argument is that there is a major imbalance between the demand and supply of organs such as hearts. Every day, 22 people on the waiting list die while waiting for a heart. As a result, the fundamental argument for offering financial incentives is the belief that allowing financial incentives will boost donation rates. This idea of course disregards the moral conflicts surrounding the idea and focuses on mere need.

2. Society:

Surprisingly, this viewpoint differed by gender, socioeconomic status, and age, with males, those from lower socioeconomic status, and 65 percent to 68 percent of those under the age of 35 favoring remuneration.

3. Autonomy:

Everyone is free to donate his body's organs according to specific guidelines and protocols. Following this principle of ethical autonomy there are few arguments in support of financial incentives for heart donation to maximize autonomy-based rights.

Arguments against financial incentives:

- Exploitation: Financial incentives could lead to exploitation of persons from lower socioeconomic classes, which is a form of abuse. It may create an unethical motive to people who believe it is their sole means of earning money. This will lead to bigger differences between individuals, as witnessed in countries where organs can be bought and sold. Living donors, for example, who need financial rewards (due to financial hardship) may alter their medical data in order to boost the likelihood of getting chosen as an organ donor.
- Decrease in altruistic value: Financial incentives could decrease donation because donors might feel that their altruistic donation is being undervalued. Donors or their families do not experience the same level of emotional appeal in their act of contribution when remuneration is offered as opposed to giving solely altruistically as a gift.

An idea to solve this ethical dilemma was to apply an ethical framework to the financial incentive offers.

This framework may be a guide to providing financial incentives. However, it does not still solve the ethical dilemma surrounding it. Even if this model is increased, certain factors should be taken into consideration. For example, if any type of payment was permitted in heart transplant donations, authorities should play a part in the process measures. This might encourage equity since the selection of organ recipients is independent of their ability to pay for the organ. As a result, additional work is needed to identify and address logistical and process concerns related with payment in order to provide protection [7]. An ethical dilemma arises when financial incentives are given in organ donation, because most religions will allow this act when it is selflessly performed, and the organ is given as a gift without the expectation of any reward; and religion is often the guide to establishing ethical principles for individuals. The widely known philosopher Immanuel Kant stated God as a fundamental requirement of ethics. Religions like Zoroastrianism, Judaism and Christianity have rules, and these are regarded as rules set by God, so naturally the argument is that they cannot be changed even if human circumstances change or ethical ideas progress [7].

Keeping financial incentives aside, there are individuals who are skeptical against organ donation anyway because they believe that their religion does not permit it, and hence it is unethical. The line of distinguishing within religion and ethics continues to be blurred, a view shared by most. However, if religious scriptures are studied thoroughly, it may be inferred that the presumed conservativeness of religion, rather than what the religion permits, may be the underlying factor against donation. So, does any religion as an ethical principle actually prohibit organ donation? In the next section, we will analyze the issue at hand using examples of some of the most popular religions [8].

8 Innocent Heart Sentenced to Life in Cheney

This was a newspaper headline following the heart transplant of former U.S. Vice President Dick Cheney. The allocation of the scarce societal resource of donor hearts to the elderly has been a cause of contention [3, 6]. It is understood that there are logistical challenges that arise when it comes to allocating organs on time to reduce ischemic damage to the heart before a heart transplantation. As a result, another patient is designated as the "better prospect." Proper referral patterns, as well as the shortage and suitability of institutions, are ethical issues associated with heart transplantation access.

A referral is required before a heart transplant may be performed. Continuation of barriers to referral, definitely prompts inquiries on fairness and equality while choosing a recipient.

More such cases are heard of. Sandra Jensen, 34, was denied a heart transplant in 1995 due to the additional chromosome and developmental retardation that she has. Paul Corby, a 24-year-old autistic man, did not initially get a heart due to his ability to care for himself although he had a supportive family to take care of him [8, 9].

As the evidence above, the allocation of hearts while the supply is scarce will remain an ethical dilemma.

Referral patterns would not establish a verdict on who is or is not a suitable candidate if there were sufficient organs for donation. There would be no waiting list if there were enough organs to match the demand for heart transplants, and everybody who wanted a heart would get one. There would be a huge reduction in the requirement for additional regulatory control if there were enough high-quality hearts available. Unfortunately, due to a scarcity of donor hearts, it appears that ethics will keep on playing a prominent part in heart transplantation. This raises the question of whether the system can be improved [10].

The answer is Yes. If we use ethics as our guiding principle, we can enhance accessibility and availability of healthcare, improve listing criteria, and introduce necessary adjustments to the regulatory system to best serve our patients.

Multiple Choice Questions:

1. **A living donor can be used as a last resort if no other suitable way exists for vital or-gan procurement?**

   (a) True
   (b) False

2. **Dead donor rule:**

   (a) irreversible cessation of circulatory functions
   (b) irreversible cessation of respiratory functions
   (c) irreversible cessation of brain death
   (d) all of the above

3. **The importance of informed consent can be reflected as the following except:**

   (a) the main principle guiding the legal requirements of vital organ donation
   (b) documented contribution of a competent individual in practicing autonomy
   (c) a legal application showing that an individual voluntarily contributed to his life decisions
   (d) an ethical proof that a patient's opinion in his healthcare is respected

4. **Informed consent:**

   (a) necessitates the individual be conscious, competent, cooperative and ready to accept any condition
   (b) the doctor, when needed, might coerce the patient's decision for the latter's own benefit
   (c) the relevant comprehension includes a complete disclosure of information related to a medical treatment of an individual with all expected risks and benefits
   (d) shows an individual's ability to willfully express his opinion respecting the doctor's autonomy

5. **Organ transplant donor:**

   (a) registered in a recognized donor system
   (b) has an organ donor card
   (c) mentioned in his will his intention to donate his organs
   (d) expressed his wish to his family members/friends before his death
   (e) all of the above
   (f) none of the above

6. **Expressed consent:**

   (a) an individual is an organ donor unless declared otherwise
   (b) an advance recorded wish to be an organ donor
   (c) the individual's family can oppose a surrogate with decision-making responsibility directed previously by the individual prior to his death
   (d) expressed consents increase the supply-to-demand ratio in the shortage of organs available for donation

7. **Presumed consent registration conflicts with the care offered to the registered patient.**

   (a) True
   (b) False

8. **Presumed consent:**

   (a) a strict version of presumed consent requires the family's approval
   (b) a relaxed version of presumed consent requires the family's approval
   (c) the donor is presumed to had registered a preliminary refusal to be considered eligible for organ donation
   (d) the individuals need and rights come first to the needs and interests of the society

9. **The success of organ donation systems require:**

   (a) a positive recognition and motivation for organ donors that aids in declaring potential candidates as eligible for organ donation regardless of any expressed registrations
   (b) a positive motivation for organ donation with the effective registration for organ donation
   (c) legal binding to inform the individual's family and take their decision and permission to recover organs
   (d) a positive motivation and presumed consent law in the form of registered objection with the ability to be changed at any point upon the individual's decision only

10. **The efficiency of presumed consent:**

   (a) respects the donor's right to autonomy
   (b) favors to increase the supply of available organs for transplantation

    (c)   compromises limitlessly the values of other individuals
    (d)   all of the above
    (e)   none of the above

11. **Individuals that do not support organ donation should take the time to register their preference because:**

    (a)   they owe the society the effort to register their objection
    (b)   their noncooperation is depriving other members of the society an organ if they need it
    (c)   the burden of communicating their objection can cost the organ donation system
    (d)   all of the above
    (e)   none of the above

12. **False positives in presumed consent can be a result of:**

    (a)   unregistered preferences for certain reason
    (b)   ignorance
    (c)   not aware of the presumed consent system
    (d)   donation information is sent through postcards and letters to citizens
    (e)   all of the above

13. **Ethical arguments against presumed consents express their objection from the point of view of the individual's autonomy in that:**

    (a)   a public declaration encourages people to conclude their opinion based on their own justifications
    (b)   it is a moral obligation for a citizen to express their objection publicly
    (c)   consent is a dichotomous variable applicable to the individual
    (d)   an individual's decision may be influenced by the fact that it is expressed publicly
    (e)   none of the above

14. **Combating the existing moral turpitude and trying to improve the laws governing organ recovery includes:**

    (a)   extensive education and collaboration among involved individuals and stakeholders
    (b)   improving consent and donation rates by recruiting healthcare coordinators that can assess in informed consent declarations
    (c)   the use of improved networks that can encourage people to donation and publicly coercing them into signing their profiles as organ donors
    (d)   a and b
    (e)   all of the above

15. **Even though the ethical prospect regarding financial incentives for organ donation is complex, a form of compensation that is legally permissible can be justified if:**

   (a) it compensates the expenses of the donor for a whole year after when the donation is to occur
   (b) it compensates the payments of the donor presumed to be a family provider for the period of the donation process and recovery that he might spend workless
   (c) it compromises gifts and purchase that account for the financial value of the donated organ
   (d) if the purpose is to mitigate the financial loss the donor might incur as a result of the donation process itself

16. **Financial incentives decrease the moral principle of organ donation and exploits people in lower socioeconomic classes leading to an imbalance in organ availability, decrease in organ donation rates and creating greater disparities between individuals:**

   (a) True
   (b) False

17. **To maintain public trust in organ donation, it is essential to:**

   (a) convey gratitude
   (b) respect the sacred nature of the human body
   (c) honor the deceased and not assign a value for his organs
   (d) b and c
   (e) all of the above

18. **Religion has different perspective on the topic of organ donation that can be reflected as:**

   (a) allowed act along as it is selflessly performed
   (b) organ donation is gifted with the expectation of a reciprocated act
   (c) organ donation is not allowed in religions such as Judaism and Christianity, unless the human circumstances change or ethical ideas progress
   (d) a and c
   (e) all of the above

19. **Heart transplantation:**

   (a) in a heart transplantation the risks are diminished in relative to the advantages of the operation, the main aim is to undergo the transplantation
   (b) depends on the conditions of the donor heart and recipient, available equipment and expertise of the doctors to perform the transplantation
   (c) the medical condition of the patient is not as essential as the importance to reduce the ischemic damages to the heart
   (d) none of the above

20. **A better candidate in a heart transplantation procedure is seeked in the following case:**

    (a) the donor heart is in great condition in a state 4 h away from the recipient's residing hospital
    (b) the recipient's condition has deteriorated 1 h before the surgery and there exists a better candidate for the heart in the hospital
    (c) the recipient showed associated cardiac conditions but with low risks of jeopardizing the operation
    (d) a and b
    (e) a and c

21. **The scarcity in available organs and the elevated heart failure demand contribute to the necessity of waiting lists and the categorization of patients according to corresponding barriers to referral in order to maintain to an extent a fair balance and equality for everyone.**

    (a) True
    (b) False

22. **Although the system of presumed consent have shown higher success rates with organ transplantation, it has not been adopted worldwide due to:**

    (a) the prevalent dilemma between the donor's autonomy and the receiver's right to live
    (b) the different policies regarding consent existent worldwide
    (c) its conflict with some religions and religious beliefs
    (d) all of the above
    (e) none of the above

23. **Organ donation registration can be encouraged through:**

    (a) simpler registration processes
    (b) spread awareness regarding organ donation
    (c) improve the laws governing organ recovery
    (d) all of the above
    (e) none of the above

24. **Informed/Expressed consent:**

    (a) an ethical and legal requirement
    (b) provides all required information to a competent individual so they can make a conscious decision
    (c) reflects the practical application of autonomy
    (d) legal documentation that an individual's opinion is respected
    (e) all of the above

25. **The principles of informed consent may not be always the ethical guide due to the fact that:**

    (a) it cannot be used with unconscious patients
    (b) it is not limited by the patient's family cooperation and orientation
    (c) it is a principle that can be only applied to living donors
    (d) a and c
    (e) all of the above

26. **In the concept of presumed consent, an individual is excused from this policy and considered objector regardless, unless stated otherwise.**

    (a) True
    (b) False

27. **An unknown person is brought to the hospital dead on arrival (DO(A)) and is found to have a tattoo on his chest that says "organ donor". Inspecting the patient's heart and organs reveals high potential for organ donation. Is it legal and ethical to procure organs from the body?**

    (a) organ recovery can be initiated if proven brain dead by a number of physicians and the body cannot be identified
    (b) organ recovery cannot be initiated unless the person is identified with no legal objection to organ donation recorded in his name or there exists a legal documentation that can assure the deceased's legal registration as an organ donor
    (c) procure organs as soon as possible to prevent ischemic damage as long as the person has a tattoo of registration as organ donor
    (d) no organ recovery can be initiated even if the tattoo says "organ donor"

28. **A Muslim individual was considered eligible for heart recovery and was found to have registered legally as an organ donor. The deceased's family object against organ recovery and threaten the doctor into a law suit. What can be done in this case?**

    (a) the doctor abides to the family's wishes and organ recovery procedure is terminated
    (b) the doctor explains the eligibility of the deceased's organs to recovery and the presence of a recipient in need of the heart trying to change the family member's minds
    (c) the doctor proceeds with the organ recovery since the deceased has a legal registration for organ donation
    (d) the doctor if proceeds with the recovery of organ will be facing a law suit in favor of the deceased's family members

29. **A heart donor was recovered in a hospital with 2 recipients on the waiting list; a 56-year-old man with terminal heart failure and a 7-year-old girl with congenital heart disease. Who is more eligible to receive the heart?**

(a) the young girl should receive the heart since she has a better prognosis for heart transplantation at a young age

(b) the transplantation council at the hospital should assign the heart to the recipient offering financial incentives

(c) the man should receive the heart since his condition is critical compared to the congenital heart disease of the little girl

(d) the man should receive the heart since after transplantation he will resume his daily life and career and attain a productive factor in the society

30. **A father rushes his wife and kid to the hospital after a car accident. The wife is later announced brain dead and the son needs an urgent heart transplantation. His mother's heart is eligible for the operation but it is found that she had registered an objection to organ donation 10 years ago. The husband claims that she had wanted to change the objection but haven't had the chance to do so yet. What is ethical to be done in this case?**

(a) recover the heart from the mother anyways for transplantation since it is for her son

(b) have the husband sign a registration on behalf of his deceased wife

(c) respect the deceased's documented objection and abide from organ procurement

(d) carry on the transplantation if the husband can provide a legal and ethical proof that his wife wanted to change her objection and register for organ donation.

Answers:

1. Answer: b

   (a) Wrong; dead donor rule exemptions include the removal of organs or tissue that would not threaten the life of the donor, examples include the removal of the second kidney or a liver lobe.

   (b) Correct; life-prolonging organs are only removed after the human donor's death.

2. Answer: c

3. Answer: a

   (a) Correct; the informed consent is the main moral principle guiding the donation of organs such as a kidney for transplant purposes and the issue is more complex in the case of life-prolonging organs.

   (b) Wrong; the process of comprehending all related risks and benefits to the patient before approving on a medical procedure and accepting the patient's decision is a respect of his autonomy.

   (c) Wrong; informed consent respects the individual's opinion and legally acknowledges his contribution to his own health voluntarily.

    (d) Wrong; informed consent provides an ethical documentation that the process was well explained to the patient and the latter had the time to consider all risks and benefits before making his own decision.

4.   Answer: c

    (a) Wrong; the individual has to be competent, conscious and adheres to his own decision voluntarily without any external pressure.

    (b) Wrong; the doctor has to explain all information related to the medical procedure with all benefits and risks without any coercion or duress.

    (c) Correct; an informed consent comprises all information regarding a medical treatment with all related risks and benefits.

    (d) Wrong; an informed consent is a principle respecting the patient's autonomy and ability to act in his own health care.

5.   Answer: e

6.   Answer: b

    (a) Wrong; an individual will not be an organ donor unless declared otherwise.

    (b) Correct; an advance directive with a recorded wish to be an organ donor; ex: driver's license.

    (c) Wrong; the presence of a surrogate with decision-making responsibility directed previously by the individual prior to his death has solely the authority to declare the deceased wishes as a candidate for organ donation or not.

    (d) Wrong; the expressed consent model is not deemed as effective in increasing the supply to match it to that of the demand.

7.   Answer: b

    (a) Wrong; organ and tissue recovery occur only after all efforts to save a life are exhausted and death is declared. The medical team involved in organ recovery is separate from the doctors previously working with the patients.

    (b) Correct; care is provided to all patients equally regardless of whether they are registered for organ donation or not.

8.   Answer: b

    (a) Wrong; in the strict version of presumed consent the donor's family is not welcome to interfere with the decision to donate.

    (b) Correct; the relaxed version of presumed consent requires the permission of the donor's family, if located, prior to any manipulation.

    (c) Wrong; a clinically and legally suitable candidate for organ and tissue recovery will be presumed to have consented to organ donation if a preliminary refusal had not been registered.

    (d) Wrong; supporters of the presumed consent model believe that individual needs and rights come second to the needs and interests of the society, the "common good".

9. Answer: d

    (a) Wrong; a positive recognition and motivation for organ donors that aids in declaring potential candidates as eligible for organ donation if no objection had been previously registered.

    (b) Wrong; a positive motivation for organ donation does not ensure an increase in the number of available organs for donation compared to the number of registered donors in the system.

    (c) Wrong; the opinion of the individual's family by some laws is not legally accepted when the individual has legally considered organ recovery and attributed it to the common good.

    (d) Correct; a positive motivation and presumed consent law can help encourage more candidates to organ donation while respecting their involvement as a personal decision.

10. Answer: a

    (a) Wrong; favors the recipient's right to live over the donor's right to autonomy.

    (b) Correct; presumed consent shows efficiency in increasing the supply of available organs for transplantation.

    (c) Wrong; compromises within limit the values of other individuals within the concept of choosing the greater good.

11. Answer: d
12. Answer: e
13. Answer: e
14. Answer: d

    (c) Wrong; social media can be used to track organ donors' profiles and encourage communication and positive motivation without the pressure or coercion exerted onto anyone's decision.

15. Answer: d

    (a) Wrong;

    (b) Wrong;

    (c) Wrong;

    (d) Correct; financial incentives are to mitigate financial loss rather than encourage for donation.

16. Answer: a
17. Answer: e
18. Answer: a

    (a) Correct; donation needs to be a selflessly performed act without the expectation of any reciprocation or reward.

    (b) Wrong; organ donation is gifted without the expectation of a reciprocated act.

    (c) Wrong; religions such as Judaism and Christianity are regarded as a rule set by God and cannot be changed even if human circumstances change or ethical ideas progress.

19. Answer: b

    (a) Wrong; in cases when the risks exceed the advantages as when the patient is too sick to undergo the transplantation, another person becomes the better candidate for the process.

    (b) Correct; the available equipment, adequacy of centers and expertise of the doctors play a crucial role in the conditions of the heart donor and recipient in the overcoming of the related challenges to heart recovery and transplantation.

    (c) Wrong; the medical state and condition of the recipient is as important as that of the heart; if any part is compromised the operation as a whole is compromised.

20. Answer:

    (a) Wrong; the heart can survive for 4 to 6 h before transplantation

    (b) Correct; the operation cannot be performed when the recipient's condition doesn't allow for the transplantation

    (c) Wrong; as long as the advantages overweight the risks of the operation, heart transplantation can be performed.

21. Answer: a

    (a) Correct; access to heart transplantation first involves a referral and the continuation of barriers to referral prompts inquiries on fairness and equity while choosing recipients.

22. Answer: d
23. Answer: d
24. Answer: e
25. Answer: e
26. Answer: a
27. Answer: a

(a) Correct; in the concept of the greater good, as long as the body abides by the brain-dead rule.
(b) Wrong; it is time consuming and a waste to hold the organ recovery process if no body identification can be produced.
(c) Wrong; a tattoo is not a legal documentation nor ethically accepted as a legal registration for organ donation
(d) Wrong; in the concept of the greater good and need for organ recovery, organs can be procured if legally and ethically accepted.

28. Answer: c

(a) Wrong; the organ recovery procedure is initiated based on the legal documentation of the patient and his opinion.
(b) Wrong; since the deceased has a legal registration for organ donation organ recovery can be initiated regardless of the family's acceptance.
(c) Correct; since the deceased has a legal registration for organ donation organ recovery can be initiated without the consent of any family member.
(d) Wrong; the doctor is legally and ethically safe as long as the deceased has a legal registration as an organ donor

29. Answer: c

(a) Wrong; the organ eligibility for transplantation takes into consideration the condition of recipients in the waitlist.
(b) Wrong; financial incentives are not an ethical consideration in transplantation waitlist.
(c) Correct; the medical condition of the recipients attains the strategy on whom to have a place on the waiting list for organs.
(d) Wrong; the social position or career of the recipient is not an ethical consideration to base an organ donation on.

30. Answer: d

(a) Wrong; recover the heart from the mother anyways for transplantation since it is for her son.
(b) Wrong; the registration cannot be signed on behalf of the donor even if proven brain dead.
(c) Wrong; when in critical similar cases it is of more importance to cherish the better good rather than the donor's wish.
(d) Correct; if proven that an organ donor registration can be applied, it is ethically and legally accepted to carry on organ recovery.

References

1. Evans RW, et al. Donor availability as the primary determinant of the future of heart transplantation. JAMA. 1986;255(14):1892–8.
2. Doig CJ, Rocker G. Retrieving organs from non-heart-beating organ donors: a review of medical and ethical issues. Can J Anesth. 2003;50(10):1069–76.
3. Abouna GM. Ethical issues in organ transplantation. Med Princ Pract. 2003;12(1):54–69.
4. Potts JT, Herdman R. Non-heart-beating organ transplantation: medical and ethical issues in procurement. 1998.
5. Bearl DW. Ethical issues in access, listing and regulation of pediatric heart transplantation. Translational Pediatrics. 2019;8(4):278.
6. Freeman RB, Bernat JL. Ethical issues in organ transplantation. Prog Cardiovasc Dis. 2012;55(3):282–9.
7. Robertson JA. Supply and distribution of hearts for transplantation: legal, ethical, and policy issues. Circulation. 1987;75(1):77–87.
8. Egan TM. Ethical issues in thoracic organ distribution for transplant. Am J Transplant. 2003;3(4):366–72.
9. Carosella ED, Pradeu T. Transplantation and identity: a dangerous split? The Lancet. 2006;368(9531):183–4.
10. Patel A, et al. Variations in criteria and practices for heart transplantation listing among pediatric transplant cardiologists. Pediatr Cardiol. 2019;40(1):101–9.

Cultural and Religious Aspects of Heart Transplantation

Jose-Maria Dominguez-Roldan, Ikram-ul-Haq, Naseer Ahmed, Visist Dhitavat, Feng Huo, Jie Zhao, and Marti Manyalich-Vidal

Abstract Organ donation and transplantation has always had an important social, cultural, and religious component apart from the scientific component. Organ donation for heart transplantation also entails the fact that since ancient times the heart has been considered a central organ of the body. Different religions and cultures have been adapting and accepting the donation of organs for transplantation, and especially cardiac donation, as a singular, acceptable fact, since they not only achieve a significant benefit for the recipient of the heart transplant, but also enable their survival. This chapter discusses the most important cultural and religious positions

The original version of this chapter has been revised. The name 'Ikran' has been corrected as 'Ikram'. The correction to this chapter can be found at https://doi.org/10.1007/978-3-031-17311-0_18

J.-M. Dominguez-Roldan (✉)
Neurological ICU, Hospital Universitario Virgen del Rocio, Seville, Spain
e-mail: jmdominguez@telefonica.net

J.-M. Dominguez-Roldan · M. Manyalich-Vidal
Donation and Transplantation Institute (DTI), Universidad de Sevilla, Seville, Spain
e-mail: marti.manyalich@dtifoundation.com

Ikram-ul-Haq
Department of Medicine, Letterkenny University Hospital, Letterkenny, Ireland

N. Ahmed
Rehman Medical Institute, Hayatabad, Phase 5, Peshawar, Pakistan

V. Dhitavat
Thai Red Cross Organ Donation Centre, Bangkok, Thailand
e-mail: visist@redcross.or.th

F. Huo
Organ Transplant Center, GHOPO, General Hospital of Southern Theater Command of PLA, Shenyang, China

ODTQC of Guangdong Province, Guangzhou, China

Council of COTDF, Beijing, China

J. Zhao
External Affairs Department of COTDF, BROAOD Belt and Road Organ Donation Capacity Improvement Cooperation Training Project, Beijing, China

H. T. Hashim et al. (eds.), *Heart Transplantation*,
https://doi.org/10.1007/978-3-031-17311-0_15

in the world regarding heart donation for transplantation, including Islamic, Buddhist, Chinese, and Catholic perspectives. Anyway, further studies and research should be conducted to determine the other religions' perspectives regarding the procedure.

Keyword Organ donation · Heart transplantation · Islamic religion · Buddhism · China · Catholic religion · Ethics · Heart donation

1 Introduction

Organ donation and transplantation has important support from all religions.

Therefore, to help citizens to understand and accept organ donation and transplantation, we need a well-organized system that guides them through the whole process and advises them regarding their final decision. The better is the system, the easiest will it be to take this decision independently of religion, because the final goal is to save lives.

My colleagues in this chapter, experts very respected worldwide, will provide an accurate perspective of their own beliefs, and provide an understanding of the principles and beliefs that support organ donation and transplantation, depending on each religion and its cultural aspects.

In my experience worldwide in organ donation and transplantation, religions have never been an obstacle to organ and tissue donation and transplantation; however, understanding and cultural practice must be educated and learnt, and this book is a way to achieve that.

We have focused on these religions and communities that have issues with the procedure of heart transplantation, so, Protestant, Orthodox Christianity, Hinduism and Judaism have not mentioned because we need to gather more information about them and many of them have not any opinion regarding the procedure.

2 Cultural and Religious Aspects of Heart Transplantation (Islamic Perspective)

2.1 Introduction

As there are no initial rulings for the same, so silence is the starting point of every discussion. Islamic Scripture is looked upon to give an explanation for some of the unexplained abstract topics regarding ownership of the body, human dignity, and prohibition of mutilation [1, 2]. These are the concepts that can be argued both ways and depend on the interpreter of the subject as there is no known ruling for organ transplantation.

For all the new inventions and development in the scientific field, a ruling is needed to act upon, and for that reason, fatwa is required which is a formal ruling or interpretation on a point of Islamic law given by a qualified legal scholar. The joint ponderings at such conferences lead to the birth of a different approach of reasoning and a novel way of arriving at religious verdicts known as *ijtihād jamāʿī* (collective legal reasoning) [3].

2.2 Islamic Perspective of Heart Transplantation

As discussed above, heart transplantation is an advancement and needs logical reasoning (*ijtihad*) in order to give a ruling on its permissibility or non-permissibility. Therefore, we have differences in opinions with regards to organ transplantation (the heart specifically and other organs in general). The following headings will discuss the positive and negative positions about the permissibility of organ transplantation.

2.3 Contrary Opinions

Starting with the opposing opinion, which can be considered as the default position on the procedures needed to preserve the bodily integrity of human beings. It advocates allowing the human body to go through its natural history to the extreme possibility without causing any mutilation or change in its structure by any invasive intrusion:

اللهِ لِخَلْقِ تَبْدِيلَ لَا عَلَيْهَا النَّاسَ فَطَرَ الَّتِي اللهِ فِطْرَةَ

> This is the natural disposition God instilled in mankind—there is no altering God's creation (Quran 30:30).

The holy scripture undoubtedly keeps the authority of everything within Allah's dominion:

قَدِيرٌ شَيْءٍ كُلِّ عَلَى وَهُوَ الْمُلْكُ بِيَدِهِ الَّذِي تَبَارَكَ

> Exalted is He who holds all control in His hands; who has power over all things (Quran 67:1).

In another verse Allah mentions human beings as property:

النَّاسِ إِلَهِ .النَّاسِ مَلِكِ .النَّاسِ بِرَبِّ أَعُوذُ قُلْ

> Say, 'I seek refuge with the Lord of people, the Master of people, the God of people'. (Quran 114:1–3).

These are a few of the verses which are considered to be the basis for the true ownership of Allah over human beings who are mere servants, stewards, and Khalifah of Allah. This is the reason why humans are not free to act on their own in terms of their bodies. Humans are accountable for the freedom given to them.

It is also understandable to some extent on their part as if there are no Government basis programs for transplantation, which can lead to an increase in demand for organs which will open the door for black market organ trade.

As mentioned in the Quran:

وَلَقَدْ كَرَّمْنَا بَنِي آدَمَ وَحَمَلْنَاهُمْ فِي الْبَرِّ وَالْبَحْرِ

> And verily we have honored the children of Adam and He has created for you all that is on the earth and ocean (Quran 17:70).

Mufti Shafi divides transplantation into three types (a) xenotransplantation, (b) artificially constructed organs, and (c) allotransplantation (live or cadaveric). According to him, the former two are permissible as human beings are the beneficiaries and the later one is not permissible because it is seen as devaluing and a violation of the divine sanctity of the human body. Heart transplantation comes under the third type so it is not permissible according to Mufti Shafi. He strengthens his opinion by quoting other scholars and jurists, for example in Hidayah of Imam Al-Marghinani in which he states:

> It is unlawful to sell the hair of a human, as it is (unlawful) to derive benefit out of it, for a human is honored and sacred, and it is not permissible to disgrace any part of a human's body [4].

Mufti Shafi sees it as impermissible even in life-or-death scenarios. He quotes the famous saying of Prophet Muhammad (PBUH): "Breaking the bone of a dead person is similar to breaking the bone of a living person." (Sunan Abu Dawood 3207) [5].

Taking this hadith as evidence Mufti Shafi states the human body is sacred and sanctified whether it is alive or dead, which puts a full stop to both live and cadaveric donation.

The second reason which leads Mufti Shafi to conclude organ transplantation is impermissible is the association between humans and Allah. He says that the human body and its organs are given to man as a loan, a mandate (*amanah*), and there is a trust between Allah and humans and we are not the owners of our bodies, as mentioned in the Quranic verse which asserts that Allah is the owner of everything in the universe:

لِلَّهِ مُلْكُ السَّمَاوَاتِ وَالأَرْضِ وَمَا فِيهِنَّ وَهُوَ عَلَى كُلِّ شَيْءٍ قَدِيرٌ

> To Allah belongs the dominion of the heavens and the earth and whatever is within them. And He is over all things competent (Quran 5:120).

2.4 Supportive Opinion

Heart in specific and organ transplantation surgery in general is a common practice in the developed world and in some of the developing countries. It is considered to be one of the best developments in today's technological world for the benefit of mankind.

2.5 Basic Concept Behind the Permissibility of Organ Transplantation

Organ transplantation is done when someone's life is on the verge of death and cannot be saved with other means, such as for end-stage organ disease, for example heart failure, which needs heart transplantation when all medical therapies are exhausted. Basic concepts which are used in the argument of permissibility are now briefly discussed.

The legal maxims/axioms used are as follows:

(i) Matters shall be judged by their objectives: (al-Umūr bi-Maqāṣidihā)

All matters are judged by their objectives and purpose. The goal and objective of heart transplantation are to cure end-stage heart disease. The procedure is not performed with the intention of mutilating, harming the dignity, or causing agony to the deceased. Rather, it is carried out with the noble intention of saving human life.

(ii) Harm must be abolished: (al-darar yuzal)

Abolishing or eliminating harm is one of the objectives of Islamic law. Heart transplantation fulfills this goal. Allah regards human life much more than anything and has promised great return for the people who are involved in saving human lives, as mentioned in the Quran:

جَمِيعًا النَّاسَ أَحْيَا فَكَأَنَّمَا أَحْيَاهَا وَمَنْ

Translation: "and if anyone saved a life it would be as if he saved the life of the whole people" (Quran 5:32).

(iii) Hardship begets facility: (al-mashaqqa tajlib at-taysīr)

Heart transplantation is a means of overcoming the difficulty a human being faces in terms of end stage heart diseases not curable with other methods. So, this problem of end stage organ failure has motivated humans to find treatment, which is transplantation, as supported by Quranic verse:

الْعُسْرَ بِكُمُ يُرِيدُ وَلاَ الْيُسْرَ بِكُمُ اللَّه يُرِيدُ

Translation: "Allah intends every facility for you He does not want to put you to difficulties" (Quran 2:185).

2.6 Adoption of the Lesser-of-Two Evils

One of the other strong arguments put forward by proponents is that of avoiding great harm or evil by selecting the lesser evil or harm. In the case of transplantation greater harm/evil is the losing the life of the patient and the lesser harm/evil is harvesting organs from the deceased; so preventing harm takes priority over preserving the body of the deceased.

It is obvious from Islamic law that it allows mankind to do the unlawful (harm) when in dire need, for example if someone is starving to death then he or she can eat those things which are unlawful (haram) under normal circumstances in order to save his or her life, provided that there are no lawful options available at that time and with the best intentions. This argument is supported by the Holy Quran as:

رَّحِيمٌ غَفُورٌ اللّهَ إِنَّ عَلَيْهِ إِثْمَ فَلا عَادٍ وَلاَ بَاغٍ غَيْرَ اضْطُرَّ فَمَنِ

Translation: "But if one is forced by necessity without willful disobedience, nor transgressing due limits—then is he guiltless. For Allah is Oft-Forgiving Most Merciful" (Quran 2:173).

Use of medical means to treat diseases is permissible in Islam, and heart transplantation is one of the ultimate treatments for heart failure. This is supported by the following saying of the Holy Prophet Muhammad (PBUH):

ع ل يه ه‍ال ل ص‍د لى النَّبِيَّ أَتَيْتُ قَالَ ،شَريكِ بْنِ أُسَامَةَ عَنْ ،عِلاَقَةَ بْنِ زِيَادٍ عَنْ ،شُعْبَةُ حَدَّثَنَا ،النَّمَرِيُّ عُمَرَ بْنُ حَفْصُ حَدَّثَنَا
تَدَاوَىأَنَّ اللهِ رَسُولَ يَا فَقَالُوا هُنَا وَهَا هَا مِنْ الأَعْرَابُ فَجَاءَ قَعَدْتُ ثُمَّ فَسَلَّمْتُ رُالطَّيْرِ رُءُوسِهِمُ عَلَى كَأَنَّمَا وَأَصْحَابُهُ و س‍لم
فَقَالَ " تَدَاوَوْا فَإِنَّ اللَّهَ عَزَّ وَجَلَّ لَمْ يَضَعْ دَاءً إِلاَّ وَضَعَ لَهُ دَوَاءً غَيْرَ دَاءٍ وَاحِدٍ الْهَرَمُ " .

Narrated by Usamah ibn Sharik:

"I came to the Prophet (ﷺ) and his Companions were sitting as if they had birds on their heads. I saluted and sat down. The desert Arabs then came from here and there. They asked: Messenger of Allah, should we make use of medical treatment? He replied: Make use of medical treatment, for Allah has not made a disease without appointing a remedy for it, with the exception of one disease, namely old age". (Sunan Abu Dawood 3855) [5].

2.7 List of Some of the Rulings (Fatwas)

Table 1 lists the issued rulings by major Islamic scholars and jurists [6].

2.7.1 Fatwas in Malaysia

Organ transplantation has been discussed since 1960 and, specifically, heart and eye transplantation were discussed in 1970; a fatwa was issued in support of the permissibility of donation and receiving an organ in 1970 by the National Fatwa Council.

Table 1 Rulings issued by major Islamic scholars and jurists (adopted from [6])

Chronological summary of official fatwas regarding organ transplant treatment

Year	Jurist/Organization	Position	Country	Summary of ruling		
				Prohibited	Permissible	Comments
1959	Hasan Mamun	Grand Mufti	Egypt		See comment	Gomeal transplants permissible
1966	Abd al-'AI Haridi	Grand Mufti	Egypt		X	Organ trading is prohibited
1967	Muhammad Shafi Uthmani	Grand Mufti	Pakistan	X		
1969	Islamic International Conference	International Conference	Malaysia		X	
1972	Algiers Supreme Islamic Council	National Council	Algeria		X	
1973	Muhammad Khatir Muhammad al-Shaykh	Grand Mufti	Egypt		See comment	Harvesting skin from unidentified corpses is permissible
1977	Supreme Council for Fatwas	National Council	Jordan		X	
1978	Senior Ulama Council	National Council	Saudi Arabia		See comment	Corneal transplants are permissible
1979	Gad al-Haq AM Gad al-Haq	Grand Mufti	Egypt		X	
1980	Fatwa from Ministry of Endowment	National Council	Kuwait		X	
1981	1st Internat'l Conf. on Islamic Medicine	International Conference	Kuwait		X	Transplants involving injuring to donor are permissible
1980	Religious Affairs Supreme Council	National Council	Turkey		X	
1982	Senior Ulama Council	National Council	Saudi Arabia		X	
1985	IFA-MWL— 8th Session	International Conference	International		X	

(continued)

Table 1 (continued)

Chronological summary of official fatwas regarding organ transplant treatment

Year	Jurist/Organization	Position	Country	Summary of ruling		
				Prohibited	Permissible	Comments
1986	Council of Islamic Jurisprudence	International Conference	Amman		See comment	Brain death equals actual death in Islamic law
1986	IFA-OIC—3rd Session	International Conference	International		See comment	Brain death equals actual death in Islamic law
1987	Muhammad Sayed Tantawi	Grand Mufti	Egypt		X	Selling organs is prohibited
1988	IFA-OIC—4th Session	International Conference	International		X	
1989	IFA-India	National Council	India		See comment	Live donation is permissible, cadaveric donation is prohibited
1994	University of al-Azhar	National Council	Egypt		X	
1994	Ahmad bin Hamad al-Khalili	Grand Mufti	Oman		X	
1996	Indonesian Council of Ulama	National Council	Indonesia		X	
1995, 1998	Yusuf al-Qaradawi	Independent Mufti	Egypt/Qatar		X	Brain death equals actual death in Islamic law

2.7.2 Fatwa of the Islamic Religious Council of Singapore

A general fatwa was issued for permissibility in 1986, followed by some specific organs like cornea transplantation in 1995; fatwas were issued in 2003 and 2004 for permissibility of heart and liver donations [7].

Fatwa of the Senior Ulama Council of Saudi Arabia.

A fatwa regarding cadaveric organ donation was issued in 1982 and living organ donation was permitted as early as 1967 [8].

2.7.3   Kuwaiti Council of Fatwa

Cadaveric organ donation was permitted in 1979 by the Kuwaiti Council of Fatwa, with or without the deceased's consent [9].

2.7.4   International Islamic Fiqh Academy (IIFA)

In 1988 IIFA issued a fatwa which allows transplantation from a deceased to an end stage disease patient provided that consent is obtained from the deceased before death, family members, or from the head of the Muslim community if the deceased cannot be identified or does not have any next of kin [9].

2.7.5   Islamic Fiqh Academy, India

A session was held in 1989 and a fatwa was issued to allow donation and transplanting organs from live or cadaveric donors provided all the cautions were taken as discussed above [10].

2.7.6   Islamic Sharia Council, UK

The Islamic Sharia Council of the UK in 1995 issued a fatwa in support of organ transplantation as a method to save the lives of patients with end-organ failure. Consent can be obtained from the donor or the legal guardian [11].

2.7.7   Fatwa of Dr. Yusuf al-Qaradawi

Dr. Yusuf al-Qaradawi, a well-known scholar from Egypt, stated in a ruling that organ donation and transplantation are permitted in dire need, provided that this act does not cause any harm to the donor or the guardians. Consent can be obtained from the donor or the family members if not instructed by the deceased. He mentioned the permissibility of donating organs to non-Muslims and receiving organs from non-Muslims and strictly prohibited its trade [12].

2.7.8   European Council for Fatwa and Research (ECFR)

ECFR was established in 1997 in Dublin, Ireland and Shaykh Yu⁻suf al-Qarada⁻w⁻ı was its first president, replaced by Shaykh Dr. ʿAbdullah al-Judai. The council is widely accepted among Muslims living in the Western world. ECFR issued its fatwa in collaboration with and quoting IFA and IIFA and allows the donation and transplantation of organs provided the same caution and rules as mentioned by all other councils.

2.7.9 Brain Death

One of the main issues which came around with transplantation is the declaration of death, because in time the organs will be of no use or there will be more chance of failure. The concept of brain death was discussed in 1985 in Jeddah, Saudi Arabia followed by Amman, Jordan in 1986, and a fatwa was issued which stated that death can occur either by the cessation of the functions of the heart and lungs or if the brain stops functioning and is verified by a specialist doctor that there is no more hope for recovery and death can be declared. At that time heart or other organs can be harvested and transplanted in patients who are in dire need.

3 Donation and Transplantation from the Cultural and Religious Perspective of Buddhism

In this section, the similarities and differences of Buddhist's religious and cultural perspectives towards organ donation and transplantation will be examined. While it can be argued that the core Buddhist teachings support the donation of organs, the variety of Buddhist sects and culture affect their perspective on organ donation. While the Pali Canon can be interpreted in favor of organ donation, local beliefs and traditions can impact how the religion is practiced and hinder organ donation. Some sects of Mahayana Buddhism refrain from disturbing the dead person's body, while local superstitions may prevent Theravada Thais from donating their organs, as it may impact their next reincarnation.

Buddhism is the fourth largest religion in the world with over 520 million followers. Buddhists across the world vary in their practices and doctrines—from new spiritual converts in the Western world to rural Thai Theravada farmers—a level of internal diversity many outside of the religion are unfamiliar with. Furthermore, religious doctrine is often subservient to the normative cultural practices and attitudes of the area. In a religion as adaptable as Buddhism, this means the religion interacting and accepting the local beliefs into the area's practice of Buddhism.

While each Buddhist sect can be distinct, core similarities between the various sects can be identified. Buddhists believe that human life is a cycle of suffering (*dukkā*) and rebirth, but that if one achieves a state of enlightenment (*nirvana*) and discards all desires, it is possible to escape this cycle forever [13]. The *Four Noble Truths*, Buddhism's core teachings, teaches the followers to overcome *dukkā* or the suffering that is caused by desires and the ignorance of the impermanence of reality. Unlike the Abrahamic religions' belief in a permanent Afterlife, Buddhism views life as impermanent: as the body dies, the soul reincarnates again and again. To help end the cycle of suffering, Buddhist teachings focus on compassion and giving. Thus, it can be seen as being in favor of organ donation as it helps others overcome their illnesses. This idea is also echoed in many Buddhist leaders advocating for organ donations [14].

Buddhism is a very adaptable and resilient religion that takes on the practices of the society it comes into contact with—Chinese Buddhism is different from the ones in Thailand, Tibet, India, or the West [15]. The variations in Buddhist practices depend on the culture it is influenced by, such as Chinese Buddhism having Confucian and Taoist philosophies as well. In practice, this means that Buddhism's idea on the dead body and souls may vary from one society to the other, as each tradition has their own scriptures and different interpretation of the core beliefs.

The first perspective comes from Mahayana Buddhism mainly practiced in East Asia: China, Japan, Korea, and Taiwan. The cornerstone of the Mahayana branch of Buddhism is the *bodhisattva*, who are spiritual practitioners that strive to liberate themselves and other sentient beings from the cycle of life and death [16]. The main teachings to reach the *bodhisattva* are the practices of the Six Perfections: giving, ethics, patience, vigor, concentration, and wisdom [17]. Many contemporary Mahayana Bhikkhī and Bhikkhunīs interpret the teachings in favor of organ donation as it is considered the highest form of giving. In the case of Bhikkhunī Cheng Yen from Taiwan, she focused on ending the dukkhā of illness and formed the Buddhist Compassion Relief Tzu Chi Foundation. Her advocacy for organ donation to help end patients' illness is well known [14].

However, in other branches of Mahayana Buddhism, Pure Land Buddhism holds a different view and does not accept organ donations as it considers the death process as an important time for the soul to embark on a peaceful journey to its new reincarnation. They strongly believe that the dead person cannot be disturbed for eight hours after death as the spiritual consciousness is still departing the body. The procurement of organs will, undoubtedly, negatively impact the dead person [18]. These views are theorized to be the influence of local Confucianism and Taoism that are prevalent in the same regions as Pure Land Buddhism [16].

Meanwhile, another perspective can be offered by Theravada Buddhism, which is the dominant belief in Thailand, Cambodia, Laos, Myanmar, and Sri Lanka. Their core scripture, the Pali Canon, is a preserved version of Gautama Buddha's teaching. It is often considered by its believers to be the most accurate version of Buddha's teaching as it is recorded and revised by Theravada councils [16]. Based on the doctrine, there is nothing in Theravada Buddhism that rejects the idea of organ donation as long as the transplantation is undertaken with goodwill and compassion.

Unlike other beliefs, Theravada Buddhism does not revere the body as a sacred vessel of the soul. Instead, it is seen as a negative aspect as it is the source of attachment to *dhukkā* and worldly affairs that prevent the reaching of *nirvana* and the end to suffering. In the Pali Canon, the body is compared to a bag of vile and dirty things (blood, phlegm, saliva, pus) and needs to be washed often. It is nothing that should be held onto longer than strictly necessary [15]. With no great love or respect for the body, the willing sacrifice of the body or internal organs to continue someone's life seems to be the ideal situation: the donor is decreasing their own *dukkā* by giving to others and letting go of the vile body. With no restrictions from the doctrine, it could even be said that the spirit is entering the reincarnation cycle more positively.

The scripture also contains stories that could be considered as support for donating your body. There is a traditional story, a Jataka tale, of the Buddha's past life before he became a Buddha. While reincarnated as a noble king, the Buddha practiced the merit of giving. After giving away his riches, he realized he can still give away his own flesh. The news of the King's decision reached far and wide and a Brahmin decided to test the King's resolve. Despite the agony, the King relinquished his eyes and left to live an astute. This great act of giving helped the Buddha to receive special eyesight that perfectly perceived his surroundings. Thus, it can be claimed that there is Buddhist precedent for using one's body to help save the lives of others.

However, the lack of restrictions in the doctrine does not mean Thai Buddhists fully accept organ donation, as many are still influenced by the local superstitions and beliefs about organ donation. Like many other countries, Thailand has a low rate of donation in an opt-in system; many factors contribute to this hesitation and one of these is superstitious beliefs. Many Thais are skeptical of organ donations and cite fears of being born without some organs in their next life.

During the long process of organ donation taking root in Thailand, Buddhism plays a role in helping to convince people, similar to the story of organ donation in many other religions. Its scriptures can be used to assuage religious individuals' fears and worries about donation. It can also help convince Buddhists to register as organ donors. As many Thais are religious and eager to make merit for a better reincarnation, this desire serves as a strong incentive for individuals and their relatives to agree to donate their organs [15], as Buddhism thinks merit comes from the intention of the donor, despite not eventually donating their organs.

From the stories above, it can be observed that Buddhist teachings and cultural attitudes to organ donation and transplantation is varied. The core Buddhist teachings' focus on the impermanence of reality and compassion does not hinder organ donations. In the scriptures, no explicit prohibitions exist and some of the scriptures show the *bodhisattva* engaging in acts of giving his body. Many contemporary religious leaders are in favor of organ donation and help advocate for widespread acceptance and dispelling myths about the procedures. However, with the diversity in Buddhist thoughts and culture, it means that organ donation may be less practiced in some areas.

4 Donation and Transplantation from a Cultural and Religious Perspective in China

4.1 Introduction

The earliest recorded organ transplantation in Chinese and global history is heart transplantation, which can be found in the classic work "Lie Zi Wen Pian." In the fif century BC, Gong Yi of the State of Lu and Qi Ying of the State of Zhao became ill and sought treatment from a legendary doctor, Bian Que. Bian Que exchanged hearts for them, and they were both healed. Bian Que's heart-exchange practice has been widely admired by the Chinese people, and it has become a source of sustenance for the public, who are filled with wonder and anticipation at the magical procedure. This became a reality in 1978 when China's first heart transplant was performed successfully in Shanghai, and the patient survived for 109 days.

With the continuous improvement of China's organ donation and transplantation system (CODTS) over the past years, the number of deceased donors from citizens (DD) in China has increased from 2,766 cases in 2015 (2.01 per million population [PMP]) to 5,222 cases in 2020 (3.70 PMP), with the highest level in 2018 at 4.53. It is worth noting that this data was only 0.03 in 2010. During the same period, heart transplantation (HTx) in China increased from 279 to 557 cases, and the average 30-day, 1-year, and 3-year survival rates after HTx were 92.6, 85.3, and 80.4% respectively [19]. The number of hospitals approved by the National Health Commission that are qualified for heart transplantation had reached 56 by the end of 2020, with three hospitals performing more than 50 cases of HTx in 2020.

Along with the quantitative growth of organ donation, organ transplantation-related technological advances, such as new surgery methods and treatment innovations in China, are also noteworthy, among which the ischemia-free organ transplant is the most impressive. The first ischemia-free liver transplantation and the first ischemia-free kidney transplantation were reported in 2017 and 2018 respectively, and the world's first ischemia-free heart transplant was performed in Guangzhou in 2021. During the six-month follow-up, the recipient of the ischemia-free heart transplant was in good health.

On the other hand, while a lack of donor organs has always been a bottleneck impeding the growth of organ transplantation around the world, the problem is particularly acute in China. China, as is well known, has a large population, and the number of patients newly diagnosed with end-stage organ failure diseases exceeds 300,000 patients each year. While organ transplantation is the only treatment for these patients, the number of organ donations in China is a drop in the ocean. To meet people's needs, it is a challenge as well as a bounden duty for the Chinese government to boost the development of organ donation. As a result, in addition to continuously improving CODTS and optimizing the Chinese model of organ donation, it is critical to research the cultural and religious factors influencing people's thinking and to effectively raise public awareness.

4.2 Influence of Chinese Traditional Values and Customs on Organ Donation

Throughout its 5,000-year history, with the three religio-philosophical traditions (Confucianism, Taoism, and Buddhism) and nine schools of thought at its core, China has developed its own culture and tradition. The interdependence, interpenetration, and mutual influence of these theories have profoundly impacted Chinese people's values and customs.

First, the belief that individuals must ensure body intactness upon death, according to Confucian focus on *xiao* (filial piety), has long been one of the most essential cultural barriers to organ donation in China. Assembled in 400 BC, *The Canonical Book of Filial Piety*, the *Xiaojing*, stated that: "our body, with hair and skin, is derived from our parents. One should not hurt one's own body in any situation. This is the starting point of filial piety". Confucius, the founder of Confucianism, once said Parents gave the body to their son. After the son dies, he also returns his body to parents, and he may be called a filial son. Neither injure his parent's body; nor disgrace his name. This may be called to protect the remains of his parents completely". Furthermore, requirements on offering sacrifice in a good manner, as recorded in the *Book of Rites,* the *Book of Ritual Rules*, and the book of *Zhou Li,* assembled around 200 BC, along with other classical literary expressions such as dying in peace, dying without illness, end one's days on one's native soil, burial brings peace to the deceased, and so on, have also affected people's attitudes toward organ and tissue donation to varying degrees.

Meanwhile, the intertwining of Taoism and Buddhism, which emphasize the immortality of the soul, *saṃsāra* (a Buddhism term, which stands for the continuous cycle of life, death, and rebirth), and so on, has resulted in unique funeral customs for various ethnic groups in various regions of China. People tend to believe that on the first seven-day period after death, the spirits of the dead will return to their home to experience for the last time the glorious world that made them hesitant to leave and then enter the cycle of reincarnation. To make the procedure easier, the dying person's soul should be led back to his hometown, and as he has been born as a whole, he should return as a whole. Relatives often hold honorable funerals with the deceased's entire body, as if they were still alive, believing that this shows the utmost respect and filial piety to the elders. And they often wear mourning garments for 49 days after their beloved one's death, to show respect and remembrance.

To complicate matters further, in some rural areas with strong traditional roots, people tend to require that relatives must die at home. Even when patients were receiving treatment in hospital, they were taken home before death. People believe that only in this manner can the remains (or ashes) of the deceased be buried in the family cemetery, and the spiritual tablets be allowed to enter the ancestral hall. It is believed that, similar to how fallen leaves return to their roots, dying at home allows the deceased's souls to return to their hometowns, which finally allows the deceased to rest peacefully and the descendants of the family to be protected by their deceased loved ones. All of these customs and practices have had a significant impact on relatives' decision-making.

4.3 Influence of People's Perception of Mortality on Organ Donation and Transplantation

Chinese society tends to abstain from talking about death. Unlike Christianity, which believes that after death one can be with God and aspire to heaven, Confucianism emphasizes: "How can one know death when one does not know life?" In the 16,000-word Analects, the term "death" appears only 38 times, mostly to teach people how to "live", such as "when one hears the Dao, one can die at night". Not only does it never talk about death positively, but it also emphasizes that "subjects on which the Master did not talk were: extraordinary things, feats of strength, disorder, and spiritual beings". In addition, the basic doctrine of Chinese Taoism is the pursuit of Dao and immortality. Another example is the "Journey to the West", which is one of the Four Great Masterpieces of China. Inside this book, the lifelong pursuit of most characters is "immortality". All of these have formed the embodiment of the taboo of death. Believing that talking about death will bring bad luck, people tend to use phrases like "Jiabeng" (death of a King), "Qushi" (leave the world)", "Xianshi" (pass away), and so on, instead of mentioning death directly. Such traditions often hinder organ donation coordinators from doing their job.

When it comes to people's perceptions of death, we have to admit the profound impact brought by the combination of the Taoist concept of health and Traditional Chinese Medicine theories. Since ancient times, the absence of breath has been widely accepted as the standard of death by the Chinese people. As stated by Zhuangzi, a representative figure of Taoism, in "Journey to the North" (Zhi Bei You), "The life of a person is also the gathering of qi; gathering of qi brings life; dispersing of qi brings death". It is commonly held that when qi (which could be translated into breath or energy) arises and gathers, life is born, and when qi disperses and is exhausted, death occurs. Since this understanding is not very accurate and scientific, coma and suspended animations sometimes might be mistaken for death as well. According to ancient texts, there have been records of loved ones waking up again during the seven-day *wake* (a Chinese *wake* means that during the seven days after death, relatives take turns to stay awake and keep an eye on the deceased's body). These concepts have further complicated the public's perception of death. Even when death has been declared with no breath and no heartbeat, the family often expects a miracle to occur.

Furthermore, Chinese traditional culture is also known as "heart culture". Mencius, another Confucian representative, believed that the "heart" is not only a biological part of humans, but also a pivotal organ capable of telling right from wrong, distinguishing between good and evil, and displaying sympathy and humility. At the same time, according to Traditional Chinese Medicine (TCM) theories, "the one who loses SHEN dies, who gains SHEN lives". SHEN, which could be translated as mind, spirit, and soul, dominates all the physical and psychological activities of human beings. TCM considers that SHEN emerges from and resides in the heart, and is a vital substance of the body. The combination of these factors has resulted in the fact that even when patients have been diagnosed with brain death, as long as their hearts are still beating, it is often difficult for their families to accept that they are dead. This kind of death perception is a substantial barrier for Chinese people's acceptance of organ donation after brain death.

In 2013, Huang Fen et al. [20] conducted a survey of the willingness of rural residents to donate organs and discovered that approximately 76% of respondents in western Hunan Province did not accept the concept of organ donation, believing that the soul of the deceased who has donated his organs could not be transcended, and thus could not rest in peace. The research results of Yang Ying et al. [21] showed that more than 50% of the population believes that traditional Chinese culture and traditions, such as people's inherent values, religious beliefs, and customs, are major barriers to enhancing people's willingness to donate organs. Additionally, lack of understanding of organ donation, lack of trust in medical staff, and fear of misunderstanding from neighborhoods are also hurdles to organ donation in China [22–24].

4.4 Advancement of People's Perception toward Organ Donation

In recent years, the Chinese government has been committed to optimizing CODTS and publicizing DD.

First of all, in order to show respect to Chinese traditional culture, which places "heart" at its core, the Chinese government has developed its own three-class criteria for human organ donation after death. That is in addition to C-I: DBD (Donation after Brain Death) and C-II: DCD (Donation after Circulatory Death), China has established C-III as DBCD, which stands for donation after brain death followed by circulatory death. DBCD is a unique donation criterion that has only been adopted in China. It not only takes into account the neurological determination of death, but also adheres to Chinese traditional culture and customs, particularly the Chinese idea of "heart" and the traditional belief that death happens when one is out of breath. The implementation of this donation criterion has played a very important role in promoting the reform of organ transplantation in China. According to the *Report on Organ Transplantation Development in China*, from 2015 to 2018, DBCD accounted for 35% of the total DD organ donations in China.

At the same time, to enhance the public's support for organ donation, at the end of 2013, the General Office of the CPC Central Committee and the General Office of the State Council issued the "Opinions on Party Members and Cadres Taking the Lead in Promoting Funeral and Interment Reform", which encourages the party members and cadres to donate their organs or bodies after death. Additionally, the Chinese government has encouraged the mass media to continuously publicize and report on common practices and touching stories of organ donation to raise public awareness and create an environment in which the entire society respects this behavior. Furthermore, government departments, social organizations, universities, hospitals, and OPOs have held a series of events, including commemorative activities for organ donors, from various levels and perspectives, which has resulted in an increased willingness to donate.

As a result of the aforementioned efforts, people's attitudes toward organ donation have greatly improved, particularly after 2015, as evidenced by the growing trend of organ donation volunteer registries in China (Fig. 1) [25]. According to the official website of the China Organ Donation Administrative Center (www.codac.org.cn/), on January 23, 2022, 4,412,286 people registered as organ donation volunteers, which is 194 times more than in 2014. According to Li et al.'s [22] study on Chinese people's views on DD, people's willingness to donate organs increased from 32 to 39% after 2015, compared to the early stage of CODTS.

Furthermore, public acceptance toward brain death in China has also improved to some extent. According to the *Report on Organ Donation and Transplantation in China,* a proportion of DBD cases to total deceased donation cases climbed from 23% during 2015–2018, to 44.33% in 2020; that of DBCD declined from 35 to 20% for the same period.

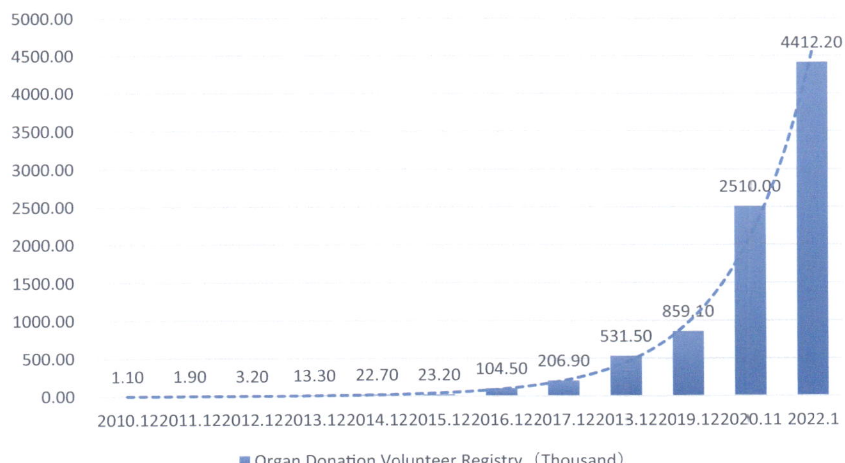

Fig. 1 Number of registered organ donation volunteers on the China Organ Donation Administrative Center's website over the years [6]

4.5 Cultural and Religious Factors as Facilitators

As organ donation and transplantation in China enter a new stage of development, it is a huge challenge to break free from the shackles of traditional culture and religion, and even to make these factors facilitators of organ donation.

In fact, Confucianism's inner meaning is broad and profound. Although it emphasizes the importance of respecting and cherishing life and the body, when faced with options such as "benevolence", "righteousness", "loyalty", and "integrity", it advocates "sacrific[ing] one's life for righteousness and benevolence", to "serve the country with loyalty", and "a person with integrity is a person who devotes his life to safeguarding the virtues". All of these sayings can be interpreted as advocating for organ donation [26].

Furthermore, Confucianism advocates that one should set one's virtue, set one's merit, and expound one's ideas in writing during one's lifetime, with virtue being the most important. Realizing the worth of life and making it immortal are concepts that are very consistent with the "relay for life" concept of organ donation.

Making full use of the mass media is also critical in popularizing these new interpretations of traditional Chinese cultures. Newspapers, television programs, and new media have all played an important role, with new media platforms such as Tiktok, Alipay, and WeChat demonstrating their enormous potential in promoting organ donation. According to data from the Chinese Love & Hope organ donation volunteer service platform (www.savelife.org.cn/), more than 80% of newly registered volunteers in 2020 and 2021 expressed their desire to donate organs via new media channels, and the trend is on the rise.

It is also critical to continue to promote educational programs about Chinese traditional culture and organ donation. Organ donation has been included in some provinces' high school textbooks or university liberal arts education curricula; as Chengdu City established the country's first real-life experience base for life education shows, life education has also been gradually gained attention across the country. Furthermore, grassroots political party organizations, communities, and other public sectors play an important role in facilitating social education. The China Organ Transplantation Development Foundation has been actively publicizing the concept of organ donation to medical institutions, social organizations, public sectors, colleges, universities, and research institutes through the Life Relay Vanguard activities. As a result of these events, over 500,000 people had registered as organ donation volunteers by 2021.

4.6 Conclusion

The influence of culture and religion on people is changing imperceptibly in an increasingly open and inclusive China. The greatest truths are the simplest, and the greatest love is boundless. To create a community of shared future for humanity,

China's diverse culture and plural society will undoubtedly improve the development of organ donation in the country.

Data concerning Hongkong, Macao, and Taiwan regions were not included in the chapter.

5 Cultural and Religious Aspects of Heart Transplantation (Catholic Perspective)

5.1 Introduction

Sometimes it is heard, or even spread in the media, that the Catholic Church is an obstacle to the donation of organs for transplants. Probably this right to free interpretation of the position of the Catholic Church is associated with a lack of knowledge, not only of the historical bases of the birth of transplantology but also of the public manifestos made by the church regarding it. Proposing that the Catholic Church is an obstacle to the diagnosis of death based on neurological criteria or to the establishment of measures to limit therapeutic effort as good clinical practice means ignoring the contents of the documents and declarations that the Catholic Church has made in recent years in relation to the transplantation of organs and tissues in human beings. The Church is not unmoved by the changes in organ procurement techniques that have developed in recent years. The Church's support for organ harvesting from brain-dead donors arises from an in-depth analysis of the clinical and ethical factors that affect this type of donation. The subsequent development of organ harvesting techniques in asystolic donors has opened a new field of discussion of various ethical and moral aspects that have not yet been resolved.

5.2 Doctrine of the Catholic Church in Relation to Brain Death and Organ Transplantation

It was in 1957, during the Congress of the Italian Society of Anesthesiology, that Pope Pius XII stated in a speech addressed to the participants in said Congress: "It is up to doctors to give a clear and precise definition of death and the moment in which death has occurred in those patients who die in a state of unconsciousness" [27]. In this speech, Pope Pius XII urged doctors to establish death criteria based on neurological criteria, given that, with the development of cardiopulmonary resuscitation techniques and artificial mechanical ventilation, in Intensive Care Units (ICUs) [28] there were patients with profound neurological damage who, according to clinical and instrumental criteria, could be considered in an irreversible and terminal situation. Previously, in 1956, the first cases of patients admitted to the ICU and artificially ventilated had already been published, in which a complete cessation of cerebral circulation was detected, which led to the suspicion of the impossibility of brain activity in these patients, although this clinical phenomenon was not associated with the person's death.

Pope Pius XII highlighted the importance of doctors in determining death, and emphasized in relation to cases in which there are doubts regarding the time of death: In case of insoluble doubt, one must resort to presumptions of law and of fact. In general, it will be necessary to presume that life remains, because there is involved here a fundamental right received from the Creator, and it is necessary to prove with certainty that it has been lost.

Pope Pius XII's call to establish new death criteria was made even before the first scientific publications appeared that referred to clinical situations of advanced neurological damage in patients connected to mechanical ventilation, such as coma depasse [29], which were not published in the medical literature until 1959. Until then, no one had established clinical criteria to diagnose the death of patients based on neurological criteria, since until then only the classic cardiocirculatory criteria had been used.

Professor Henry Beecher defined the first criteria for establishing a person's death based on neurological criteria and they were published in *JAMA* magazine in August 1968. That article specified some of the motivations that led to the development of that consensus. One of them was to avoid therapeutic futility in patients with irreversible neurological damage admitted to ICUs, and another, as also explicitly stated in the published article, the possibility that some of these patients, who met the criteria for global brain death, could become organ donors. It should not be forgotten that a few months earlier, in December 1967, the world's first heart transplant had been performed. It should be noted that the aforementioned article from the Harvard Medical School presented as the main element that triggered the consensus on brain death, the content of the speech that Pope Pius XII had made years before and as the only bibliographic reference included in that article was the aforementioned speech by Pope Pius XII. Evidence such as the ones mentioned is a clear proof of the attitude of the Catholic Church regarding brain death, organ donation, and correct clinical practice in patients at the end of life.

The support of the Catholic Church for organ donation was not only shown in the initial stages of organ transplantation, but has continued to manifest itself over the years. This support has covered both activities to promote organ donation in small Catholic groups (acts organized by communities of believers, parishes, etc. in support of organ donation), as well as through the demonstrations carried out by popes, as stated by John Paul II: The Gospel of life is to be celebrated above all in daily life, which must be filled with love of dedication to others. Beyond these exceptional moments, there is a daily heroism, of gestures of sharing, large or small, that builds an authentic culture of life.

The explicit support of the Catholic Church for the donation of organs from deceased in a state of brain death has been reinforced with the document prepared at the initiative of the Pontifical Academy of Sciences, entitled "Why the concept of brain death is valid as a definition of death" [6], in which it is stated: "brain death is the death of the person", and "most of the arguments against the criterion of brain death are not tenable and constitute incorrect deviations if they are examined from a neurological perspective". Pope John Paul II to the Participants of the 1989 Pontifical Academy of Sciences indicated: The problem of the moment of death has serious implications at the practical level, and this aspect is also of great interest to the Church. In practice, there seems to arise a tragic dilemma. On the one hand there is the urgent need to find replacement organs for sick people who would otherwise die or at least would not recover. In other words, it is conceivable that in order to escape certain and imminent death a patient may need to receive an organ which could be provided by another patient, who may be lying next to him in hospital, but about whose death there still remains some doubt. Consequently, in the process there arises the danger of terminating a human life, of definitively disrupting the psychosomatic unity of a person. More precisely, there is a real possibility that the life whose continuation is made unsustainable by the removal of a vital organ may be that of a living person, whereas the respect due to human life absolutely prohibits the direct and positive sacrifice of that life, even though it may be for the benefit of another human being who might be felt to be entitled to preference.

A particularly praiseworthy example of these gestures is the donation of organs, carried out in an ethically acceptable way, in order to offer a chance for health and life to the sick who sometimes have no other hope (Evangelium Vitae, No. 86) or the manifesto on organ donation and transplants carried out by Pope Benedict XVI [30]. The Pontifical Academy for Life held in 2008 an international congress titled "A Gift of Life, Considerations on Organ Donation". In that event Pope Benedict XVI stated, it is useful to remember that the various vital organs can only be extracted ex cadavere [from a dead body], which possesses its own dignity and should be respected ... It is good then, that achieved results receive the common consensus of the entire scientific community in favor of looking for solutions that give everyone certainty. In an environment such as this, the minimum suspicion is not allowed, and where total certainty has not been reached, the principle of caution should prevail. For this, it is useful to increment interdisciplinary research and study in such a way that the public is presented with the most transparent truth on the anthropological, social, ethical, and legal implications of a transplant. In these cases, respect for the life of the donor should be assumed as the primary criterion, in such a way so that the extraction of organs only takes place after having ascertained the patient's true death [31].

The Catholic Church emphasizes the fact that all precautions must be taken to prevent other interests from conditioning the diagnosis of death, and likewise that the parameters of brain death must not be understood or used as an alternative definition of death: death of the person. The Catholic Church insists on the fact that in the donation of organs from brain-dead donors: (1) the retrieval of vital organs from living people must be avoided; (2) a false diagnosis of death in unconscious people, in a vegetative state, must be prevented; and (3) organ harvesting should be avoided in patients with severe neurological disabilities.

To avoid these dangers, the Catholic Church advises that before donating organs for transplants, the following conditions must be met: (1) the donor must be in a situation of proven death, and also meet the legal requirements for death. (2) The deceased donor must have expressed their wish to donate in advance (informed consent). In the absence of prior consent from the donor, the consent of the next of kin is admissible, provided that the deceased had not previously expressed his opposition to the donation. (3) The donor's body must be treated with the same respect as it was before death. The Catechism of the Church (cf. Compendium of the Catechism of the Catholic Church, n. 476) explains that "organ transplantation is morally acceptable with the consent of the donor and without excessive risks for him" (this last statement referring to a living donor). Also, and in relation to the donation of organs from deceased donors, the catechism is explicit, although it highlights the relevance of evidencing death: For the noble act of organ donation after death, one must have full certainty of the actual death of the donor. For this reason, in the context of verifying the death of the donor, there cannot be the slightest suspicion of doubt, and when complete certainty of death has not been reached, the precautionary principle must prevail and, consequently, not establish the diagnosis of death [32].

One more piece of evidence of the relevance that the positive opinion of the Church has on the donation of organs for transplantation, and recognizing that there are many factors (social, health, economic, social justice, etc.) [8] that influence donation, is the fact that in most of the countries in the world with a high rate of organ donation for transplants, the rate of the Catholic population is very high, such as Spain, France, Italy, Portugal, Austria, or the United States [33].

References

1. Ebrahim AF. Organ transplantation: contemporary Sunni Muslim legal and ethical perspectives. Bioethics. 1995;9(3–4):291–302.
2. Sachedina A. Islamic biomedical ethics: principles and application. New York: Oxford University Press;2011.
3. Alexandre C. Facts, values, and institutions: notes on contemporary Islamic legal debate. Am J Islam Soc Sci. 2017;34.
4. Shafi M, Tanshit al-Azhan fi 't-Tarqi' bi A'da al-Insan ya'ni Insani Aza ki Paivankari, Karachi: Darul Isha'at;1967. p. 30 (Hussaini).
5. Al-Kawthari M, Organ Donation and Transplantation. n.d. 2004. www.daruliftaa.com.
6. Abū Dā'ūd Sulaymān ibn al-Ash'ath ibn Isḥāq al-Azdī al-Sijistānī, Sunan Abu-Dawood,855 AD.
7. Organ Donation among Muslims: An Examination of Medical Researchers' Efforts to Encourage Donation in the Muslim Community R, Shoaibhttps://hdl.handle.net/2027.42/85315.
8. Islamic Religious Council of Singapore. Pemindahan Organ di dalam Islam. Singapore: Islamic Religious Council of Singapore; 2007. pp. 10–11.
9. Purport of the Senior Ulama Commission. Decision No. 99, dated 06–11–1402 H. In Directory of the Regulations of Organ Transplantation in the Kingdom of Saudi Arabia. (n.d.). Jeddah: Saudi Center for Organ Transplantation. p. 46.
10. Mohammed Ali Albar Op. cit. (2010). p. 105.
11. Ebrahim AFM. Organ transplantation: an Islamic ethico-legal perspective. In: FIMA Year Book 2002. Islamabad: Federation of Islamic Medical Associations; 2002. pp. 76–78.
12. Howitt R. Islam and Organ donation: a guide to organ donation and Muslim beliefs. London: NHS Blood and Transplant; 2009.

13. Al-Qaradawi Y. Op. cit. (1995). pp. 367–37.
14. Donner SE. Self or no self: views from self psychology and Buddhism in a postmodern context. Smith Colle Stud Soc Work. 2010;80(2–3):215–27.
15. Liu J. Organ Donation after death in Mahāyāna Buddhist perspective. J Int Assoc Buddh Univ (JIABU). 104–119.
16. Hongladarom S. Organ transplantation and death criteria: Theravada Buddhist perspective and Thai cultural attitude.
17. Tai MC. An Asian perspective on organ transplantation. Wien Med Wochenschr. 2009;159(17–18):452–6.
18. Payutto P. The Pali Canon: what a Buddhist must know, 2nd ed. Sahadhammik Press;2010.
19. Lecso PA. The Bodhisattva ideal and organ transplantation. J Relig Health.
20. Huang JF. The report on organ donation and transplantaion in China. Beijing: Tsinghua University Press; 2019/2020.
21. Huang F ZJ, LIu JQ, et al. [Investigation on knowledge, attitude and willingness of organ donation among rural residents]. Chin J Public Health. 2013;29(03):417–419.
22. Yang YHH, Qiu HZ. Analysis on the influence of Chinese traditional culture and concept on organ donation intention. Chin J Tissue Eng Res. 2014;18(05):803–8.
23. Li XMJ, Gao R, et al. The general public new views on deceased organ donation in China. Medicine (Baltimore). 2020;99(50): e23438.
24. Xi LXLK, Jiang W, et al. Understanding public opinion regarding organ donation in China: a social media content analysis. Sci Prog. 2021;104(2):00368504211096.
25. Wu YER, Li L, et al. Cadaveric organ donation in China: a crossroads for ethics and sociocultural factors. Medicine (Baltimore). 2018;97(10): e9951.
26. China Organ Donation Administrative Center. [Act out of love, borr. in the sun-ten years report of China organ donation (2010–2020)]. https://www.codac.org.cn/contents/cpublication/20201013/044524834.htm.
27. Pope P XII. The prolongation of life. Pope Speak. 1958;4:393–398.
28. A definition of irreversible coma. Report of the Ad Hoc Committee of the Harvard Medical School to Examine the Definition of Brain Death. JAMA. 1968;205(6):337–40.
29. Mollaret P, Goulon M. Le coma depasse. Revue neurologique. 1959;101:3–15.
30. Benedetto XVI. Un dono per la vita. Considerazioni sulla donazione di organi. Accessed 24 Feb 2016. thwvvcb-xis.
31. De Paula IC. Los parámetros de lamuerte cerebral desde el punto de vista de la moral católica. Persona y bioética 2000;5(1112):65–71
32. Dominguez-Roldan JM, Aznar J. Aproximación ética al diagnóstico de muerte bajo criterios neurológicos y cardiocirculatorios. Reflexiones sobre el posicionamiento de la Iglesia Católica sobre la donación de órganos para trasplante. Medicina e Morale 2017/2: 147–159.
33. International Registry in Organ Donation and Transplantation Accessed on 24 Feb 2022. http://www.irodat.org.

Bridging Strategies for Heart Transplantation

Ahmed Gamal Abouarab, Mohammed Mustafa Mohammed,
Karim Heweidy, and Abdelrahman Mohamed Nasreldin

Abstract The necessity of hemodynamic stabilization in end-stage heart failure patients awaiting heart transplantation is undebatable. End stage heart failure is a serious condition that requires heart transplantation as a destination therapy in most of the cases, and heart transplantation continues to be the gold standard long-term treatment for those cases. However, patients' constantly lengthy waiting lists together with the limited availability of suitable organ donors remain the main challenging problems hindering transplantation. The limited availability of donors continuously opens the way for investigating and studying different methods till the transplantation is ready to go. Different strategies have been developed in hope of bridging this gap and ameliorating many of the symptoms; some strategies are even being tested as a definitive therapy for replacing the failed innate heart completely. Nevertheless, a lot of research is still being made in this area. Choosing the optimum strategy for the best post-implant outcomes and the least complications can be a difficult task. All strategies mentioned are useful and will provide benefit to the patient if used on the right patient with the right indications. For instance, long-term Milrinone provides the best outcomes compared to other strategies, but only if used in the right group of patients with special characteristics.

Keywords Bridging strategies · Heart transplantation · total artificial heart · Extracorporeal Membrane Oxygenation · Left ventricular assist device

1　The Total Artificial Heart (TAH)

The total artificial heart (TAH) is a pneumatically-powered artificial mechanical circulatory support that replaces the patient's innate failed ventricles and is approved for bridging biventricular failure patients to heart transplantation. So generally, TAH

A. G. Abouarab (✉) · K. Heweidy · A. M. Nasreldin
Faculty of Medicine, Ain Shams University, Cairo, Egypt
e-mail: ahmedgabouarab@gmail.com

M. M. Mohammed
Faculty of Pharmacy, Cairo University, Cairo, Egypt

© The Author(s), under exclusive license to Springer Nature Switzerland AG 2022　　　295
H. T. Hashim et al. (eds.), *Heart Transplantation*,
https://doi.org/10.1007/978-3-031-17311-0_16

is meant for patients who need biventricular support such as those with biventricular failure who are not candidates for LVAD as those patients generally have bad outcomes with LVAD compared to patients with isolated left ventricular failure. Another indication for TAH is end stage heart failure accompanied by conditions that are not well managed by LVAD. Such conditions include hypertrophic, restrictive, or infiltrative cardiomyopathies. They also include patients requiring massive repair on top of the primary heart failure condition such as aortic aneurysms, congenital heart disease, large LV thrombus, or post-infarction VSD [1].

Although there are no randomized control trials comparing different types of ventricular support in terms of efficacy, multiple retrospective studies comparing them have been conducted. One study compared TAH with two different LVADs and results were as follows: 75% effectiveness rate for TAH in bridging to transplantation and 57 and 38% effectiveness rates for the two different LVADs. Another study compared the TAH with extracorporeal and para-corporeal bi-ventricular assist devices and actually showed no significant difference between successful bridging to transplantation rates. However, there was a very significant difference in stroke rates between them as follows: 16% of TAH bridged patients reported strokes compared to 61% for extracorporeal and 57% for the para-corporeal bi-ventricular assist devices. Another study was made on 66 patients bridged with TAH for a median of 87.5 days. Results show that 76% were successfully bridged to transplantation, and 14% died while on TAH [1].

Although approved for bridging to transplantation, the TAH has a lot of complications that are reported regularly. Other notable complications that were also reported frequently include renal failure and chronic anemia. Oliguric renal failure was reported after TAH placement in about 15% of patients who had no previous renal dysfunction. It is hypothesized that upon removal of the ventricles, type B natriuretic peptide decreases significantly which in turn precipitates oliguric renal failure. This hypothesis was tested by administering low doses of nesiritide (the type-B natriuretic peptide) upon ventriculectomy and dramatic increase in urine output was seen after with no hemodynamic instability. Although reliable on the short term, the efficacy of nesiritide is yet to be proven on the long term. Post-implantation severe anemia was also a remarkable complication that is attributed to many causes. The first cause is severe hemolysis caused by mechanical shear stress and by the pneumatically powered diaphragms. The second cause that attributed to severe anemia is the inflammation-induced anemia which is due to the device materials, as shown by elevated C-reactive protein levels. The third cause is inadequate hematopoiesis as evidenced by the reduced reticulocyte index. Interestingly, hematocrit levels returned to the baseline levels after TAH removal and heart transplantation. In conclusion, TAH is a reliable bridging strategy but the unfavorable complications that come with the TAH render its use on the long term and thus other options are considered [1].

2 Left Ventricular Assist Device (LVAD)

LVAD is indicated for patients with congestive heart failure refractory to maximal medical therapy and conventional therapy, patients with ejection fraction less than 25%, or patients with reduced functional capacity as measured by maximal oxygen consumption Vo2 < 14 mg/kg/min. On the other hand, patients with limited life expectancy, severe comorbidities, hematological conditions such as active bleeding or infection, anatomical defects as congenital heart disease, large VSD, or hypertrophic cardiomyopathy, hemodynamic instability like severe independent right-sided HF or significant irreversible aortic insufficiency, and psychosocial problems are all contraindicated to have the LVAD. The survival rates are 81% and 70% in the first and second years, respectively [2].

Although the survival rate and quality of life are promising, the wide range of adverse effects stands as an obstacle in the prevalence of this approach. The 8th annual INTERMACS report states that 60% of the patients are re-hospitalized at least once in 6 months post-implantation and the rate increases from 65 to 80% after 1 year. But the most common complication is bleeding, especially gastrointestinal bleeding, which affects 15% to 30% of all device patients. Managed by re-suturing and proton pump inhibitors, GIB can also require multiple transfusions that may cause antibody reactions and increase the risk of donor rejection and transplant delay. Besides bleeding comes pump thrombosis which affects the survival rate post implantation. Its incidence increased dramatically from 2.2% in 2011 to 8.7% in 2013, but recent trials showed that strict surgical implantation techniques, anticoagulant regimens, and pump speed protect against the risk of pump thrombosis. The most debilitating adverse effect affecting around 13 to 30% of the patients is stoke, which is more prevalent among women with the ischemic etiology being more common than the hemorrhagic one. Moreover, more than 30% of the patients suffer from aortic insufficiency 2 years post-implantation. Finally, infection is a major complication to the LVAD with soft tissue infections around the outlet being the most common one with a prevalence rate of 15.4%. Infections by Gram positive rods are the most common, but Gram-negative rods, fungi, and mycobacterium are also identified [2].

In conclusion, LVAD became an important option in the treatment of end-stage heart failure patients with many people now undergoing it in an upward trend [2].

3 IABP (Intra-Aortic Balloon Pump)

As the mechanical circulatory support systems are evolving, IABP (Intra-aortic balloon pump), which was first conceptualized in 1960s, is the method under spotlight. Being rapidly and easily substituted, comparatively cheap, and minimally invasive, indications for such treatment modality are growing making it a valuable mechanical option for transient hemodynamic support [3].

The statistical data shows that 80% of the population studied hasve succeeded to undergo heart-transplantation without further support, 18% of the population cases worsened after initial benefit, and 2% died. The IABP post-transplant mortality rate was minimal and similar to the control groups after 30 days, 1 year, and 3 years. The rate of success of IABP used as a bridge to transplantation was high with minimal complications [3].

In conclusion, the IABP potential as a successful bridging-to-transplantation method is demonstrated through statistical data of the study as it stabilizes the deteriorated heart failure and reverses kidney and liver disease. Assuming the availability of cardiac donors, IABP's hemodynamic stabilization, few and manageable complications, short- and long-term survival, high similarity to already stable patients, IABP is a great feasible option for bridging.

4 ECMO (Extracorporeal Membrane Oxygenation)

ECMO (Extracorporeal Membrane Oxygenation) is a technique that is currently used as a bridge to heart transplantation as it helps gaining time to stabilize the patients till a decision is made; however, the outcomes, survival rates, and adverse events of this technique is still undergoing further studies for optimum stabilization procedure [4].

ECMO was first initiated in the pediatric population. The outcome of bleeding-related complications is determined by the chosen method where the central methods, unlike the peripheral, produce more unfavorable events such as the need for blood transfusion and higher rates of reoperation. Furthermore, the organs that need to be bypassed determine how ECMO circuits are set up [4].

ECMO complications mark a great obstacle to its use. Complications include lack of balance between bleeding and anticoagulation, heparin-induced thrombocytopenia, progression of preexisting renal failure, bleeding from preexisting surgical sites, disseminated intravascular coagulation, and limb ischemia. The bleeding and anticoagulation imbalance is a great challenge in using the ECMO technique; the interaction of blood with non-endothelial surfaces causes inflammation, prothrombosis, and dilution of coagulation factors due to blood exchange. The complex balance between the two states requires an optimum protocol to handle such situations [4].

Recent studies show poor early and midterm post-transplantation survival rates with ECMO compared to other mechanical techniques such as continuous-flow left ventricular assist devices (CF-LVAD) making the preposition of the ECMO bridging technique as a questionable priority. Although using ECMO more often may reduce the patients' wait list mortality, it increases the post-transplant mortality leading to organ waste [4].

Although ECMO may seem an attractive method of bridging to transplant, the complications, poor survival outcomes in certain studies, and mainly the limited literature made only on small numbers of patients make the use of such techniques as bridge-to-transplant highly debatable [4].

5 Long-Term Milrinone

Long-term inotropic therapy is becoming more prevalent in maintaining the heart baseline functions; however, the use of such agents has not been fully evaluated and is still undergoing studies [5]. Milrinone, a potent noncatecholamine inotrope, acts by inhibiting phosphodiesterase-III. Dobutamine, one of the inotropic enhancers, causes down-regulation of β-adrenoreceptors in severe congestive heart failure patients, making adrenoreceptor agonists less effective than milrinone which spares β-adrenoreceptors and catecholamines [6, 7]

Multiple Choice Questions:

(1) **The IABP catheter is applied to a cardiac patient**

    (a) Post-operative only
    (b) 1-week post heart transplantation operation
    (c) 2 weeks post heart transplantation operation
    (d) The IABP catheter is kept intact through transplantation and maintained into early post-operative.

(2) **IABP catheter is used in all except**

    (a) Cardiogenic shock
    (b) Circulatory support in patient undergoing heart surgery
    (c) Septic shock
    (d) Improve hepatic and renal function

(3) **IABP catheter is used in**

    (a) Bridging to transplantation method
    (b) Treatment of VSD
    (c) Treatment of atrial fibrillation
    (d) Treatment of pulmonary hypertension

(4) **TAH stands for:**

    (a) Total Artificial Heart
    (b) Technical Adjuvant Heart
    (c) All of the above
    (d) None of the above

(5) **The most common complication of TAH is**

    (a) Stroke

    (b) Infections
    (c) Bleeding
    (d) Renal failure

(6) **Post-implantation severe anemia is caused by:**

    (a) Severe hemolysis
    (b) Inflammation-induced anemia
    (c) Inadequate hematopoiesis
    (d) All of the above

(7) **The Effectiveness rate TAH showed by one study is:**

    (a) 32%
    (b) 45%
    (c) 75%
    (d) 95%

(8) **Indications of TAH include:**

    (a) CVP > 18 mmHg
    (b) RV ejection fraction < 20%
    (c) Ventricular Tachycardia
    (d) All of the above

(9) **The survival rate of LVAD Patients in the first year is:**

    (a) 25%
    (b) 50%
    (c) 70%
    (d) 81%

(10) **Contraindications for LVAD include all of the following except:**

    (a) limited life expectancy
    (b) infection
    (c) active bleeding
    (d) middle age adults

(11) **The most common complication for LVAD procedure is:**

    (a) Infection
    (b) stroke
    (c) Pump thrombosis
    (d) GIT bleeding

(12) **The most common infections to occur are caused by:**

    (a) Gram + ve rods

    (b) Gram –ve rods

    (c) Fungi

    (d) Protozoa

(13) Ischemic stroke is caused:

    (a) secondary to hypertension

    (b) secondary to endocarditis

    (c) due to hemorrhagic conversion of ischemic infarcts

    (d) due to embolic causes such as thrombotic deposition at the pump

(14) ECMO stands for:

    (a) Endocardial membrane outflow

    (b) Extracorporeal membrane oxygenation

    (c) All of the above

    (d) None of the above

(15) ECMO cannulation can be done peripherally through:

    (a) Femoral artery

    (b) Popliteal artery

    (c) Brachial artery

    (d) Axillary artery

(16) Studies conducted in France showed the survival rate one-year post transplantation to range from:

    (a) 20% to 30%

    (b) 35% to 40%

    (c) 50% to 70%

    (d) 80% to 90%

(17) ECMO complications include which of the following:

    (a) DIC

    (b) Limb ischemia

    (c) Bleeding from preexisting surgical sites

    (d) All of the above

(18) Taiwan stated that the survival rate to a hospital discharge is:

    (a) 51%

    (b) 65%

    (c) 73%

    (d) 87%

(19) Milrinone acts by:

    (a) Stimulating phosphodiesterase 3

  (b) Inhibiting phosphodiesterase 3
  (c) Stimulating phosphodiesterase 2
  (d) Inhibiting Phosphodiesterase 2

(20) **Milrinone:**

  (a) Increases AMP concentration in smooth and myocardial cells
  (b) Decreases AMP concentration in smooth and myocardial cells
  (c) Increases ATP concentration in smooth and myocardial cells
  (d) Decreases ATP concentration in smooth and myocardial cells

(21) **The terminal half- life for Milrinone is:**

  (a) 2 to 3 days
  (b) 2 to 3 h
  (c) 1.5 to 2 days
  (d) 1.5 to 2 h

(22) **The success rate of Milrinone is around:**

  (a) 10%
  (b) 50%
  (c) 60%
  (d) 80%

(23) **The number of the patients in the conducted trial in the success and failure group, respectively, is:**

  (a) 117 and 33
  (b) 100 and 50
  (c) 80 and 70
  (d) 70 and 80

(24) **Milrinone is:**

  (a) Inotropic
  (b) Chronotropic
  (c) Dromotropic
  (d) Lusitropic

ANSWER KEY:

  1. D
  2. C
  3. A
  4. C
  5. B
  6. D
  7. C

8. D
9. D
10. D
11. D
12. A
13. D
14. B
15. A
16. C
17. D
18. C
19. B
20. A
21. D
22. D
23. A
24. A

References

1. Cook JA, Shah KB, Quader MA, Cooke RH, Kasirajan V, Rao KK, Smallfield MC, Tchoukina I, Tang DG. The total artificial heart. J Thorac Dis. 2015;7(12):2172–80. https://doi.org/10.3978/j.issn.2072-1439.2015.10.70.Erratum.In:JThoracDis.2017Mar;9(3):E342.PMID:26793338; PMCID:PMC4703693.
2. Han JJ, Acker MA, Atluri P. Left ventricular assist devices. Circulation. 2018;138(24):2841–51. https://doi.org/10.1161/CIRCULATIONAHA.118.035566 PMID: 30565993.
3. Gjesdal O, Gude E, Arora S, Leivestad T, Andreassen AK, Gullestad L, Aaberge L, Brunvand H, Edvardsen T, Geiran OR, Simonsen S. Intra-aortic balloon counterpulsation as a bridge to heart transplantation does not impair long-term survival. Eur J Heart Fail. 2009;11(7):709–14.
4. Nair N, Gongora E (2019) Extracorporeal membrane oxygenation as a bridge to cardiac transplantation. https://doi.org/10.5772/intechopen.84935
5. Assad-Kottner C, Chen D, Jahanyar J, Cordova F, Summers N, Loebe M, Merla R, Youker K, Torre-Amione G. The use of continuous milrinone therapy as bridge to transplant is safe in patients with short waiting times. J Card Fail. 2008;14(10):839–43. https://doi.org/10.1016/j.cardfail.2008.08.00. Epub 2008 Nov 5. PMID: 19041047
6. Canver CC, Chanda J. Milrinone for long-term pharmacologic support of the status 1 heart transplant candidates. Ann Thorac Surg. 2000;69(6):1823–6. https://doi.org/10.1016/s0003-4975(00)01313-8 PMID: 10892930.
7. Lee EC, McNitt S, Martens J, Bruckel JT, Chen L, Alexis JD, Storozynsky E, Thomas S, Gosev I, Barrus B, Goldenberg I, Vidula H. Long-term milrinone therapy as a bridge to heart transplantation: Safety, efficacy, and predictors of failure. Int J Cardiol. 2020;15(313):83–8. https://doi.org/10.1016/j.ijcard.2020.04.055 Epub 2020 Apr 19 PMID: 32320777.

Heart Memory and Feelings

Ali Talib Hashim, Ahmed Sattar Albayati, and Ethar Nazal

Abstract This chapter encounters the question, "is the heart related to the memory or not". According to heart transplantation studies, there are multiple changes in the personality of the receiver that favors the traits of the donor. In addition to that the chapter tackles a comparison between the common definition of the memory and the cellular memory, in which both have the ability of encoding, storage, and retrieval. In addition to that the exosomes (proteins) play a role in information transfer between the organs and body cells, adding to our understanding of different shapes of memories within the human body. Neuroplasticity, on the other hand, plays a major role in the memory as well. It has shown that heart transplantation recipients have showed the ability to retrieve information believed to be stored in the intra-cardiac nervous system. Moreover, the neurotransmitters play a key role in the process as they represent the main medium for information transfer between the neurons. Heart memory evidences are rising in number as the medicine is taking new approaches toward technology and research. It was proven that multiple forms of memory were found on cellular and neurological levels. Evidences are derived from heart transplantation studies and molecular sciences, in which all points to the theory of "multiple forms of memory".

Keywords Heart memory · Heart feelings · Neurocardiology · Immune system

A. T. Hashim (✉)
Golestan University of Medical Sciences, Gorgan, Iran
e-mail: talibhashim42@gmail.com

A. S. Albayati
College of Medicine, University of Baghdad, Baghdad, Iraq

E. Nazal
Kharkiv National Medical University, Kharkiv, Ukraine

© The Author(s), under exclusive license to Springer Nature Switzerland AG 2022
H. T. Hashim et al. (eds.), *Heart Transplantation*,
https://doi.org/10.1007/978-3-031-17311-0_17

1　Introduction

We think that the heart is just a pump for blood that receives and transfers blood and oxygenates it. But many studies developed especially after heart transplantation surgeries that found that the behavior of the recipients has changed into donor's behavior in some situations and issues [1–3] (see Fig. 1).

Emotions which are controlled by the brain have some sources in the heart so we call it heart feelings. These feelings can be transferred with the heart to the new recipients that can act like the donor [4, 5].

Heart memory is a very important factor in exploring these ideas, as the brain has a memory, the heart also does. The development of specific signs and symptoms in certain situations under the control of autonomic nervous system is also a contributing factor [6, 7].

According to heart transplantation studies, there are multiple changes in the personality of the receiver that favors the traits of the donor. In addition to that the chapter tackles a comparison between the common definition of the memory and the cellular memory, in which both have the ability of encoding, storage, and retrieval. In addition to that the exosomes (proteins) play a role in information transfer between the organs and body cells, adding to our understanding of different shapes of memories within the human body. Neuroplasticity, on the other hand, plays a major role in the memory as well. It has shown that heart transplantation recipients have showed the ability to retrieve information believed to be stored in the intra-cardiac nervous system [3, 8]. Moreover, the neurotransmitters play a key role in the process as they represent the main medium for information transfer between the neurons. Heart memory evidences are rising in number as the medicine is taking new approaches toward technology and research. It was proven that multiple forms of memory were found on cellular and neurological levels. Evidences are derived from heart transplantation studies and molecular sciences, in which all points to the theory of "multiple forms of memory" [5, 9].

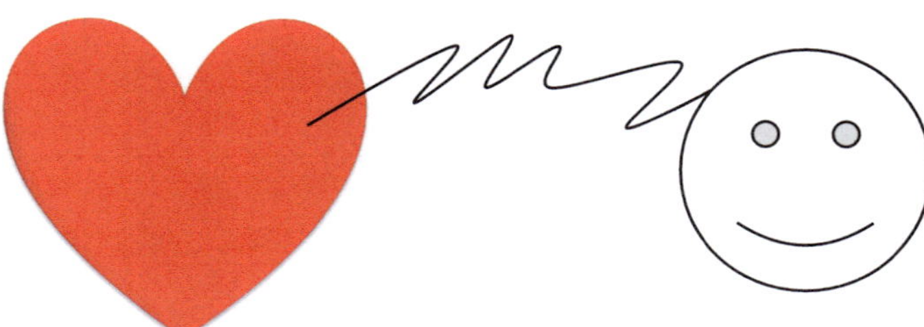

Fig. 1　Heart memory sketch

2 Heart Memory

Hear memory means that the heart can remember either everything or part of things. So, when the transplanted heart is being implanted into the new recipient, it will keep its programming for the previous body. This does not cancel the effects of the recipient's brain and immune system.

Heart memory also can be determined by electrocardiography (ECG), where some changes are not resolved and persists even after healing or treating the cause, such as T-wave changes in STEMI [10, 11].

Some emotional thoughts in the heart can be kept in the heart cells and the heart being transferred, it will transfer these feelings to the new person that can affect his original thoughts and feelings [2–4].

Keeping the memory with the heart may have consequences on the recipients, like, for instance, when the donor is a criminal and emotionless, this may affect the recipient negatively and may affect his mind and thoughts. So, it is important to study these effects carefully and perform more studies and researches on these topics to control these feelings and keep the recipient safe from any changes [8].

3 The Role of Genes

The genes (see Fig. 2) may have a role in keeping the heart memory going from patients to another with heart transplantation. RNA and DNA composition and proteins alternation in the cardiomyocytes have their special sequences that may differ from human to human. So, after transplantation, they keep their own sequences that will keep the same function for the transplanted heart so when the heart has a memory of feeling, these feelings will be kept and transferred to the recipients where they will be expressed again [7, 10].

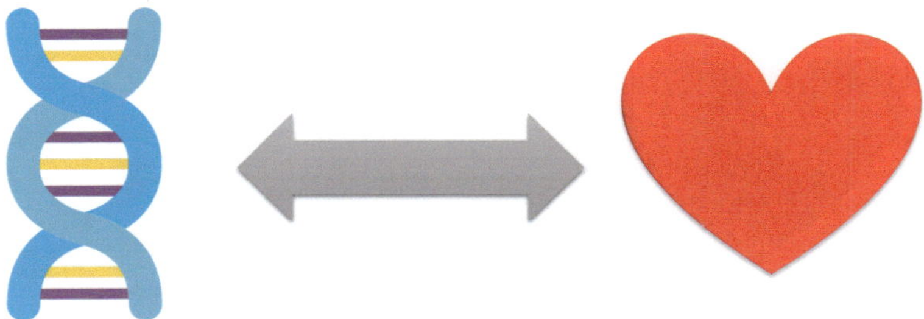

Fig. 2 The effects of the genes on the heart

4   The Role of Nerves

The heart, like any other organ in the body, is supplied by the nervous system. So, these nerves that supply the heart may affect its memory as well. We are not sure about the effects of the recipients on the new heart but many studies approved the effects of the heart on the recipients [3, 8, 9] (Fig. 3).

Multiple Choice Questions

1. **Which of the following is the most effective in the heart memory?**

    a.   Genes
    b.   Nerves.
    c.   Cardiomyocytes.
    d.   All of the above.

    Answers: d

2. **Which of the following is mostly non-understood by the medicine?**

    a.   The heart has a memory.
    b.   The effects of the transplants heart on the recipients.
    c.   The effects of the recipients on the transplanted heart.
    d.   b and c.

    Answer: d

3. **RNA and DNA have no role in heart memory.**

    a.   True.
    b.   False.

    Answer: b

4. **Heart memory is very important to be studied because its consequences on the recipient's patients can be negative.**

    a.   True.
    b.   False.

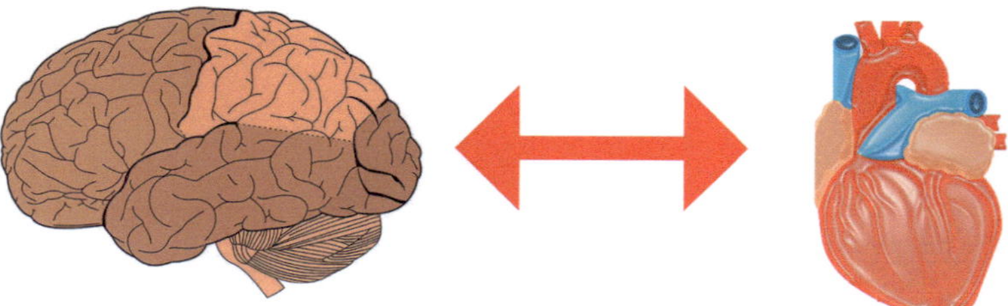

Fig. 3 The effects of the nervous system on the heart

Answer: a

5. **Nerves can affect the heart memory.**

    a. True.
    b. False.

Answer: a

6. **The brain has an effect on the heart memory, so there may be changes occurring after the transplantation either from the recipients or from the donors.**

    a. True.
    b. False.
    c. Unknown.

Answer: c

References

1. Iversen S, Kupfermann I, Kandel ER. Emotional states and feelings. Princ Neural Sci. 2000;4:982–97.
2. Chasteen AL, et al. How feelings of stereotype threat influence older adults' memory performance. Exp Aging Res. 2005;31(3):235–60
3. Liester M. Personality changes following heart transplantation: the role of cellular memory. Med Hypotheses. 2020;135: 109468.
4. Shewey D. In memory of my feelings. Film Comment. 1990;26(3):11.
5. Rosen M. The heart remembers. Cardiovasc Res. 1998;40(3):469–82.
6. Koivunen AR. Redistributing feelings: migrant memories in Finnish Blood, Swedish Heart (Mika Ronkainen, Finland-Sweden 2012). Montreal, Canada: Society for Cinema and Media Studies Conference (SCMS), March 25–29, 2015;2015
7. Gow M. Transient feelings: creative response. Netw Knowl: J MeCCSA Postgrad Netw. 2021;14(1):121–4.
8. Cirillo M. The memory of the heart. J Cardiovasc Dev Dis. 2018;5(4):55.
9. Rosen M, Binah O, Marom S. Cardiac memory and cortical memory. Circulation. 2003;108(15):1784–9.
10. Wistrich AJ, Rachlinski JJ, Guthrie C. Heart versus head: do judges follow the law of follow their feelings. Tex L Rev. 2014;93:855.
11. O'Hara F. In memory of my feelings: a selection of poems. The Museum of Modern Art;2005

Correction to: Cultural and Religious Aspects of Heart Transplantation

Jose-Maria Dominguez-Roldan, Ikram-ul-Haq, Naseer Ahmed, Visist Dhitavat, Feng Huo, Jie Zhao, and Marti Manyalich-Vidal

Correction to:
Chapter "Cultural and Religious Aspects of Heart Transplantation" in: H. T. Hashim et al. (eds.), *Heart Transplantation*, https://doi.org/10.1007/978-3-031-17311-0_15

In the original version of the book, the following belated corrections have been incorporated:

The author name "Ikran ul Haq" has been changed to "Ikram-ul-Haq" in the Frontmatter and in Chapter 15.

The chapter and the book have been updated with the change.

The updated original version of this chapter can be found at
https://doi.org/10.1007/978-3-031-17311-0_15

Index

© The Editor(s) (if applicable) and The Author(s), under exclusive license
to Springer Nature Switzerland AG 2022
H. T. Hashim et al. (eds.), *Heart Transplantation*,
https://doi.org/10.1007/978-3-031-17311-0

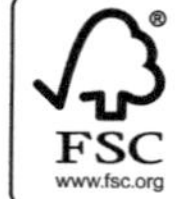